GENDER, WOMEN, AND THE TOBACCO EPIDEMIC

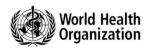

World Health Organization

WHO Library Cataloguing-in-Publication Data
Gender, women, and the tobacco epidemic / edited by Jonathan M. Samet and
Soon-Young Yoon.

1.Smoking - epidemiology. 2.Women's health. 3.Women. 4.Tobacco - adverse effects.
I.Samet, Jonathan M. II.Yoon, Soon-Young. III.World Health Organization.

ISBN 978 92 4 159951 1   (NLM classification: QV 137)

© World Health Organization 2010

The designations employed and the presentation of the material in this publication do
not imply the expression of any opinion whatsoever on the part of the World Health
Organization concerning the legal status of any country, territory, city or area or of its
authorities, or concerning the delimitation of its frontiers or boundaries. Dotted lines on
maps represent approximate border lines for which there may not yet be full agreement.

The mention of specific companies or of certain manufacturers' products does not imply
that they are endorsed or recommended by the World Health Organization in preference
to others of a similar nature that are not mentioned. Errors and omissions excepted, the
names of proprietary products are distinguished by initial capital letters.

All reasonable precautions have been taken by the World Health Organization to verify
the information contained in this publication. However, the published material is being
distributed without warranty of any kind, either expressed or implied. The responsibility
for the interpretation and use of the material lies with the reader. In no event shall the
World Health Organization be liable for damages arising from its use.

The named authors alone are responsible for the views expressed in this publication.

Printed in Manila, Philippines.

Table of Contents

Preface

Dr Margaret Chan, Director-General of the World Health Organization (WHO), stated in her Foreword to the 2009 WHO report on women and health*:

> *The Millennium Development Goals and other global commitments have focused primarily on the entitlements and needs of women. The current financial crisis and economic downturn make this focus even more urgent: protecting and promoting the health of women is crucial to health and development – not only for the citizens of today but also for those of future generations.*

A rise in the number of women smokers around the world will have enormous adverse effects on households' financial status and family health. While the epidemic of tobacco use among men is in slow decline in some countries, use among women in some countries is increasing. However, in India and in several other countries, women also use other forms of tobacco, such as chewing tobacco. Unless innovative and sustained initiatives are undertaken, the number of female users of tobacco is predicted to rise over the next several decades as a result of increased prevalence, as well as population growth.

This monograph is part of WHO's continued efforts to curb an epidemic of tobacco use affecting girls and women of all ages. It originated from a previous WHO monograph, *Women and the Tobacco Epidemic – Challenges for the 21st Century*, published in 2001. That monograph presented scientific papers commissioned by WHO in preparation for the 1999 WHO Conference on Tobacco and Health, Making a Difference to Tobacco and Health: Avoiding the Tobacco Epidemic in Women and Youth, held in Kobe, Japan. Since then, new data, changes in tobacco control legislation, and issues have emerged that warrant a new publication.

---

* *Women and Health: Today's Evidence, Tomorrow's Agenda.* Geneva, World Health Organization, 2009.

Much progress has been made on the issue of gender, women, and tobacco since 1999. Most significantly, the WHO Framework Convention on Tobacco Control (WHO FCTC), now endorsed by 168 signatories and with more than 170 Parties, emphasizes the need for a gender perspective. The Preamble states:

> **Alarmed** *by the increase in smoking and other forms of tobacco consumption by women and young girls worldwide and keeping in mind the need for full participation of women at all levels of policy-making and implementation and the need for gender-specific tobacco control strategies,*

> **Emphasizing** *the special contribution of nongovernmental organizations and other members of civil society not affiliated with the tobacco industry, including health professional bodies, women's, youth, environmental and consumer groups, and academic and health care institutions, to tobacco control efforts nationally and internationally and the vital importance of their participation in national and international tobacco control efforts,*

> **Recalling** *that the Convention on the Elimination of All Forms of Discrimination against Women, adopted by the United Nations General Assembly on 18 December 1979, provides that States Parties to the Convention shall take appropriate measures to eliminate discrimination against women in the field of health care.*

In addition, Article 4 of the Guiding Principles of the WHO FCTC specifically mentions gender, noting "the need to take measures to address gender-specific risks when developing tobacco control strategies".

WHO has given high priority to strengthening global action on the gender, women, and tobacco issue in its own programmes, including an operational project in Viet Nam. In the WHO Western Pacific Region, all five-year Action Plans on tobacco or health since 1990, including the 2010–2014 Plan, have emphasized the importance of preventing a rise in tobacco use among women. In 2010,

Gender and Tobacco with an Emphasis on Marketing to Women is the theme of the WHO campaign for World No Tobacco Day.

Progress has also been made in mobilizing non-governmental organizations (NGOs), foundations, and the scientific community in support of activities concerned with gender, women, and tobacco. For example, the International Network of Women Against Tobacco (INWAT), founded in 1990 to address issues of tobacco and women, has grown steadily and now has members in more than 80 countries. INWAT regularly distributes reports and newsletters and in 2006 published *Turning a New Leaf: Women, Tobacco and the Future*. *The Tobacco Atlas*, now published by the American Cancer Society and the World Lung Foundation, places a special emphasis on girls and women. A gender perspective has been integrated into many American Cancer Society tobacco projects. The CHEST Foundation, based in the United States of America, developed a Speaker's Kit on Women and Girls—an educational tool addressing the dangers of tobacco use—which has been produced in many Asian languages. World and regional conferences on tobacco and health now strive for gender equality in their committees, chairs, and speakers, and they include the topic of gender, women, and tobacco in their programmes.

The publication of this monograph is opportune. The numbers of women who use tobacco and who are exposed to second-hand smoke (SHS), especially in poor communities, are expected to increase in the coming decades, for the following reasons:

- The female population in low- and middle-income countries is predicted to increase; thus, even if smoking prevalence remains low, the absolute numbers of women smokers will increase.

- Girls' and women's spending power is increasing, so cigarettes are becoming more affordable for them.

- The social and cultural constraints that have prevented many women from smoking are weakening in some countries.

- Women-specific health education and quitting programmes are rare, especially in low- and middle-income countries.

- In countries where rates of smoking are increasing among men, women will be increasingly exposed to the hazards of SHS.

- The tobacco companies are targeting women, using well-funded, alluring marketing campaigns.

In her editorial for INWAT, Dr Gro Harlem Brundtland, the former Director-General of WHO and a lifelong anti-tobacco advocate, concluded:

> *We need a broad alliance against tobacco, calling on a wide range of partners such as women's organizations to halt the relentless increase in global tobacco consumption among women. There is a special need for gender-sensitive health education and quitting programmes. There is also a need to involve more women in senior, decision-making positions in the tobacco control movement, on editorial boards of medical journals which include tobacco issues, on WHO expert panels, and in nongovernmental organizations that deal with tobacco issues.*

In keeping with this urgent call, this monograph helps to assess the current situation, identifies gaps in research, and offers solutions that must be heeded to prevent an epidemic of the gravest order.

Dr Judith Mackay

Senior Advisor, World Lung Foundation/Bloomberg Initiative
Senior Policy Adviser, Tobacco Free Initiative,
World Health Organization

Acknowledgements

Jonathan M. Samet and Soon-Young Yoon edited this monograph and coordinated the team of scientists who contributed their expertise to these chapters: *Summary and Overview* by Jonathan M. Samet and Soon-Young Yoon; *A Gender Equality Framework for Tobacco Control* by Natasha Jategaonkar and Soon-Young Yoon; *Prevalence of Tobacco Use and Factors Influencing Initiation and Maintenance Among Women* by Benjamin J. Apelberg, Mira Aghi, Samira Asma, Elisabeth Donaldson, Chng Chee Yeong, and Rose Vaithinathan; *Impact of Tobacco Use on Women's Health* by Virginia Ernster; *Second-Hand Smoke, Women, and Children* by Jonathan M. Samet, Margaret A. Hawthorne, and Gonghuan Yang; *The Marketing of Tobacco to Women: Global Perspectives by* Nancy J. Kaufman and Mimi Nichter; *Addiction to Nicotine* by Janine C. Delahanty, Carlo C. DiClemente, and Miranda M. Garay; *Quitting Smoking and Beating Nicotine Addiction* by Miranda M. Garay, Carlo C. DiClemente, and Janine C. Delahanty; *Pregnancy and Postpartum Smoking Cessation* by Carlo C. DiClemente, Janine C. Delahanty, and Miranda M. Garay; *How to Make Policies More Gender-Sensitive* by Nicola Christofides, Virginia B. Bowen, and Michelle J. Hindin; *Taxation and the Economics of Tobacco Control* by John Tauras, Rowena Jacobs, Frank Chaloupka, Hugh Waters, and Ayda Yurekli; *Women's Rights and International Agreements* by Charlotte C. Abaka and Pramila Patten; and *The International Women's Movement and Anti-Tobacco Campaigns* by Mabel Bianco, Margaretha Haglund, Yayori Matsui, and Nobuko Nakano.

The World Health Organization (WHO) would like to thank the Ministry of Health, Labour and Welfare of Japan for its support in the preparations for and final publication of this monograph, as well as in papers originally commissioned for the WHO monograph *Women and the Tobacco Epidemic—Challenges for the 21st Century*, first published in 2001.

Hiroko Minami, Judith Mackay, and Yumiko Mochizuki-Kobayashi shared their technical expertise. Douglas Bettcher, Director of the WHO Tobacco Free Initiative, provided invaluable guidance, along with WHO staff and consultants Vera da Costa e Silva, Katherine DeLand, Dongbo Fu, Anne-Marie Perucic, Armando Peruga, Vinayak Prasad, Kerstin Schotte, Gemma Vestal, and Ayda Yurekli. Contributions were made by the WHO Framework Convention on Tobacco Control Secretariat and other related WHO units, including Information, Evidence and Research, in collaboration with Tonya Nyagiro, Peju Olukoya, and Elena Villalobos of the Gender, Women and Health department. Sun Goo Lee helped coordinate communications in collaboration with the chief editors, and Gauri Khanna provided technical assistance for data review. Elizabeth Tecson gave administrative support in finalizing the document. Janet DeLand edited the final text with help from Athena Foong, Richard M. Smith, and Barbara Campanini. Finally, the editors would like to acknowledge Jonathan Soard, who masterfully prepared the cover and layout design for this volume.

World Health Organization

A Message from Dr Margaret Chan

Director-General, WHO

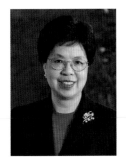

We need to strongly support women's leadership in tobacco control, and we must act now. As the 2009 WHO report on women and health noted, tobacco use is one of the most serious avoidable risk factors for premature death and disease in adult women and is responsible for about 6% of female deaths worldwide. Without action to reduce smoking, deaths among women aged 20 years and over may rise from 1.5 million in 2004 to 2.5 million by 2030; almost 75% of these projected deaths will occur in low- and middle-income countries. Furthermore, second-hand smoke is a killer, and there is no safe level of exposure. In regions where the majority of smokers are men, millions of women and children suffer from exposure to second-hand smoke. Most alarming, the rates of smoking are increasing among youth and young women in several regions of the world. Where tobacco use is still relatively low among women and girls, an opportunity exists for preventing increased uptake and future premature deaths.

Let us remember that tobacco poses a threat to achieving the United Nations Millennium Development Goals (MDGs). The MDGs are about reducing poverty, as well as achieving gender equality. They recognize that poor health anchors large populations in poverty. They also acknowledge that better health allows people the opportunity to find their way out of poverty. Still, there is an alarming trend that links poverty with tobacco use. Poor families are more likely to include smokers than richer families. Poor families spend a substantial part of their total expenditures on tobacco—often more than they spend on education or health care. According to the World Bank, the use of tobacco results in economic losses of billions of dollars each year—and most of those losses occur in developing countries. Cost-effective tobacco control strategies can work. Bans on tobacco advertising, increased tobacco taxes, graphic labels on tobacco packaging, controls on smuggling and counterfeiting, and legislation to create smoke-free environments in all public places and workplaces have helped. Enforcing and enacting such measures with women's full participation is sound social and economic development policy.

WHO is committed to improving women's health and promoting women's leadership and chose Gender and Tobacco with an Emphasis on Marketing to Women as the theme of its 2010 World No Tobacco Day. As I have often said, the challenges are different for women. That is why women need special attention in health agendas. As caregivers in the home, they are an important resource. They are also susceptible to special health problems and have a heightened risk of premature mortality. Also, many women do not have adequate access to health services, even though continuity of care is essential over a life-course. Part of the solution is to empower women to leverage their resources and creativity. We have seen example after example of women who are given the right encouragement and an enabling environment making changes, not only in their own lives, but in the lives of their families and communities.

This monograph makes an important contribution to our scientific understanding of tobacco use among women. It also provides an analytical framework for promoting a gender perspective in policy-making. We have added an important new tool in the effort to scale up technical and other assistance at country level. On 27 February 2005, the WHO Framework Convention on Tobacco Control (WHO FCTC) entered into force. Currently, more than 170 Parties have ratified the Convention. Its Preamble recognizes women's leadership as key to achieving the goal of tobacco control. Most important, it supports a principle central to achieving gender equality in health—that women's right to health is a human right.

Sex appeal?
No, second-hand
smoke.

SMOKING
IS UGLY

WWW.WHO.INT/TOBACCO

Protect women from
tobacco marketing and smoke.

31MAY:WORLDNOTOBACCODAY

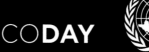

World Health
Organization

WORLD HEALTH ORGANIZATION 2010. DESIGNED BY NOVA S/B

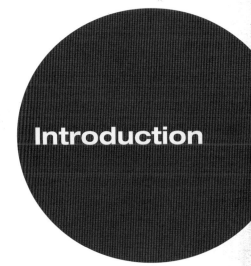

Introduction

Make
every day
World No
Tobacco Day.

www.who.int/tobacco

31 MAY

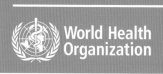 World Health
Organization

1. Summary and Overview

Background

In 1999, in collaboration with the Japanese Ministry of Health, Labour and Welfare, the World Health Organization (WHO) hosted a meeting in Kobe, Japan, entitled Making a Difference to Tobacco and Health: Avoiding the Tobacco Epidemic in Women and Youth. More than 500 participants from 50 countries met to consider issues related to gender equality and tobacco. The Conference proved to be a turning point in the tobacco control movement, as it brought together multiple stakeholder groups concerned with gender and tobacco. It provided a much needed forum for health scientists and other professionals to open a dialogue with leaders representing local authorities, youth, women, and human rights.

The participants at the Kobe Conference cited a number of reasons for the need to consider gender and gender equality in national and international programmes and strategies. Among the points emphasized were:

- Women and girls, particularly among the poor, are often invisible in health statistics. Information is lacking on epidemiological statistics and risks and level of health knowledge. The emphasis given to men reflects gender discrimination and the inequality underlying many tobacco control programmes.

- When women are held responsible for reproductive health, they may be blamed for their addiction to tobacco and its negative impact on their children. Much less medical attention has been paid to the negative health effects of paternal smoking on fertility and the health of the fetus. Cessation programmes for fathers are seldom provided as part of reproductive health services.

- The majority of victims of second-hand smoke (SHS) are women and children, exposed in their homes through the smoking of men. Curtailing exposure to SHS needs to be given a higher priority to protect women's and children's rights to a safe and smoke-free environment in homes and public places.

Tobacco control programmes seldom recognize women as potential leaders. Unless women are empowered they cannot fully participate in tobacco control programmes.[1]

Much of the success of the Kobe Conference was due to the persuasive power of sound evidence. With the help of a grant from Japan, WHO convened a scientific working group for one year prior to the Conference. The results of the scientific working group were first published in the 2001 WHO monograph *Women and the Tobacco Epidemic—Challenges for the 21st Century*. Nearly 10 years later, gender, women, and tobacco policies must take into account new epidemiological patterns, social and economic trends, and political challenges. For example, a landmark in international law is the WHO Framework Convention on Tobacco Control (WHO FCTC), which went into force in 2005 and has been ratified by more than 170 countries. The WHO FCTC is a multilateral evidence-based treaty that provides the legal framework for countries to reduce the supply and demand for tobacco, in addition to supporting women's rights to health as a human right.

For this monograph, an international team of scholars and experts reviewed the most current research to provide an overview of tobacco control issues related to gender, with a focus on women. Interdisciplinary teams included researchers and activists in public health, medicine, nursing, and dentistry, as well as anthropology, psychology, economics, law, journalism, and gender studies. The concerns of tobacco control policy-makers, educators, public health advocates, and economic planners, as well as youth and women leaders, are addressed. Special attention is paid to policies that affect women throughout their life-course. A gender analysis should provide information on why specific programmes are working for men and not for women. However, due to a lack of data, particularly regarding poor women and men in developing countries, it is not possible to perform a comprehensive analysis at this time. Rather, this monograph presents available research findings and data, identifies gaps to be addressed, and suggests directions for future study.

The monograph has four sections: Tobacco Use and Its Impact on Health; Why Women and Girls Use Tobacco; Quitting; and Policies and Strategies. Topics covered include determinants of starting to use tobacco, exposure to SHS, the impact of tobacco use on health, the nature

World Health Organization

of addiction and cessation, and treatment programmes, as well as policy issues involving economic and tax measures, gender analyses, and human rights.

Tobacco Use and Its Impact on Health

Tobacco Use

What are some of the salient findings? Globally, the prevalence of smoking is higher for men (40% as of 2006) than for women (nearly 9% as of 2006), and males account for 80% of all smokers. In most countries around the world, men—being more likely than women to smoke—are also almost two times more likely to die from smoking. However, data from several industrialized and developing countries show that men's smoking rates may have peaked and are now in slow decline. Programmes should include efforts to sustain this downward trend, particularly among adolescent boys. At the same time, much more attention needs to be paid to the increasing numbers of women who use tobacco.

As noted in Chapter 3, Prevalence of Tobacco Use and Factors Influencing Initiation and Maintenance Among Women, there is wide regional variation in smoking prevalence among both males and females. In the Americas and Europe, the prevalence of female smoking is high, around 17% and 22%, respectively. The disparity between male and female smoking prevalence is greater in other regions of the world. For example, male smoking prevalence is near 37% in South-East Asia and 57% in the Western Pacific, while prevalence among women is around 4% to 5%. Globally, boys are more likely than girls to smoke. However, in half the countries surveyed by the Global Youth Tobacco Survey (GYTS), there is no sex difference in rates of youth smoking, indicating that tobacco use among girls may be increasing in some countries. If the rates of use of any form of tobacco—e.g. water pipes, cheroots, chewing tobacco, snuff—were to be included, the figures would be much higher. These disparities reflect differing social norms, cultural traditions, and socioeconomic and demographic factors.

Women who smoke tend to do so in part for different reasons than those of men smokers. The roots of tobacco uptake for women and girls often include cultural,

psychosocial, and socioeconomic factors, including body image and peer pressure. In the Asian and Pacific countries where smoking has become a symbol of women's liberation, many young women are turning to tobacco as a sign of freedom. Others take up the habit because of a popular belief that smoking keeps them slim. Regardless of the reason for starting to smoke, addiction sets in quickly, as a cigarette is a carefully designed nicotine delivery system that provides sufficient nicotine to establish and maintain dependence on tobacco.

Less is known about traditional tobacco use, such as the use of khaini, mawa, or betel quid and bidis among subgroups of women. Similarly, a new trend of increased use of water pipes by women requires more attention. However, data from India suggest the need for much more research on local practices. The prevalence rates of smoking and chewing tobacco vary widely by region in India, and in many areas women are more likely to use oral tobacco products than to smoke. Reasons for starting may reflect local beliefs and cultural practices. For example, some Indian women believe that chewing tobacco can cure toothaches or can be useful during childbirth.

Studies in many countries indicate that most tobacco use begins in early adolescence. The age of starting to use tobacco has important implications. Adolescents who begin smoking at a younger age are more likely to become regular smokers and are less likely to quit than those who start later. Socioeconomic status (SES) has been implicated in the risk for onset of smoking among adolescents. In some countries, young people with more spending money have higher levels of tobacco use, in both uptake and frequency of smoking. In developing countries, the lack of health education programmes results in girls having little knowledge of the harmful effects of tobacco use. More research is needed on the gender influences leading to unequal access to health education and information by girls and boys.

Several studies in the United States of America and in Canada have found that girls have lower self-esteem than boys and that low self-esteem is associated with smoking among girls. Another significant determinant in high-income countries is the belief that smoking can reduce appetite and control body weight. Parental smoking, peer smoking, and exposure to smoking in movies can also influence tobacco use, although further research is needed in low-income countries, where differences in social

World Health Organization

norms, family life, and culture influence behaviours. In countries where the rate of tobacco use (and particularly cigarette smoking) by women and girls is still relatively low, programmes are needed to prevent increased uptake and future premature deaths and disabilities.

Impact on Health

Chapter 4, Impact of Tobacco Use on Women's Health, concludes that women who use tobacco face virtually the same risks that men face and even greater risks for some diseases. Many women are still unaware of the full scope of risks caused by the many toxic and carcinogenic compounds in tobacco smoke: tobacco smoke contains more than 4000 chemicals, hundreds of which are toxic or carcinogenic. The reasons for both men and women failing to get accurate health information concerning sex-specific impacts of tobacco use on health need further study, followed by intervention.

Current research, largely from industrialized countries, indicates cause for alarm. Lung cancer mortality rates among women in the United States have increased approximately 800% since 1950. By 1987, lung cancer had surpassed breast cancer to become the leading cause of cancer death among women in the United States. Women who smoke have higher risks for many cancers, including cancers of the mouth, pharynx, oesophagus, larynx, bladder, pancreas, kidney, and cervix, as well as for acute myeloid leukaemia. And there is a possible link between active smoking and premenopausal breast cancer.

Smoking also affects reproductive health. Women who smoke are more likely than non-smokers to experience infertility and delays in conceiving. Maternal smoking during pregnancy increases risks of prematurity, stillbirth, and neonatal death and may cause a reduction in breast milk.

Women who smoke are at increased risk of developing potentially fatal chronic obstructive pulmonary disease (COPD), which includes chronic bronchitis and emphysema. In industrialized countries, the prevalence of COPD is now almost as high in women as it is in men. In addition, smoking is a cause of coronary heart disease (CHD) in women, for whom risk increases with the number of cigarettes smoked and the duration of smoking. The risk of CHD is even higher among women smokers who use oral contraceptives. Among postmenopausal women,

current smokers have lower bone density than non-smokers and an increased risk of hip fracture.

There are many gaps in the data about the health impact of tobacco use on girls and women of all ages and throughout the life-course. Much more research is needed on the ways women—particularly in developing countries—use a variety of tobacco products, including snuff, chewing tobacco, and traditional forms of rolled tobacco. Finally, high-quality, population-based cancer incidence data are needed on health risks for women who work in the informal sectors of tobacco growing, production, and marketing.

Second-Hand Smoke

In 2004, second-hand smoke (SHS) was estimated to have caused about 600 000 premature deaths per year, (28% of which were among children). Of the 430 000 adult deaths, about 64% were among women. Although by 2008, an additional 154 million people worldwide had been covered by comprehensive smoke-free laws, nearly 90% of the world's population is not protected, and laws do not limit exposure to SHS in homes where women and children are exposed through the smoking of male family members. Second-hand tobacco smoke contributes about 1% of the total global disease burden; in the United States, the economic costs total about US$ 19.3 billion per year.[2] Chapter 5, Second-Hand Smoke, Women, and Children, sounds the alarm for those women and children who are exposed to smoke and its health hazards even though they do not use tobacco themselves. SHS jeopardizes women's health, especially in countries and cultures where many women do not have the power to negotiate smoke-free spaces, even in their own homes.

Progress has been made in improving indicators of SHS exposure, including biomarkers such as levels of cotinine in blood, urine, or saliva, which are direct measures that can be used to estimate exposure. In industrialized countries, nearly half of the children and adolescents are exposed to SHS. In China, which accounts for one third of the world's cigarette consumption, the tobacco epidemic is almost entirely a male phenomenon. A 2002 national survey reported that less than 3% of women in China smoked. However, more than half of the women of reproductive age were regularly exposed to SHS.

World Health Organization

There is now sound scientific evidence that SHS causes illnesses and deaths among women and children. Women whose male partners smoke have increased rates of lung cancer and increased risk for CHD. Paternal smoking may have effects on sperm and may lead to postnatal health problems, including increased risk for sudden infant death syndrome (SIDS), reduced physical development, and possibly increased risk for childhood cancer. Studies from China show that paternal smoking alone can increase the incidence of lower respiratory illness in children. Maternal smoking during pregnancy reduces birth weight substantially and is a causal factor for SIDS. Exposure to SHS results in lower respiratory tract illnesses, chronic respiratory symptoms, middle-ear disease, and reduced lung function in children.

> *The tactics that have been used in marketing tobacco in the United States and other industrialized nations for decades now threaten women in the developing world.*

Studies have found that smoke-free legislation increases cessation rates and reduces consumption. It also decreases SHS exposure and brings immediate health benefits. For example, a study in Scotland measured salivary cotinine levels in schoolchildren and found that the average concentration decreased by 30% after smoke-free legislation was put in place. Still, many governments have not taken or enforced adequate public health measures to protect women and children against exposure to SHS. Lack of enforcement is particularly relevant in developing countries where legislation prohibiting tobacco use in public places may not be strictly enforced. Since there is no safe level of exposure to SHS, the chapter's recommendations include enactment and strong enforcement of 100% smoke-free indoor workplaces and public places and smoke-free child-care settings, which would remove a major source of SHS exposure for infants and children. Special campaigns that are culturally appropriate are also needed to address the problem of SHS in the home, a major locus of exposure for women and children.

Why Women and Girls Use Tobacco

Marketing, Advertising, and Promotion

Even though the health hazards of tobacco use are known, women are becoming increasingly addicted to it. One of the powerful influences driving changing rates of tobacco use is industry advertising and sponsorship. The tobacco industry has long fostered the false idea that tobacco is linked to women's empowerment by suggesting that cigarette smoking symbolizes high fashion, freedom, and "modern" styles and values, and that it even promises weight reduction.

Chapter 6, The Marketing of Tobacco to Women: Global Perspectives, leaves little doubt that the tobacco industry considers female consumers to be a lucrative market. In the United States, 11% of total advertising and promotion expenditures in 1996 came from the tobacco industry; in 2005, US$ 13.11 billion was spent on tobacco advertising and promotions. The tactics that have been used in marketing tobacco in the United States and other industrialized nations for decades now threaten women in the developing world. In many countries recently affected by free trade agreements, the tobacco industry has targeted a flood of savvy marketing strategies towards women. Large companies sponsor events such as women's tennis tournaments and disco dances to create a public image of smoking as a promoter of health and relaxation. "Female brands", "light" cigarettes, low prices, easy availability, and free samples help these marketing strategies succeed among young women.

Tobacco companies rank among the 10 top marketers in several Asian countries. Research in Asia, including Indonesia, Sri Lanka, Viet Nam, China, India, and the Philippines, indicates that massive advertising combined with changing gender roles and women's increased earning power produces a favourable environment to advance sales. British American Tobacco (BAT), Japan Tobacco, and the China National Tobacco Corporation have substantial shares in this market. In India, where it may not be culturally "correct" for women to buy cigarettes openly, companies have offered to deliver them to the home.

Modern marketing seeks to attach symbolic meaning to brands, associating products with psychological and social

World Health Organization

needs in a coordinated strategy that surrounds the consumer with stimuli. A cigarette brand has become the ultimate "badge product", because it is like a name badge that sends a message every time it is seen, projecting a distinctive identity. Brand images may appeal to consumers' social insecurities by appearing to propose solutions to identity problems. In addition, advertising is used to reduce fears about tobacco use and to associate products with dazzling blue skies and mountains, happiness, and healthy sports activities. Consumer culture is visual, and images of modern, Western-style women play a dominant role in developing countries. In the global consumer culture, having the right body becomes part of a woman's identity, and this ideal type is used extensively in advertisements. In the Philippines and Viet Nam, posters advertising cigarettes typically portray big-busted foreign women wearing scanty clothing. Prominent themes appealing to Asian women include weight control, stress relief, and independence. Surprisingly, women also represent 50% of the market share of brands that use images of masculinity, e.g. Marlboro and Camel.

Promotions aim for immediate action on the part of the consumer. Discount coupons may be especially effective for reaching poor women and youth, and clothing promotions create "walking billboards". Sponsorships of entertainment, sporting events, and fashion shows embed advertising within the events. In an era of globalized media, such sponsorships can reach audiences across borders and can touch millions of children, youth, and women in their homes. One study estimated that 25% of young people 12 to 17 years of age watch auto racing on television, and women constitute 39% of NASCAR's audience. Sponsorship of dance and art events, women's organizations, campaigns against domestic violence, schools, scholarships, beauty contests, and youth sports events has linked tobacco companies with social causes, as well as fun. Of particular concern has been the tobacco industry's use of film and music sponsorships, because these are known to influence tobacco initiation and uptake among children and youth. The Internet offers a still unregulated opportunity to market tobacco products to women and youth.

Addiction

Chapter 7, Addiction to Nicotine, points out that nicotine's effects on a user vary with the tobacco product and the way nicotine enters the body. Women use a variety of combustible tobacco products, including roll-your-own cigarettes, cigars, bidis, and kreteks, as well as water pipes and pipes. The nicotine content of tobacco products varies widely according to form and brand. More women than men smoke "light" or "ultra-light" cigarettes (63% vs 46%), often in the mistaken belief that "light" means "safer". In fact, "light" smokers engage in compensatory smoking, inhaling more deeply and more often in an effort to achieve the desired amount of nicotine. Further study is needed on factors driving consumer preferences for smokeless tobacco, such as chewing tobacco and the moist and dry snuff that are gaining in popularity.

Contrary to popular belief, all tobacco products can be deadly and addictive, regardless of their form or disguise. While cigarettes are the most efficient product for delivering nicotine into the body, the nicotine content in water pipes and cigars has been shown to be significantly higher than that in manufactured cigarettes. Tobacco companies have recently introduced potentially reduced-exposure products for which information on potential risks is lacking.

Nicotine affects women's physiology and mood differently from the way it affects men's. For example, rates of nicotine metabolism are significantly higher in women smokers who use oral contraceptives and those who are pregnant. Tobacco-related health risks for women include osteoporosis and increased risk of fracture, early menopause, and sexual and reproductive health problems. Nicotine replacement therapy (NRT) is useful for cessation, but women have higher sensitivity to nicotine than men have. Key barriers that may make quitting more difficult for women than for men include poverty, depression, lack of social support, and fear of weight gain. Appetite suppression is a critical aspect of the appeal of smoking for many women and girls in some socioeconomic groups. Research indicates that in some countries, girls who use tobacco tend to have relatively stronger attachments to peers and friends than do boys who smoke. The girls also tend to overestimate smoking prevalence in their environment, are less knowledgeable about nicotine and addiction, and usually have parents or friends who smoke. More research is needed on the process of initiation into smoking, transitions from experimentation to addiction, and risk and protective factors for girls and women in different cultural settings and in developing countries.

Models of addiction provide useful frameworks for designing interventions and offer a point of departure for preventing and treating addiction, taking into consideration behavioural and psychological factors, social and environmental influences, and marketing. It is important to remember that there are multiple pathways to overcoming addiction. Often overlooked are some obvious guidelines, e.g. that treatments should address women's specific concerns and that the single most effective method is to quit in the early stages of use.

Quitting

Beating Nicotine Addiction

Chapter 8, Quitting Smoking and Beating Nicotine Addiction, emphasizes the fact that most smokers and tobacco chewers are addicted tobacco customers, not satisfied consumers. Studies in Canada, the United Kingdom, Australia, and the United States show that nearly 9 out of 10 smokers say they regret smoking, with women more likely to express regret about smoking than men.

Women seem to be less successful at quitting smoking than men, although there are scant global data on this issue. Because women are more prone to depression, and depression increases the risk of relapse, this is a special concern for women. Some studies indicate that adolescent girls and women are more concerned about weight gain than men are and may resume smoking to avoid it. Also, pregnant women may prefer individual counselling over group counselling, especially if they anticipate disapproval of their smoking by others. Women-only groups may be required for intervention. The social and economic status of women smokers is also relevant, as poor, less-educated women are significantly less likely to quit.

At the moment, there does not appear to be sufficient evidence of clinically important differences between men and women to guide treatment. More research is needed on use by women of non-nicotine medications such as bupropion, varenicline, and other emerging therapies. Pregnant women should attempt cessation with non-pharmacological modalities before using NRT. There is insufficient evidence about the long-term benefit of the use of interventions to help smokers reduce but not quit tobacco use.

Determining the best way to help smokers quit requires better knowledge of their behaviour as consumers of cessation methods and services, determinants of their preferences, and the role of costs. Studies among pregnant women indicate that 82% want behavioural support, and 77% want self-help materials. In one study, two thirds of the women thought that if their partner, family, or friends quit smoking, it would be easier for them to quit. In some cultures, tobacco cessation professionals may be involved, while in others, spiritual leaders and faith healers may be consulted. All interventions need to be adapted for particular subgroups, specific cultures, and countries.

Models of behavioural change such as the Social Cognitive Theory/Social Learning Theory, Health Belief Model, and the Theory of Planned Behaviour have been applied to tobacco control with varying degrees of success. The Transtheoretical Model of intentional behaviour change is the most multidimensional of the behaviour-change theories and appears to be the most predictive. It views smokers as moving through a series of stages: precontemplation, contemplation, preparation, action, and maintenance. This stage-based approach has been used to help providers of support determine clients' readiness for change. Research supports the notion that cessation success can be predicted by the stage of change. Relapse back to tobacco use is expected after a period of abstinence and recycling through the stages.

Large numbers of tobacco users have been able to quit on their own or with minimal assistance. For those requiring assistance, combining behavioural and pharmacological treatments may increase quitting success, particularly for heavy smokers. Interventions that easily reach women at home include quit lines, Internet smoking cessation sites, and counselling. Women are especially likely to benefit from combination therapy, and psychosocial support seems to offer benefits. It is important to remember that comprehensive tobacco control measures—including bans on smoking in public places and appropriately high taxation—all contribute to higher cessation rates.

Pregnancy and Postpartum Cessation

Chapter 9, Pregnancy and Postpartum Smoking Cessation, concludes that for female users of tobacco and their partners, pregnancy represents an opportunity to

World Health Organization

quit. The smoking cessation guidelines calling for 5 As (Ask, Advise, Assess, Assist, and Arrange for follow-up) should be used in gynaecological office practice. Emphasis should be given to the benefits of cessation *before* women become pregnant. Benefits of quitting include reduced frequency of low-birth-weight and pre-term births and of pregnancy complications, as well as improved health of the mother. A significant reduction (more than 50%) in smoking, with the associated decrease in exposure of the fetus during pregnancy, can significantly increase birth weight. For national health-care systems, cessation by women can also result in significant savings.

In the early 1990s, when the smoking prevalence among the female population in the United States was higher than 20%, the rate for women in obstetric care was estimated to be 13.6%. These figures, however, do not reflect the wide range of smoking rates among pregnant women, nor do they identify the subgroups having particularly high rates. For example, cigarette smoking is generally less prevalent among Afro-American, Hispanic, and Asian women in the United States across all age ranges, while prevalence rates are high among less-educated non-Hispanic whites.

There are multiple opportunities for intervention prior to, during, and after pregnancy, each with varying challenges. A key to success is ensuring that partners and family members support quitting during pregnancy and through the critical transition to the postpartum period. As partner smoking is probably the single most important facilitator of women's continued smoking, quitting programmes should also focus on paternal smoking. As with SHS, men have important responsibilities in helping to improve the health environment and behavioural outcomes related to women and tobacco.

Research undertaken primarily in industrialized countries has refined the approaches to effective interventions. These findings may be applicable in other settings, although further research is needed on their applicability in developing countries. For example, subgroups of pregnant women display different quitting behaviours. The non-smokers may actually include many previous users of tobacco. Indeed, information on pre-pregnancy quitting is likely to be inaccurate, as women who stop smoking prior to becoming pregnant may report themselves as never-smokers. For this group, which may relapse to smoking after pregnancy, it is important to maintain positive, tobacco-free health behaviour. In countries where access to obstetric and gynaecological care may be limited, midwives, elders, modern medical professionals, and indigenous health-care providers should be trained to promote quitting in early adulthood.

Pre-pregnancy quitters typically sustain cessation throughout the pregnancy and may be smoke-free for their entire life. Newly pregnant spontaneous quitters are often highly motivated to protect their babies. It is noteworthy that pregnant women in cultures where extended families may be heavily involved in managing the pregnancy often have lower smoking rates. However, the return to smoking for spontaneous quitters during the postpartum period may exceed 50% and may be as high as 80%. For this reason, more attention needs to be paid to relapse prevention services for women in the postpartum period.

Women who continue to smoke during pregnancy are typically less-educated, unemployed, and of lower SES. They also often live in more smoke-filled home environments. Studies in the United States, the United Kingdom, Sweden, Australia, and Canada indicate that cessation counselling in brief periods can be effective early in pregnancy. The cost–benefit ratio for an intervention that achieved a 15% smoking cessation rate, compared with the 5% cessation rate of usual practice, would be US$ 11 in savings for each US$ 1 of investment. Women who continue to smoke later in pregnancy find it particularly difficult to quit, and promoting cessation is even more difficult with women who have already had a child and smoked during the prior pregnancy.

Interventions should be based on the premise that there is no safe level of exposure to nicotine for the fetus. Health-care providers should encourage male partners who are smokers to support and not undermine a partner's cessation during pregnancy and in the postpartum period. One interesting attempt to do so was Project PANDA, which sent video and print materials tailored to the male perspective on pregnancy and child care. Cessation in light of impending fatherhood and emphasis on the dangers of SHS were also included. Evaluation indicated that 28% of the men who received the materials were not smoking at three months postpartum, compared with 14% of the control-group men. The use of NRTs should be envisaged only as a harm-reduction strategy for women who are heavy smokers and who continue to smoke during pregnancy. Additional studies are needed to evaluate pharmacotherapy options.

Pregnancy provides an opportunity for change that affects the entire family. Most of the benefits of smoking cessation during pregnancy have focused on the fetus and the child. However, programmes can also help to improve the health of mothers and fathers. Smoking cessation interventions designed to reach mothers and fathers, using gender-sensitive approaches, should be integrated in family-planning programmes and in pregnancy testing, both at home and in clinic offices.

Policies and Strategies

A Gender Framework and Gender-Sensitive Policies

A gender framework for tobacco control focuses attention on the social, cultural, and economic factors underlying tobacco use among women throughout the life-course. "Gender" is defined as the social, economic, and cultural construct of the relations between men and women, and, as such, it underlies the social construction of tobacco promotion, consumption, treatment, and health services. Gender inequality contributes to women's lack of participation in health policy decision-making. Gender inequality is embedded in institutions at many levels, from the household to macroeconomic structures. As WHO has noted, "Many of the main causes of women's morbidity and mortality—in both rich and poor countries—have their origins in societies' attitudes to women, which are reflected in the structures and systems that set policies, determine services and create opportunities".[3] Furthermore, the exclusion of girls and women of all ages on the basis of race, caste, ethnicity, religion, or disability is a serious obstacle to successfully implementing gender-sensitive tobacco control policies.

Chapter 2, A Gender Equality Framework for Tobacco Control states that a gender analysis differs from a "women and development" approach in that it acknowledges how gender roles, norms, and relations affect both women and men. Masculinities (the social construct around what being a man is) can be counterproductive or even destructive for men. For example, one reason for rising rates of tobacco use among men has been the targeted marketing that promotes smoking as macho, healthy, sexually attractive, and trend-setting. Yet men have important proactive roles in engaging in women's rights to health. As the majority

of the world's smokers, men are mainly responsible for women's involuntary exposure to SHS. As more men join the gender equality movement, stronger support for women's human rights as a cornerstone for tobacco control is in sight.

Implementing the WHO FCTC through a gender perspective should be understood as part of a country's political and development agenda. If the tobacco epidemic among women and girls continues to spread, it will contribute to rising health-care costs and will use valuable resources needed for social development. It will also make achieving the United Nations Millennium Development Goals (MDGs) on improving maternal health and reducing poverty more difficult. The WHO FCTC Preamble recognizes that applying a gender equality framework to tobacco control is integral to effective implementation of its Articles. Provisions concerned with SHS, packaging and labelling, health warnings, and bans on advertising, promotion, and sponsorship, as well as improving national research, are all relevant to women's concerns.

At a theoretical level, the WHO Regional Office for South-East Asia (WHO/SEARO) model of health behaviour can be used to analyse the effects of gender inequality throughout the health system and can help map interrelationships between tobacco control and broader social, cultural, and economic processes. A gender equality framework suggests that comprehensive tobacco control requires applying a gender analysis to many sectors outside health—including finance, trade, and agriculture—all of which influence tobacco use among women. The economic costs of the death and disability of a male head of household due to tobacco use are high for poor households, and they affect women and men disproportionately.

There are a number of strategic actions that can help make a difference. Governments must improve coordination with national agencies and stakeholders for women's affairs, provide adequate financing, and apply indicators for gender equality in national planning. Gender mainstreaming of policies is more likely to succeed if gender experts are included at senior policy levels. Budgeting for gender equality requires development of sensitive, cost-effective indicators and baseline data disaggregated by age as well as by sex.

The WHO FCTC is the pre-eminent global tobacco control instrument; it contains legally binding obliga-tions for its Parties, sets the foundation for reducing both

World Health Organization

demand and supply of tobacco, and provides a comprehensive direction for tobacco control policy at all levels.[2] In its global tobacco reports on tobacco control, WHO launched and analysed the MPOWER package, introduced to assist in the country-level implementation of effective measures to reduce the demand for tobacco, contained in the WHO FCTC.[2,4] Although the MPOWER measures, which correspond to one or more Articles of the WHO FCTC, do not explicitly refer to a gender equality perspective, seen through a women's rights lens they can be interpreted as follows:

1. **M**onitor tobacco use *by gender* and *ensure that* prevention policies *are gender-sensitive* (Article 20 of the WHO FCTC).

2. **P**rotect *girls and women of all ages* from tobacco smoke (Article 8 of the WHO FCTC).

3. **O**ffer help to assist *women in quitting* tobacco use (Article 14 of the WHO FCTC).

4. **W**arn *women and girls* about the dangers of tobacco *through gender-sensitive information and communication strategies* (Articles 11 and 12 of the WHO FCTC).

5. **E**nforce bans on tobacco advertising, promotion, and sponsorship *by empowering women to identify and counter these influences* (Article 13 of the WHO FCTC).

6. **R**aise taxes on tobacco, *with the active participation of women leaders* (Article 6 of the WHO FCTC).

According to Chapter 10, How to Make Policies More Gender-Sensitive, the gender bias inherent in many existing health policies and tobacco control programmes must be challenged. Data from South Africa, China, Sweden, and the United Kingdom indicate varied forms of gender policies, according to Kabeer's typology of gender-related policies. Among these, gender-blind policies, which may appear to be unbiased, are often, in fact, based on information derived from men's activities and assume that all persons have the same needs and interests as men.

Tobacco control should aim to improve gender-redistributive policies that recognize women's exclusion and disadvantage in terms of access to social and economic resources, as well as decision-making. Gender-redistributive policies include provision of microcredit loans to women to help empower them and transform gender relations—measures that some health advocates believe must be taken if women's health is to improve. Tobacco control policies need to keep the goal of gender-sensitivity in mind while implementing measures to reduce consumption. The design of policies may be gender-neutral, yet the policies may affect women and men very differently. Thus, all policies, health services, and programmes must be monitored and evaluated, using gender indicators as well as conventional health indicators. Data and indicators should be disaggregated by sex where appropriate.

Economics and Taxation

Taxes that increase the price of tobacco and reduce its affordability are very effective in reducing both paternal and maternal smoking prevalence, thereby reducing the negative consequences of smoking on maternal and child health. Chapter 11, Taxation and the Economics of Tobacco Control, points out that tobacco control programmes must pay increasing attention to economic policies concerned with trade, taxation, tobacco production, and price (Article 6 of the WHO FCTC). Tobacco control is not likely to cause the estimated 33 million people engaged in tobacco farming worldwide—many of whom are women and children—to lose their jobs in the short run. Agricultural policies should therefore take into account evidence that tobacco control will have minimal negative impact on long-run economic growth, employment, or the foreign trade balance.

Rapid urbanization and changes in lifestyle and diet mean that scarce resources are now being used for treatment of noncommunicable diseases, potentially limiting the resources available for prevention. A study in the United States found that smoking-attributable neonatal costs totalled almost US$ 367 million (in 1996 dollars). The calculated annual costs to New York City related to infants' developmental delays caused by prenatal exposure to SHS amounted to US$ 99 million. In China, direct costs of smoking in 2000 were estimated to be 3.1% of national health expenditures. At the household level in Indonesia, where smoking is most common among the poor, 15% of the total expenditure of the lowest income group is on tobacco, while the poorest 20% of households in Mexico spend nearly 11% of their income on tobacco. Productivity losses for smokers and their caregivers—including lost wages because of time off from work—represent a substantial cost to society.

The costs of SHS exposure are particularly relevant to a gender perspective on tobacco control, because women and children are the majority of the world's involuntary smokers. A study in Minnesota estimated the cost of direct medical treatment for conditions related to SHS to be US$ 228.7 million (in 2008 dollars), equivalent to US$ 62.68 per capita annually. A report from the American Society of Actuaries calculated that US$ 2.6 billion was spent for medical care for lung cancer and heart disease caused by exposure of non-smokers to SHS in the United States.

There is solid evidence that taxation of all forms of tobacco is highly effective in reducing consumption, particularly among youth and low-income groups, among which prevalence is often highest. Increases in cigarette taxes could be a powerful tool for protecting poor women in developing countries, because higher taxes are known to have a significant negative effect on maternal smoking rates. Increased taxes also help to prevent former users from re-starting and can lead current users to try to quit. Studies in the United States, the United Kingdom, and Canada have concluded that the overall price elasticity of demand ranges from –0.5 to 0.25, implying that a 10% increase in the price of cigarettes will decrease overall cigarette consumption in these countries by between 2.5% and 5.0%. Young people are found to be much more price-sensitive than adults in low-, middle-, and high-income countries, according to studies in Nepal, Ukraine, Myanmar, and the Russian Federation.

The share of taxes in the price of cigarettes varies from more than 80% to less than 30%, with many lower-income countries having the lowest tax rates. Taxes could be increased to 65–75% of the retail price of cigarettes, the level in several countries. However, tax increases need to be applied symmetrically across all types of tobacco products in a manner that equalizes the retail sales of the various types; taxes also must keep up with inflation in order for their real value not to be eroded. Concerns about tobacco taxation, such as efficiency and equity related to low-income smokers and threats of smuggling, should be addressed. Earmarking a portion of the revenue generated from tobacco taxes for tobacco control programmes reinforces the effects of the taxes on consumption.

Studies indicate that individuals from lower-income groups respond more to price changes than do persons with higher incomes, more education, and higher SES. Furthermore, evidence from many countries, including Indonesia, Malaysia, Turkey, Viet Nam, and China, shows that changing per capita income significantly affects smoking prevalence, as well as cigarette demand. One study in Turkey found that income elasticity declined with household income level. The evidence suggests that to reduce consumption by a desired amount, the percentage increase in price must be higher if income is increasing. The data on impact by gender and age are not conclusive as to whether females are more price-sensitive than males. Also, much more research is needed on the costs and impact of taxation policies related to the wide variety of smoked and smokeless tobacco products used by girls and women of all ages.

International Agreements and the International Women's Movement

Mobilization and leadership can make a difference. Chapter 13, The International Women's Movement and Anti-Tobacco Campaigns, provides an historic perspective on regional and international movements and traces women's groups' activities in reproductive health and consumer rights, as well as anti-tobacco activities.

Around the world, nongovernmental organizations (NGOs) are doing their share. The Framework Convention Alliance (FCA), a coalition of NGOs and individuals representing nearly 300 organizations from more than 100 countries, helps to organize an international social movement in support of the WHO FCTC. The FCA is exemplary in the attention it gives to monitoring gender issues in the WHO FCTC and in its good record of gender balance in its top leadership. Throughout the WHO FCTC negotiations, its women's caucus worked to ensure that women's human rights were an integral part of the treaty. Organizations of women health professionals—physicians, nurses, and scientists—in alliance with the media, have initiated community-based programmes that contribute to women's involvement in tobacco control. Groups such as the International Network of Women Against Tobacco (INWAT) and the US National Organization of Women have pioneered community-based strategies.

The Women's Environment and Development Organization, in collaboration with WHO and the Campaign for Tobacco-Free Kids, organized a meeting of their networks to plan activities on women and tobacco. Other groups, such as REDEH/CEMINA in Brazil and the Latin American Women's Health Network, have carried out public information campaigns in China, the Lao People's Democratic Republic, Thailand, Bangladesh, Saint Kitts, and Argentina, and campaigns are being planned in 20 countries.

Gender must be mainstreamed in tobacco control, fully utilizing international agreements and human rights policies. The groundwork has been laid. As Chapter 12, Women's Rights and International Agreements, points out, many tobacco-growing countries, including China, Malawi, Zimbabwe, and Indonesia, have signed the women's "bill of rights" known as the Convention on the Elimination of All Forms of Discrimination against Women (CEDAW). CEDAW, the most important legally binding international document on the human rights of women, has been ratified by more than 185 countries. It is unique because it addresses deep-rooted and multifaceted gender inequality, emphasizing both public- and private-sphere relations and rights, and it specifically underlines the difference between de jure and de facto equality of women. The CEDAW Committee has concluded that governments' compliance with Article 12 and General Recommendation 24 of CEDAW—both concerned with health—is central to ensuring that women have equal access to health information and services. Other Articles in CEDAW that are supportive of the WHO FCTC include Article 1, which deals with discrimination against women working in the informal sector, such as bidi workers; Article 14, which is concerned with rural women; and Article 11, on women's right to the protection of health in work conditions.

The international community can use legally binding treaties to guide implementation of important policy documents such as the Beijing Platform for Action. The follow-ups to the Fourth World Conference on Women, such as Beijing Plus Ten, the International Conference on Population and Development, and other social and economic accords, are all relevant to ensuring women's rights to health. The international women's health movement, in partnership with governments and the United Nations, has succeeded in strengthening partnerships at these forums. Tobacco control leaders should build on this momentum.

Issues for Advocacy

Although there are major gaps in data and research concerning gender, women, and tobacco, particularly in developing countries, this shortcoming should not justify inaction. Current research suggests several issues for advocacy and action. First, eliminating exposure to SHS is a high priority, because it affects the majority of women throughout their life-course. Women's empowerment is key to achieving smoke-free homes and should be included in campaigns against SHS. As a first step, women and girls need to be better informed about the hazards of SHS to themselves, as well as to fetuses, children, and family members.

Second, men have an important role in protecting women's rights to health. As the majority of the world's smokers, they are primarily responsible for women's involuntary exposure to SHS. As fathers, they can protect the health of fetuses, infants, and girls. As partners, they can encourage pregnant women who quit to stay tobacco-free. As politicians, businessmen, and media leaders, men can take greater responsibility for supporting tobacco control policies that benefit women, such as enforcing total bans on advertising and promotion of tobacco products across all media. Finally, as health planners and health-care providers, their support is critical to making health systems work better for girls and women.

Third, a couples approach to tobacco use during pregnancy and the transition to the postpartum period may be the most effective means for improving the health of the entire family, including infants. Victimization of pregnant women who use tobacco can be a major barrier to their quitting smoking. Non-reporting of tobacco use, lack of support by family members and partners, and failure of doctors to ask about paternal smoking all contribute to increased health risks for pregnant women. Assuring that reproductive health services are women-friendly is also important.

Fourth, as noted in the 2009 WHO report on *Women and Health*,[3] a life-course approach is needed to fully comprehend the impacts of tobacco on the health of girls and women of all ages. A life-course perspective can deepen understanding of the implications of exposure to tobacco smoke in childhood, through adolescence, during the reproductive years, and beyond, to old age. Such an approach can help map out the interrelationships between social and biological determinants of women's and men's health, linking exposures even before conception to risk for chronic disease in adulthood. There has been little investigation of the later-life consequences of early-life exposures to tobacco smoke. Much more research is needed on how the age of starting to smoke regularly might affect both male and female children's growth and the subsequent risk of diseases caused by smoking.

Finally, gender-sensitive tobacco interventions that include a focus on women's rights should take place in the context of comprehensive tobacco control and as part of a development strategy to reduce poverty. For example, curbing tobacco use is essential for the achievement of the MDGs that concern improving maternal health. Furthermore, such an approach must recognize the diversity of women's and men's needs that may vary by age, ethnicity, economic status, and levels of education. Poor urban and rural women are disproportionately affected by the tobacco epidemic. In many countries, women of lower SES who also have less access to quitting resources have the highest rates of tobacco use. In developing countries, rural women working in tobacco production, manufacture, and marketing receive unequal and inadequate compensation for their labour and job insecurity. Poor families can least afford expenditures on tobacco that take away income that could be used for food, education, and health care. The social costs of the death of a male head of household due to tobacco use are high for widows, who often have unequal access to productive employment and social services.

Gains Made and Looking Ahead

WHO has taken the lead in the effort to coordinate a global strategic response to the tobacco epidemic. As already noted, the WHO FCTC is a powerful tool for change. It promotes women's participation and a gender-sensitive approach to tobacco control. Its Preamble supports women's right to participate fully in decision-making at all levels as a human right. Gender equality should be applied in the interpretation and implementation of all Articles in the WHO FCTC. The future challenge is to ensure that women leaders know their rights under the WHO FCTC and are mobilized at the grass-roots level.

Many governments and municipalities have initiated effective tobacco control measures. In 2004, Ireland became the first country in the world to implement national legislation that banned smoking in all indoor workplaces, including restaurants and bars. Uruguay and New Zealand have each implemented a national ban on smoking in all indoor workplaces, public transport, and public places; both countries also demonstrate high levels of enforcement of and compliance with the legislation. Seven mostly low- and middle-income countries implemented comprehensive smoke-free policies in 2008, covering an additional 154 million people. Panama passed a new advertising ban in 2008. Despite all these changes, nearly 90% of the world's population remains uncovered by comprehensive tobacco legislation.[2] Much more can be done by raising taxes; enforcing a ban on deceptive terms such as "low tar", "light", and "mild"; and improving health warnings to prevent initiation of tobacco use by women and girls.

In the past decade, WHO has continued to strengthen its gender policy, surveillance, resource mobilization, and human resources. A grant from Bloomberg Philanthropies, along with an additional grant from the Bill and Melinda Gates Foundation, has greatly increased resources devoted to fighting tobacco use where it is highest—in the developing world—and has given a boost to WHO's country-level work. In collaboration with the National Cancer Centre in Japan, WHO held an operational planning meeting in 2009 for gender and tobacco projects, with the aim of speeding up gender mainstreaming. Practical implementation plans were developed in Viet Nam to move from policy to action. Recommendations were made on ways to apply a gender analysis to project implementation on interventions such as gender-based health warnings; tax increases; smoke-free environments; bans on advertising, promotion, and sponsorship; and education and communications.[5]

Country-specific data disaggregated by sex have been reported in the *WHO Report on the Global Tobacco Epidemic, 2008: The MPOWER Package* and the *WHO Report on the Global Tobacco Epidemic, 2009: Implementing Smoke-Free Environments*. Other WHO activities have contributed to improving scientific evidence as a basis for policy formulation and programme implementation on gender, women, and tobacco. Important new information about gender differences in tobacco use is provided by the GYTS, which focuses on tobacco use in youth 13 to 15 years of age; the Global School Personnel Survey (GSPS), which collects information from school personnel concerning their use of tobacco; the Global Health Professions Student Survey (GHPSS), which collects data on tobacco use and cessation counselling among health-profession students; and the Global Adult Tobacco Survey (GATS), which monitors tobacco use among adults as part of the Global Tobacco Surveillance System (GTSS).

WHO has worked collaboratively with other partners, including the International Development Research Centre (IDRC), to hold scientific consultations on gender and tobacco. It also continues to work with human rights bodies, such as CEDAW, and NGOs, including the International Network of Women Against Tobacco. At the Eighth United Nations Ad Hoc Interagency Task Force on Tobacco Control meeting, representatives from United Nations agencies such as UNFPA, UNICEF, and the World Bank reviewed ways to strengthen interagency collaboration on gender, women, and tobacco. *Sifting the Evidence: Gender and Tobacco Control,* published by WHO in 2007, provides a summary policy guide and reflects WHO's concern with ensuring that the WHO FCTC process makes gender a central part of its implementation. In the WHO report *Women and Health—Today's Evidence, Tomorrow's Agenda*, the importance of tobacco control to support women's health throughout the life-course is highlighted.[3] The 2010 theme of the WHO World No Tobacco Day was Gender and Tobacco with an Emphasis on Marketing to Women. The international campaign highlighted the tobacco industry's misleading tactics in marketing tobacco products to women and girls. It also focused on women's right to smoke-free environments in the workplace and home.

Future efforts to curb the rising epidemic of tobacco use among women and girls must be built on solid evidence. However, improvements are needed in national databases, particularly in developing countries, and research targeting women and tobacco must be undertaken. Gender bias is pervasive, with the result that data concerning tobacco use or prevalence of tobacco-related diseases among girls and women throughout the life-course are often unavailable or outdated. Moreover, the data that are available may not be disaggregated to identify differences by income, ethnicity, or occupation. Considerable improvements in methodologies are needed to evaluate the impact of tobacco control policies—including trade, tax, and economic policies—on women's health. As the international community struggles to protect the public from SHS and curb rising rates of tobacco use among women and girls, a renewed commitment to women's right to health as a human right is more important than ever.

References

1. *Report of the WHO International Conference on Tobacco and Health, Kobe – Making a difference in tobacco and health.* Geneva, World Health Organization, 1999.
2. *WHO report on the global tobacco epidemic, 2009: implementing smoke-free environments.* Geneva, World Health Organization, 2009.
3. *Women and health: today's evidence, tomorrow's agenda.* Geneva, World Health Organization, 2009.
4. *WHO report on the global tobacco epidemic, 2008: the MPOWER package.* Geneva, World Health Organization, 2008.
5. *WHO operational planning meeting for gender and tobacco projects: meeting report 21–23 July 2009.* Geneva, World Health Organization, 2009.

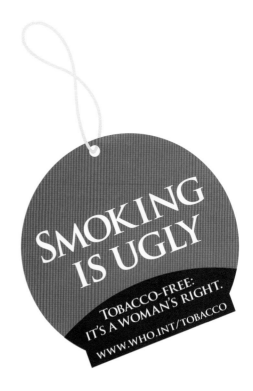

THE TOBACCO INDUSTRY CATCHES YOU YOUNG

BREAK
THE TOBACCO
MARKETING NET

BAN ALL TOBACCO ADVERTISING,
PROMOTION AND SPONSORSHIP

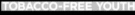
TOBACCO-FREE YOUTH

WORLD NO TOBACCO DAY, 31 MAY
www.who.int/tobacco/wntd

World Health
Organization

2. A Gender Equality Framework for Tobacco Control

Introduction

The epidemiological patterns of tobacco-related diseases and deaths are largely shaped by the social and cultural meanings associated with tobacco use that drive initiation and cessation. Of these, gender is generally the least understood by policy-makers, yet the tobacco industry continues to use gender imagery as a basic marketing tool. Clearly, it is essential to clarify the concept of gender and its relevance to the design and implementation of tobacco control. Questions to consider include: Why is a gender analysis important to women and tobacco control policies? How can gender equality be mainstreamed into tobacco control policies and budgeting? Which indicators can best monitor progress?

The objectives of this chapter are to identify the scope of gender analysis—with a focus on women's rights—for tobacco control and to outline a working action-oriented framework that shows linkages to the wider context of social and economic development. Examples of how such analysis affects tobacco control laws are provided, and guidelines for translating it into institutional and financial arrangements are discussed.

In the simplest terms, "gender" is used to describe characteristics of women and men that are socially constructed, while "sex" refers to those that are biologically determined. In human society, biology is not destiny. People are born female or male but must learn to be girls and boys, then women and men. Learned behaviour makes up gender identity and helps shape gender roles. As noted in the World Health Organization (WHO) report *Women and Health,* both "sex and gender have a significant impact on the health of women and must be considered when developing appropriate strategies for health promotion.... Gender inequality, both alone and in combination with biological differences, can increase women's vulnerability or exposure to certain risks".[1] Data on the patterns of tobacco use by gender are not the same as sex-disaggregated data. It is necessary to perform gender analysis of such data to expose the social, cultural, and economic inequalities determined by the social norms, roles, and expectations of men and women.

Social relations such as gender hierarchies constantly change as old forms dissolve and are recreated.[2] This is illustrated by the impact that death and disability resulting from tobacco use has on gender roles. The disability of a male head of household puts an unequal burden on women, because of women's central role in the care economy—the sector that contributes to family welfare through provision of unpaid services such as health care, cooking, clothing, and managing the household. Women are the backbone of unpaid care work. Time-use surveys indicate that women spend twice as much time as men on unpaid care work in addition to their own paid jobs.[2] As a result, women have longer working days on average than men have. This unequal division of labour has important implications for challenges facing women during financial crises. Traditionally, the family functions as the surrogate safety net. However, when cuts in public spending on social services occur, stresses are placed on women in their roles as household managers and caregivers.

A human rights perspective that upholds women's dignity and freedom and right to health is fundamental to remedying gender inequality. As noted in the World Bank's *Global Monitoring Report, 2007: Millennium Development Goals,* gender equality does not necessarily mean equality of "outcomes" for males and females.[3] Rather, it means "equal access to the opportunities that allow people to pursue a life of their own choosing and to avoid extreme deprivation in outcomes". Equality of rights refers to gender equality under either customary or statutory law. Discrimination is apparent in the frequent invisibility of women in national tobacco control statistics, as well as the common exclusion of women in research protocols. Equality of resources means equality of opportunities that result from investments made in women's health, including investments for subgroups such as rural women. To achieve such equality, appropriate allocation of resources is required to educate women about the health hazards of tobacco use and second-hand smoke (SHS).

Men and Gender Roles

A gender equality approach differs from a "women and development" approach in that it acknowledges the ways gender roles can also affect men. The construct of

World Health Organization

masculinity often puts men at risk of harmful health behaviours and consequences that can be destructive for them.[1] In tobacco control, the most obvious gender factor—that being born male is the strongest predictor for tobacco use—is often overlooked. Historically, in many cultures, tobacco was integrated into the fabric of a social and ritual life that was dominated by men. Indeed, tobacco use was viewed as a male prerogative in the United States and Europe until the early 20th century. One reason for rising rates of tobacco use among men has been the targeted marketing that promotes smoking as macho, healthy, sexually attractive, and trend-setting.

Integrating a gender perspective into tobacco control requires an analysis of how biological, social, economic, and cultural factors influence health risks and outcomes and lead to different needs for males and females.

Men have important roles and responsibility to help promote women's rights to health. As the majority of the world's smokers, men are primarily responsible for women's involuntary exposure to SHS. This is elaborated in the chapter in this monograph on SHS, women, and children. In some countries, including China and Viet Nam, women bear the greatest burden from exposure to men's smoking. Fathers have the ability to help protect the health of fetuses, infants, and girls. They can also encourage pregnant partners who quit smoking to stay tobacco-free. As the chapter on pregnancy and postpartum smoking cessation notes, partner smoking is the single greatest predictor of whether or not a pregnant woman will quit smoking.

However, gender norms and roles can change. An example of changing gender roles is the way in which the rising rates of tobacco use among girls and women will ultimately affect men's family responsibilities. When men die, families usually experience a downturn in economic security. However, deaths of mothers can affect the entire family's quality of life.

In some areas, such as rural Africa, a woman's death means that other family members must take over caregiving roles such as child care and caring for the elderly. A woman's death also may deprive the family of basic necessities such as the provision of water and food.[2]

Recognition of the important interaction between social policy, family life, and gender roles is making headway, with men's support. The involvement of men in national campaigns for equal responsibility of men and women has proven successful in many health-related areas, including violence against women and HIV/AIDS.[4] Similarly, male United Nations officials and government leaders have supported gender, women, and tobacco activities and are strong advocates for gender equality. As businessmen and leaders, men have assumed greater responsibility for supporting tobacco control policies such as enforcing a total ban on advertising and promotion and mandating graphic warnings on tobacco products—all of which help girls and women quit smoking. Male health planners, doctors, and nurses can help ensure access to high-quality, women-friendly health services and can serve as role models for young medical students. As more men join in the gender equality movement, stronger support for women's human rights as a cornerstone for tobacco control is in sight.

The Scope of Gender Analysis and Social and Economic Development

Integrating a gender perspective into tobacco control requires an analysis of how biological, social, economic, and cultural factors influence health risks and outcomes and lead to different needs for males and females.[1] In this effort, the health sector must provide strong leadership. However, tobacco control must also involve many other sectors, because patterns of tobacco use are affected by a variety of socioeconomic and cultural trends. Policies in financial, agricultural, and trade sectors influence tobacco production, marketing, and consumption. Equally significant, tobacco use can affect social and economic development. For example, when governments must spend millions of dollars to treat tobacco-related diseases, fewer public funds are available to invest in poverty reduction. The collection of data and the conduct of research on gender-related factors should extend across all relevant sectors.[5,6] A holistic approach can provide the scientific evidence needed to ensure that policies will be successful among both men and women and that programmes will address gender-specific issues.

What should be the scope of a gender analysis for tobacco control? Which strategies work? In many countries, the traditional public health strategy is based on the Health Belief Model, which views a person's beliefs and perceptions as the primary influence on tobacco uptake (see the chapter on quitting smoking and overcoming nicotine addiction). Public information campaigns, along with Knowledge, Attitude, and Practice surveys, are the standard tools used to change health behaviour. However, while single-strand interventions such as school health programmes have had some impact, information alone cannot always empower people to make decisions that protect their own health. Rather, a wide spectrum of interventions at multiple levels—consistently applied—is needed to reverse the tobacco epidemic.

A holistic approach is consistent with the concept developed by a team of scientists at the World Health Organization South-East Asia Regional Office (WHO/SEARO) who are concerned with broadening the scope of health behaviour research. They note that the conventional public health approach errs in focusing primarily on individuals, without reference to the social, economic, and political structures that also determine behaviour.[7] For example, to address the question of whether rural women know that tobacco leaves can cause green tobacco sickness (GTS), the conventional health education approach would be to ensure that rural women learn about health hazards and how to protect themselves. In contrast, a gender-sensitive approach would take into account the logical corollary that poor women must also be enabled to change their behaviour through economic empowerment. Unless they have money to buy protective gloves, there is little likelihood that their condition will change. While this scenario may appear obvious, the same issue of empowerment affects other situations. Any woman living in a patriarchal household knows the problems she faces in asking her husband to quit smoking in the home. Threats of domestic violence are common, yet these are seldom considered relevant to tobacco control.

A gender equality approach to tobacco control must also analyse how health cultures can influence health-promoting behaviour (see Figure 2.1). For example, a pregnant woman may be aware that smoking during pregnancy can cause low birth weight. However, she may never mention her tobacco use to a doctor for fear of being stigmatized or blamed. Similarly, the professional health culture that influences the attitudes of health-care providers can be important in determining the health behaviour of patients. The carriers of health messages must be regarded as knowledgeable, trustworthy, and, ideally, available for follow-up. They must also take responsibility for asking pregnant women whether or not they have a history of tobacco use. In many developing countries, they must also avoid the common assumption that pregnant women are tobacco-free.

The scope of a gender equality framework must be holistic and inclusive at multiple levels and must consider the social interrelationships between local health and processes.

Professional health cultures also influence traditional health practitioners such as midwives, herbalists, and shamans. It is widely recognized in developing countries that health professionals have considerable influence over self-care and the management of family health. Much more attention must be paid to actively involving them in the design of tobacco control information, education, and communication strategies.

Another weakness in conventional approaches is the tendency of health-systems analysis to focus primarily on the professional health culture—the behaviour of nurses and doctors and the delivery of information or health services—while ignoring the broader context of government policies, international trade, and socioeconomic development[7] that influences their practice. Recent trends in globalization and international trade agreements illustrate how macroeconomic policies can influence the behaviour of health-care providers, as well as patients. Free trade agreements have led to a flood of imported cigarettes and highly sophisticated marketing that targets audiences

World Health Organization

in poor developing countries. Low prices, poor enforcement of tobacco control legislation, and the absence of gender-specific tobacco control policies all contribute to the rise in tobacco use among women and girls. Doctors must increasingly treat women with tobacco-related diseases and disability, an endeavour that requires specialized knowledge about sex-specific risks. Structural adjustment programmes that require payment for health services severely curtail the frequency of visits to health centres, negatively affecting both providers and users.

The scope of a gender equality framework must therefore be holistic and inclusive at multiple levels and must consider the social interrelationships between local health systems and international processes. Figure 2.1, adapted from a WHO/SEARO model showing the importance of the social and economic environment to health-promoting behaviour,[7] illustrates this point. Lay and professional health cultures are mapped out through an historical process. Factors such as the organization of households and communities, perception of health needs, health-care-seeking behaviour,

and acceptance of tobacco control messages all contribute to changing the health behaviour of women seeking health care. The professional health culture also affects the behaviour of tobacco control professionals and health workers. The perception of health needs and interventions (or the absence of services and information) contributes to the success or failure of tobacco control in reaching women.

At a structural level, tobacco control policies should take into account the fact that gender inequality is embedded in social and economic institutions, including those at the global level. As a United Nations Research Institute for Social Development report stated, "Gender inequalities are deeply entrenched in all societies, and are reproduced through a variety of practices and institutions".[2] Furthermore, the exclusion of women on the basis of race, caste, ethnicity, religion, or disability is a serious obstacle to successfully implementing gender-sensitive tobacco control policies.

The WHO FCTC is the pre-eminent global tobacco control instrument; it contains legally binding

Figure 2.1. Health-Promoting Behaviour / Spheres of Influence

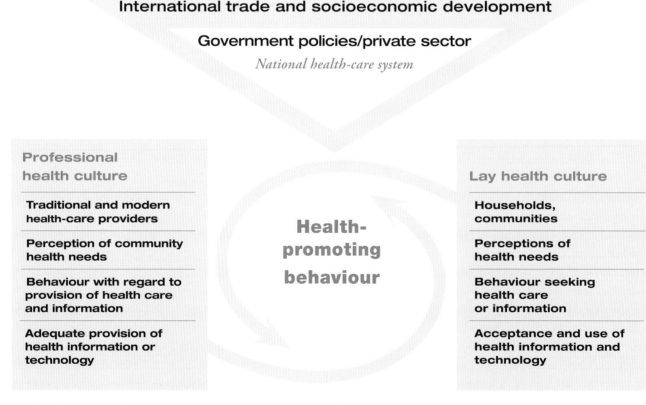

Source: Adapted from *Concepts of Health Behaviour Research.* New Delhi, WHO Regional Office for South-East Asia, 1986.

obligations for its Parties, sets the foundation for reducing both demand and supply of tobacco, and provides a comprehensive direction for tobacco control policy at all levels. In its global tobacco reports on tobacco control, WHO launched and analysed the MPOWER package,[8] introduced to assist in the country-level implementation of effective measures to reduce the demand for tobacco, contained in the WHO FCTC. Although the MPOWER measures, which correspond to one or more Articles of the WHO FCTC, do not explicitly refer to a gender equality perspective, seen through a women's rights lens they can be interpreted as follows:

1. **M**onitor tobacco use *by gender* and *ensure that* prevention policies *are gender-sensitive* (Article 20 of the WHO FCTC).

2. **P**rotect *girls and women of all ages* from tobacco smoke (Article 8 of the WHO FCTC).

3. **O**ffer help to assist *women in quitting* tobacco use (Article 14 of the WHO FCTC).

4. **W**arn *women and girls* about the dangers of tobacco *through gender-sensitive information and communication strategies* (Articles 11 and 12 of the WHO FCTC).

5. **E**nforce bans on tobacco advertising, promotion, and sponsorship *by empowering women to identify and counter these influences* (Article 13 of the WHO FCTC).

6. **R**aise taxes on tobacco, *with the active participation of women leaders* (Article 6 of the WHO FCTC).

It is evident that the scope of a gender equality framework for tobacco control must be an integral part of a country's political and development agenda. Indeed, there is growing evidence that tobacco hampers sustainable development. As noted in the chapter on taxation and the economics of tobacco control, the use of tobacco results in a net loss of billions of US dollars per year. Many costs of tobacco use, including its negative impact on the environment, affect economic development. Multinational companies gain the most, while male and female tobacco farmers and women who work in tobacco production receive only a small percentage of the profits. Rural women must also cope with the possible negative

impact of tobacco production on food production and the environment due to deforestation. In brief, tobacco has a negative impact on the health of economies as well as on the health of people.

The Millennium Development Goals

In 2000, the United Nations Member States pledged to dramatically decrease poverty, hunger, disease, and illiteracy within 15 years by meeting eight key targets. A global consensus was reached, involving heads of state, government representatives, and the private sector, as well as the active participation of civil society. These social and economic targets, known as the Millennium Development Goals (MDGs), do not explicitly refer to tobacco, but they are relevant to understanding how gender equality in tobacco control fits into the future of social and economic development.

Gender equality has been highlighted as a cross-cutting issue that is imperative for achieving all MDG targets.

Central to gender and tobacco concerns is the goal of promoting gender equality and empowering women (MDG 3). Gender equality has been highlighted as a cross-cutting issue that is imperative for achieving all MDG targets.[8] Furthermore, six of the eight MDGs are related to health, underscoring the fundamental role of health in poverty reduction and economic progress.[9]

The first MDG is to eradicate extreme poverty and hunger. Data from many countries show that regardless of a country's level of development, poor people are the most likely to smoke.[10] Poverty is itself a gendered issue: the majority of the more than 1 billion people in the world who live in poverty are women. Furthermore, the number of women living in poverty is increasing disproportionately to the number of men, particularly in developing countries.[3]

 World Health Organization

Tobacco and poverty are interrelated, as tobacco use diverts income from being used for food, medicine, and education, thereby increasing poverty among its users. One study estimates that a portion of the money currently spent on tobacco in Bangladesh could save 10.5 million children in the country from malnutrition. Research in other countries confirms similar findings: many poor households in Indonesia, Myanmar, and Nepal spend between 5% and 15% of their disposable income on tobacco, sometimes more than the amount spent on health care or education.[10,11]

> *The WHO FCTC's acknowledgement of CEDAW is important, because CEDAW is the most lucid legal blueprint of women's social, economic, and political rights, including rights to health.*

Cultivation of tobacco also does not contribute to sustainable livelihoods. Approximately 5 million hectares of land around the world are used for tobacco cultivation. It has been estimated that use of this land to produce food could feed 10 to 20 million people.[10] Tobacco is increasingly being grown in developing countries and is often mistakenly perceived as a profitable cash crop. However, the net returns to local farmers are generally low, because of the declining prices paid to tobacco producers and the high costs of loans required to purchase pesticides and fertilizers. By the end of the growing season, local farmers often owe more to tobacco companies than they earn.[12] Furthermore, the calculated returns generally fail to take into account the exploitation of labour by women and children, which, although essential to tobacco farming and manufacturing, is undervalued and often unpaid.[12] Since girls' education tends to be considered unimportant in many areas of the world,[13] the production of tobacco means that MDG 2 (achieve universal primary education) is also threatened.

MDG 4 (reduce child mortality) and MDG 5 (improve maternal health) are both also linked to the impact of tobacco use. Exposure to tobacco smoke has negative health effects, but children and women, including pregnant women, often do not have the power to negotiate smoke-free spaces.[14] Furthermore, family spending on tobacco results in less money available for health care.[10] Because structural adjustment and the global financial crisis have severely increased health costs, poor women have less access to cessation methods, health information, and health services.

MDG 6 is to combat HIV/AIDS, malaria, and other diseases. Tobacco use has been associated with increasing the morbidity of existing illnesses. Gender inequality and poverty further increase vulnerability to the socio-economic impacts of HIV/AIDS, tuberculosis, and other illnesses. About 58% of Africans living with HIV/AIDS are women. They are infected at younger ages than men—on average, by 6 to 8 years.[15] There is evidence that people with subclinical tuberculosis who smoke are more likely to progress to clinical tuberculosis, which increases the likelihood that they will both infect others and die prematurely. Similarly, it has been shown that smokers infected with HIV develop full-blown AIDS in less time than non-smokers do.[10]

In addition to tobacco use, tobacco production causes diseases among agricultural workers. Nicotine absorbed through the skin during tobacco harvest and curing causes GTS. Symptoms include headache, nausea, vomiting, dizziness, and diarrhoea. The pesticides used in tobacco farming can also cause illness and may have particularly severe effects on children, because of their small size and less-mature development.[10] There is some indication that chronic exposure to pesticides can lead to birth defects in the children born to women who work in tobacco farming, although this is another area in need of further research.[12] GTS and other illnesses related to tobacco growing tend to be more common in developing countries, where the regulation of tobacco companies for the protection of farmers may be weak or poorly enforced.[16]

Tobacco production and consumption are incongruous with MDG 7 (ensure environmental sustainability). Tobacco growing requires huge amounts of fertilizer and pesticides—as many as 16 applications during a three-month growing period[12]—and the chemical runoff from the fields pollutes local waterways. Tobacco also requires curing, using wood that causes losses of 200 000 hectares of forest each year.[17] The environmental impact of tobacco is due, in part, to the waste generated from its consumption.[18,19] The ecological stresses of tobacco production and consumption have particular implications for women, as women are often responsible for providing food and collecting water and firewood for the family. Rural women in particular suffer from the negative impact of tobacco on food production and the environment.[12]

Finally, MDG 8 (develop a global partnership for development) recognizes the need for each country to enhance and coordinate initiatives at the national level, while also calling upon industrialized and developing countries to establish partnerships in order to ensure joint progress towards each of the targets.[10] Implementation of the WHO FCTC is a prime example of the way regional and international partnerships can work together to ensure women's rights to health.

A Gender Equality Perspective on the WHO Framework Convention on Tobacco Control

The WHO FCTC is a powerful legal instrument to help stakeholders such as governments, scientists, health professionals, and community leaders achieve the highest possible standards of tobacco control. Ratified by more than 170 countries, the WHO FCTC affects more than 80% of the world's population and obliges governments to bring their national legislation into line with its agreements. The goal is to "protect present and future generations from the devastating health, social, environmental and economic consequences of tobacco consumption and exposure to tobacco smoke" (Article 3). The treaty offers an opportunity to strengthen tobacco control through a broad range of measures, from bans on promotion and advertising and improving package labelling to monitoring of the tobacco industry and anti-smuggling legislation. To translate the Articles into action, the WHO FCTC process requires that guidelines be developed for each Article, spelling out how laws are to be formulated, implemented, and evaluated.

Applying a gender equality framework to tobacco control is integral to achieving the goals of the WHO FCTC. The Preamble states that Parties to the treaty are *"alarmed* by the increase in smoking and other

forms of tobacco consumption by women and young girls worldwide and keeping in mind the need for full participation of women at all levels of policy-making and implementation and the need for gender-specific tobacco control strategies". Under the Guiding Principles, Article 4.2d notes that strong political commitment is necessary, taking into consideration "the need to take measures to address gender-specific risks when developing tobacco control strategies".

The treaty further acknowledges that women's and girls' right to health is a human right as agreed upon in the Convention on the Elimination of All Forms of Discrimination against Women (CEDAW); the International Covenant on Economic, Social and Cultural Rights; and the Convention on the Rights of the Child: *"recalling* Article 12 of the International Covenant on Economic, Social and Cultural Rights, adopted by the United Nations General Assembly on 16 December 1966, which states that it is the right of everyone to the enjoyment of the highest attainable standard of physical and mental health".

The WHO FCTC's acknowledgement of CEDAW is important, because CEDAW is the most lucid legal blueprint of women's social, economic, and political rights, including rights to health. Adopted in 1979 by the United Nations General Assembly, it had been ratified by 186 countries by 2009. As the chapter in this monograph on women's rights and strengthening international agreements notes, the CEDAW Committee emphasizes that lack of sex-disaggregated health data and inadequate provision of services constitute failure to fulfil a country's obligations to uphold women's health rights. CEDAW also mandates that women be active decision-makers and given chances to express their political rights equally with men. In tobacco control, this implies that women must be enabled to be leaders at international as well as community levels.

In the following, we provide an interpretation of the Articles of the WHO FCTC through a gender equality lens. This is not an exhaustive inventory; rather, it is a starting point for further research.

Article 11.1a requires Parties to ensure that the packaging and labelling of tobacco products do not promote the product by any means that are "false, misleading, deceptive or likely to create an erroneous impression about its characteristics, health effects, hazards or emissions" and specifically lists "low tar", "light", "ultra-light", and "mild" as terms that may be prohibited. Misleading terms such as these have traditionally been targeted at women, beginning in 1927 with a Philip Morris cigarette that was advertised as being "mild as May".[20] Article 11.1b requires Parties to the WHO FCTC to place health warnings on tobacco product packaging, with optional use of pictures or pictograms. Article 11.3 states that the warnings must appear in the principal language(s) of the country.

Health warnings can be made most meaningful by ensuring that they are placed on the packaging of all tobacco products, not only cigarettes, because women in some countries use tobacco in other forms.

To maximize the effective implementation of Article 11, countries must broaden legislation beyond banning specific terms and must further prohibit colours, graphics, and other design characteristics that could imply that one tobacco product is less harmful than another. Such legislation has been introduced in Bangladesh, Slovakia, and elsewhere, and strict enforcement of the provisions is needed.[21] Health warnings can be made most meaningful by ensuring that they are placed on the packaging of all tobacco products, not only cigarettes, because women in some countries use tobacco in other forms. Further, since the majority of illiterate adults are women,[22] picture-based health warnings are an important component of gender-specific tobacco control strategies.

Article 8.2 requires Parties to adopt and implement, at the national level, effective measures that provide for "protection from exposure to tobacco smoke in indoor workplaces, public transport, indoor public places and, as appropriate, other public places" and to actively promote the adoption and implementation of such measures at other jurisdictional levels. Tobacco smoke affects women in their homes and in workplaces outside their homes, even women who are not active smokers. Further, exposure to second-hand tobacco smoke is often in addition to exposure to other pollutants that damage the lungs (e.g. fumes from cooking fuels) and thus further harms women's health.[23] By enacting and enforcing legislation that requires indoor workplaces, public transport, and indoor public places to be free of tobacco smoke, Parties to the WHO FCTC can do much to protect women's health. It is also important to educate and empower both women and men to establish smoke-free environments at home.

Under Article 13, each Party to the treaty must, in accordance with its constitution or constitutional principles, implement a comprehensive ban of tobacco advertising, promotion, and sponsorship. A country that cannot undertake a comprehensive ban because of its constitution or constitutional principles must still apply restrictions on all tobacco advertising, promotion, and sponsorship. As described above, the tobacco industry has long incorporated a gender analysis into its marketing strategies, and thus an effective tobacco control response must also take gender into account. In implementing a comprehensive ban, Parties to the WHO FCTC should seek to ban or apply restrictions on as many forms of tobacco advertising, promotion, and sponsorship as possible. Legislation and policies should specifically address marketing strategies that target women and girls.

Parties to the WHO FCTC are required under Article 20 to "develop and promote national research and to coordinate research programmes at the regional and international levels in the field of tobacco control". Research should address the determinants and consequences of tobacco consumption and exposure to tobacco smoke, as well as the identification of alternative crops. The Parties are required to establish "national, regional and global surveillance of the magnitude, patterns, determinants and consequences of tobacco consumption and exposure to tobacco smoke" and to promote and strengthen training and support for all people engaged in tobacco control activities, including research and evaluation. To address gender-specific issues, research should investigate differences in the determinants and consequences of tobacco consumption and exposure to tobacco smoke for girls and women, as well as boys and men, at all ages throughout the life-course.

Article 12 of the WHO FCTC requires Parties to promote and strengthen public awareness of tobacco control issues. This means that each Party must adopt and implement measures to promote public awareness about "the health risks of tobacco consumption and exposure to tobacco smoke", "the benefits of cessation of tobacco use and tobacco free lifestyles", and "the adverse health, economic, and environmental consequences of tobacco consumption". In addition, Article 12 requires Parties to provide public access to information on the tobacco industry that is relevant to the objectives of the WHO FCTC; adopt and implement measures that promote tobacco control training and awareness programmes to specific persons (such as health workers, media professionals, and educators); and promote awareness and participation of agencies and organizations not affiliated with the tobacco industry in developing and implementing tobacco control programmes and strategies.

Women's participation and leadership in the implementation of Article 12 are key. Health professionals and others working in tobacco control should establish reciprocal relationships with women's organizations to increase the prominence of tobacco control on women's health and women's rights agendas.[24] Counteradvertising that debunks the false claim that tobacco use enhances women's empowerment and that exposes tobacco industry marketing tactics to youth may be effective in promoting reduction of tobacco use. Finally, tobacco control activists should engage with leaders working in social justice and human rights movements to create synergy between gender equality and sustainable health development.

Mechanisms and Indicators

Implementing appropriate institutional and financial mechanisms is essential to translating principles of gender equality and human rights into action in tobacco control programmes. The following are suggested guidelines:

1. *Harmonize government sectors to work effectively with national machineries and nongovernmental organizations (NGOs) to achieve gender equality.*

Tobacco control can gain ground on gender equality through improved harmonization of policies and programmes across sectors. Unfortunately, in many countries, national resources that can be mobilized for gender equality and tobacco control are currently underutilized. For example, the expertise of national machineries for gender equality and women's affairs are seldom tapped

for tobacco control, even though all countries that have signed on to the WHO FCTC and agreed to the MDGs have such institutional mechanisms. In 181 countries, these national machineries for gender equality are responsible for assuring gender mainstreaming and are mandated to implement the principles of women's rights to health as a human right, as embodied in the Beijing Platform for Action (1995). Mechanisms such as the Ministry for Women and Youth Affairs in Ghana and the Ministry for Women's Affairs and Social Development in Nigeria work intersectorally, often coordinating reports to CEDAW and the Convention on the Rights of the Child. Additional resources are being tapped in civil society. Many national machineries for gender and women's affairs have strong network partnerships among NGOs, youth groups, the media, unions, and education leaders.

2. *Use a two-pronged approach to gender mainstreaming.*

At the 2008 meeting of the United Nations Commission on the Status of Women, experts agreed that gender equality is losing ground in national programmes. Under the guise of "gender mainstreaming", gender programmes have faced serious reductions in financial resources.[25] The meeting participants recommended a two-pronged strategy that ensures a separate identity for gender equality and that also mainstreams gender equality into all legislation and fiscal policies, as well as decision-making. Such a strategy has been developed by Hivos, a prominent Dutch international NGO. In its evaluation process, programmes that appoint a junior-level or part-time gender expert are considered to be failing to abide by their gender mainstreaming policy.[26] In tobacco control, gender mainstreaming is more likely to succeed if gender experts at senior policy levels are provided with adequate resources to develop their own gender equality programmes. Such units can also act as monitoring bodies to measure the success or failure of gender mainstreaming. Setting high standards and providing adequate resources help to ensure that all programmes take gender equality guidelines seriously, that sound technical advice is provided, and that programmes are monitored and evaluated to measure results.

3. *Strengthen the data and indicators used in gender-responsive budgeting.*

Budgeting for gender equality in tobacco control requires development of sensitive, cost-effective indicators

Figure 2.2. Indicators for Gender Equality in Tobacco Programmes

1. *The omission of women in national statistics reflects an unequal allocation of resources between men and women.*
   Are data collected on the prevalence of all forms of tobacco used by women as well as men, including cigarettes, chewing tobacco, bidis, and water pipes? Do these data reflect the needs of girls and women of all ages who face multiple exclusions based on race, caste, ethnicity, religion, or disability?

2. *Rural women and poor urban women face particular hardships.*
   Are data and country-specific information available on women's roles in tobacco production and marketing as well as those of men?

3. *Gender-specific strategies are needed to ensure that women are equally informed about their legal rights.*
   Are adequate steps taken to ensure that women are informed about their rights under national tobacco control legislation and under the WHO FCTC?

4. *Communications, information, and media programmes must ensure that policies and programmes are gender-sensitive.*
   Are package warnings and/or public advertisements gender-specific and designed to reach women as well as men?

5. *Pregnant women are often criticized if they smoke, but maternal and child health services do not provide adequate information about the dangers of tobacco and services to help avoid risk.*
   Are adequate measures being taken to inform and empower women in response to the dangers to their health and the health of their children from tobacco use and exposure to SHS during pregnancy?

6. *Women's access to health information about occupational safety is a basic human right.*
   Are women who are involved in tobacco processing and manufacture adequately informed about the dangers of tobacco use and handling? Are precautions taken to protect them from health hazards such as tobacco dust, pesticides, and physical strain?

7. *Maternal and child health services are often gender-biased and do not address the equal responsibility of fathers for children's health.*
   Do maternal and child health services also target fathers in campaigns to quit smoking for the sake of mothers' and children's health?

8. *The WHO FCTC aims to ensure that women are able to voice their concerns and take leadership roles.*
   Are the Parties to the treaty ensuring the full participation of women at all levels of policy-making and implementation of programmes related to tobacco control?

9. *Gender mainstreaming requires all programmes to state gender-specific objectives.*
   Are specific objectives concerning gender equality stated in tobacco control policies?

10. *Resources should be allocated to ensure a separate identity for gender equality, as well as for mainstreaming.*
    Are adequate resources allocated for gender-specific interventions?

11. *Gender expertise is needed at senior policy levels to ensure adequate technical oversight.*
    Are senior-level gender experts working at the policy level?

and baseline data. As already stated, it is necessary to monitor the social, economic, and political conditions for women as well as men, particularly for those who face multiple exclusions. Equally important is tracking the distribution of financial resources between women and men. Gender-responsive budgeting at the national level is currently being implemented in many countries, including Tunisia and Norway. In Norway, the Ministry of Children and Equality conducts annual surveys on the amounts of money spent on men and on women. Reports of these surveys are required of all line ministries (including health) and are compiled in a fiscal budget annex.[27]

Gender-responsive budgeting in tobacco control requires development of indicators for gender equality. Figure 2.2 presents examples of such indicators. This list is neither exhaustive nor conclusive; rather, it is a starting point for an important research effort.

Conclusion

Although gender-blind policies are still widespread, a comprehensive approach to tobacco control is gaining ground. The WHO FCTC sets an ambitious goal to

World Health Organization

advance a gender as well as human rights perspective in the implementation of its Articles. At a theoretical level, the WHO/SEARO model of health behaviour can be used to analyse the effects of gender inequality throughout the health system and to help map interrelationships between tobacco control and broader social, cultural, and economic processes. A gender equality framework suggests that changes in policies must occur in many sectors outside health—including finance, trade, and agriculture—if tobacco control policies are to have an equal impact for women and for men.

An important tool for advancing tobacco control programmes is the WHO MPOWER package, but it, too, should be analysed through a gender equality lens. Governments must improve coordination with national machineries for women's affairs, provide adequate financing, and apply indicators for gender equality in national planning. There is more at stake than changes in health behaviour. The price for ignoring more than half of the world's population—i.e. women—is high. If the tobacco epidemic continues to accelerate, aggravating financial instability and undermining sustainable development, the MDGs will be in jeopardy.

References

1. *Women and health: today's evidence, tomorrow's agenda.* Geneva, World Health Organization, 2009.
2. *Gender equality—striving for justice in an unequal world.* Geneva, United Nations Research Institute for Social Development, 2005.
3. *Global monitoring report 2007: Millennium Development Goals.* Washington, DC, The World Bank, 2007.
4. *The equal sharing of responsibilities between women and men, including caregiving in the context of HIV/AIDS.* Moderator's summary, expert panel at the 52nd session of the United Nations Commission on the Status of Women, New York, 25 February–7 March 2008.
5. *Platform for action*, Paragraph 48. The United Nations Fourth World Conference on Women, Beijing, September 1995. New York, NY, United Nations (http://www.un.org/womenwatch/daw/beijing/platform/poverty.htm, accessed 5 December 2009).
6. *Gender and tobacco control: a policy brief.* Geneva, World Health Organization, 2007.
7. *Concepts of health behaviour research.* New Delhi, World Health Organization Regional Office for South-East Asia, 1986 (Regional Health Paper No. 13).
8. *WHO report on the global tobacco epidemic, 2008: the MPOWER package.* Geneva, World Health Organization, 2008.
9. *Empowering women key to achieving UN Millennium Goals* (press release), New York, NY, United Nations News Centre, 19 November 2007 (http://www.un.org/news, accessed 30 December 2007).
10. Da Costa e Silva VL. Preface. In: Esson KM, Leeder SR. *The Millennium Development Goals and tobacco control: an opportunity for global partnership.* Geneva, World Health Organization, 2004.
11. *The contribution of tobacco control measures to the (health-related) United Nations Millennium Development Goals (MDGs).* Geneva, World Health Organization, 2009 (unpublished discussion paper).
12. Esson KM, Leeder SR. *The Millennium Development Goals and tobacco control: an opportunity for global partnership.* Geneva, World Health Organization, 2004.
13. Khalfan M, Waverley L. From the fields to the consumer. In: Greaves L, Jategaonkar N, Sanchez S, eds. *Turning a new leaf: women, tobacco, and the future.* Vancouver, British Columbia Centre of Excellence for Women's Health (BCCEWH) and International Network of Women Against Tobacco (INWAT), 2006.
14. Greaves L, Tungohan E. Engendering tobacco control: using an international public health treaty to reduce smoking and empower women. *Tobacco Control*, 2007, 16:148–150.
15. *The world health report 2004—Changing history.* Geneva, World Health Organization, 2004.
16. Ezzati M, Lopez AD. Estimates of global mortality attributable to smoking in 2000. *The Lancet*, 2003, 362:847–852.
17. Hickey E, Chan Y. The story of the Huichol Indians. In: *Tobacco, farmers, and pesticides: the other story.* San Francisco, CA, Pesticide Action Network (PAN) North America and San Francisco Tobacco Free Coalition, 1998. (http://www.panna.org/files/tobacco.pdf, accessed 31 December 2007).
18. *Tobacco and the environment fact sheet.* London, Action on Smoking and Health (ASH) UK, July 2004. (http://www.thestopsmokingman.co.uk/tobacco-environment.html, accessed 31 December 2007).
19. *International coastal cleanup (ICC): a day at the beach.* Washington, DC The Ocean Conservancy, 2004. (http://www.preventcigarettelitter.org/files/downloads/coastal_cleanup.pdf, accessed 30 December 2007).
20. Ernster V, et al Women and tobacco: moving from policy to action. *Bulletin of the World Health Organization*, 2000, 78: 891–901.
21. Cunningham R. Package warnings and labelling. In: Jategaonkar N, ed. *Civil society monitoring of the Framework Convention on Tobacco Control: 2007 status report of the Framework Convention Alliance.* Geneva, Framework Convention Alliance, 2007.
22. *Gender equality fact sheet: state of world population 2005.* UNFPA, 2005. (http://www.unfpa.org/swp/2005/presskit/factsheets/facts_gender.htm accessed 28 December 2007).
23. *Global strategy for the diagnosis, management and prevention of COPD.* Global Initiative for Chronic Obstructive Lung Disease (GOLD) Gig Harbor, WA, Medical Communications Resources, Inc., 2007 (http://www.goldcopd.org, accessed 31 December 2007).
24. Balbach ED, Herzberg A, Barbeau EM. Political coalitions and working women: how the tobacco industry built a relationship with the Coalition of Labor Union Women. *Journal of Epidemiology and Community Health*, 2006, 60 (Suppl. 2):ii27–ii32.
25. *Final report of the expert group meeting on financing for gender equality and the empowerment of women.* New York, NY, United Nations Division for the Advancement of Women, 2007.
26. *Report gender baseline measurement 2005.* The Hague, Hivos, 2005.
27. *Guide to gender equality assessment and discussion in ministry budget propositions.* Oslo, Norwegian Ministry of Children, Equality and Social Inclusion, 2007.

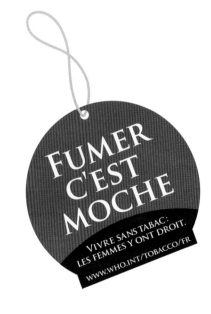

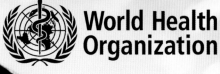

31**MAY:**WORLD**NO**TOBACCO**DAY**

World Health Organization

Glamour?
No, mouth cancer.

Protect women from
tobacco marketing
and smoke.

CHEWING
TOBACCO
IS UGLY

WWW.WHO.INT/TOBACCO

© WORLD HEALTH ORGANIZATION 2010. THE IMAGES OF WOUNDS, LESIONS OR ULCERATIONS ARE REAL AND SUPERIMPOSED ON THE IMAGE OF THE MODEL. DESIGNED BY NOVA S/B.

Tobacco Use and Its Impact on Health

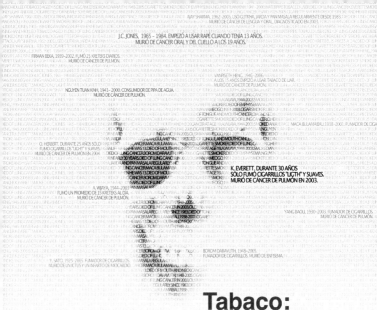

J.C. JONES, 1965 – 1984. EMPEZÓ A USAR RAPÉ CUANDO TENÍA 13 AÑOS.
MURIÓ DE CÁNCER ORAL Y DEL CUELLO A LOS 19 AÑOS.

K. EVERETT, DURANTE 30 AÑOS
SÓLO FUMÓ CIGARRILLOS "LIGTH" Y SUAVES.
MURIÓ DE CÁNCER DE PULMÓN EN 2003.

Tabaco:
mortífero en todas
sus formas

EL TABACO CAUSA
5 MILLONES DE MUERTES ANUALES
PODRÍA OCURRIRTE A TÍ.

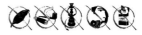

31 de Mayo Día Mundial Sin Tabaco

Organización Mundial de la Salud

MINISTERIO DE SANIDAD Y CONSUMO

3. Prevalence of Tobacco Use and Factors Influencing Initiation and Maintenance Among Women

Introduction

Tobacco consumption has fallen substantially over the past 30 years in many industrialized countries as a result of increasing awareness of the hazards of tobacco use and the implementation of aggressive and effective tobacco control policies. In contrast, over the same time period, tobacco consumption has been increasing in the developing world; developing nations now consume the greatest share of the world's cigarette production.[1] Just as global tobacco consumption is shifting between industrialized and developing countries, the tobacco pandemic is spreading to women in a variety of settings. Historically, smoking by women in industrialized countries increased during the last century, lagging behind the rise in men by about 20 to 30 years.[2] This rise among women can be attributed to weakening social, cultural, and political constraints, coupled with women's earning power and targeted marketing by tobacco companies. Today, the prevalence of smoking among women in some countries remains high, while surveillance data from other countries provide warning of increasing use among youth, particularly girls.

This chapter discusses the prevalence of tobacco use among women and girls and explores the factors that influence the initiation and maintenance of their tobacco use. The factors that motivate women to continue smoking are quite different from those that encourage young girls to start. Factors driving initiation are complex and varied,[3] not only between industrialized and developing countries, but also between different groups within a country. Maintenance of tobacco use results from nicotine addiction, lack of awareness of risk, and difficulty in quitting, which is driven by diverse psychosocial and environmental factors, as well as dependence.[4,5]

In many countries, manufactured cigarettes are the predominant form of tobacco used by both men and women. For this reason, much of the available prevalence data focuses on cigarette smoking. However, in some countries, e.g. India and Indonesia, chewing tobacco and other smoked products (e.g. bidis, kreteks, and water pipes) are used by many women. We use case-studies of particular countries to highlight women's use of smokeless tobacco and other tobacco products. The predominance of examples of initiation and maintenance in industrialized countries is not deliberate but is a reflection of the more limited research in developing countries. The types of influences and their importance in shaping youth behaviour in the industrialized world are likely to differ from those in developing countries, depending on social and cultural norms, socioeconomic conditions, and the political context of a country. Where available, representative studies from developing countries are used in this chapter to highlight potential similarities and differences in factors that influence young people to take up smoking.

Prevalence and Trends

Prevalence of Smoking

In 2006, more than 1 billion smokers in the world consumed about 5.7 trillion cigarettes.[1,6] An additional 700 billion bidis are consumed annually in India alone.[7] There is wide variation in smoking prevalence among both males and females from one region to another. Globally, the prevalence of smoking is higher for men (40% in 2006) than for women (nearly 9% in 2006), and males account for 80% of all smokers (nearly 1 billion).*

Table 3.1 provides regional estimates of smoking prevalence in 2006. In the Americas and Europe, the prevalence of female smoking is high, around 17% and 22%, respectively. The disparity between male and female smoking prevalence is greater in other regions of the world. For example, male smoking prevalence is near 37% in South-East Asia and 57% in the Western Pacific, while prevalence among women is around 4% to 5%. These patterns reflect differing social norms, cultural traditions,

---

* Unpublished data elaborated by the World Health Organization Tobacco Free Initiative (WHO TFI), based on *WHO Report on the Global Tobacco Epidemic, 2009: Implementing Smoke-Free Environments.* Geneva, World Health Organization, 2009.

 World Health Organization

and demographic factors. Socioeconomic influences must also be considered.[8]

Recent global estimates of smoking prevalence by age group are limited. The trends in smoking prevalence by age are always dynamic and reflect a combination of age, period, and cohort effects. In most settings, smoking initiation usually occurs during adolescence, and prevalence increases until early or middle adulthood, beyond which smoking declines with age. This decline with age reflects the cumulative impact of smokers quitting and smokers dying prematurely over time. Trends by age within a country are based on changes in the rate and age of initiation and patterns of smoking cessation, which change over time as a result of the interplay between pro-tobacco and anti-tobacco forces.

In addition to differences in prevalence by gender and age group, there is significant variation by income status. As seen in Table 3.2, the majority of the world's smokers (81%) are in low- and middle-income countries. Smoking prevalence among males in middle-income countries (45%) is higher than that among males in high-income countries (32%), while the reverse is true for females (7% in middle-income countries and 18% in high-income countries). These

data may be affected by some underreporting of smoking among women, particularly in countries where it is socially and culturally unacceptable for women to smoke.

A generally consistent finding is that rates of both daily and current smoking are higher among men than among women, as shown in Table 3.3. However, there is considerable variation among countries. In some countries, such as the United States and the United Kingdom, the rates among men and among women are nearly equal, and in some, such as Sweden, the rates among women are even higher than those among men. In some Asian countries, only a small percentage of women smoke, while the majority of men are smokers. These differences reflect different stages of the smoking epidemic in each country,[2] as well as the influence of social norms, cultural traditions, and socioeconomic and demographic factors.

In addition to the generally lower prevalence of smoking among women, women tend to smoke fewer cigarettes per day than men. Table 3.4 presents estimates of the number of cigarettes smoked per day by male and female smokers in a sample of countries. These data are compiled from various sources, using different survey designs and

Table 3.1. Smoking Prevalence and Number of Smokers Among Adults (Age 15 and Older), by WHO Region and Gender, 2006[a]

WHO Region	Smoking Prevalence (%)[b]			Total Smokers (millions)	% of All Smokers[b]
	Male	Female	Overall		
African Region (AFR)	16	2	9	41	4
Region of the Americas (AMR)	27	17	22	145	12
Eastern Mediterranean Region (EMR)	30	4	17	60	5
European Region (EUR)	44	22	32	238	21
South-East Asia Region (SEAR)	37	4	21	248	21
Western Pacific Region (WPR)	57	5	31	430	37
World / Total	40	9	24	1 164	100

Source: Based on *WHO Report on the Global Tobacco Epidemic, 2009: Implementing Smoke-Free Environments.* Geneva, World Health Organization, 2009.

[a]   These estimates are not age-standardized (i.e. the effects of the underlying age structures across countries are not removed) and should be used with caution when making comparisons of smoking prevalence across regions. For this reason, these estimates differ to those published in WHO's *World Health Statistics Report, 2010.*

[b]   All estimates have been rounded off.

World Health Organization

smoking definitions, but they indicate the differences in smoking behaviour between men and women.

Differences in smoking prevalence between young male and female smokers are less evident. Data from the Global Youth Tobacco Survey (GYTS) for 13- to 15-year-old students suggest a similar pattern of smoking among boys and girls in many areas of the world. Table 3.5 shows the prevalence of cigarette and other tobacco-product use by sex and region. The GYTS data presented include 29 Member States in AFR (19 national and 10 subnational); 34 Member States and four territories in AMR (25 national and 13 subnational); 21 Member States and two geographical regions in EMR (17 national and six subnational); 28 Member States and one United Nations administered province in EUR (28 national and one subnational); 10 Member States in SEAR (eight national and two subnational); and 18 Member States, two territories, one special administrative region, and one commonwealth in WPR (19 national and three subnational).[22] Although boys are significantly more likely than girls to smoke cigarettes in AFR, EMR, SEAR, and WPR, significant differences were not observed by gender in AMR and EUR.[22] Boys were found to be significantly more likely than girls to use other tobacco products overall and in AMR, EUR, and SEAR; however, significant differences by gender were not observed in AFR, EMR, or WPR.[22]

No differences in cigarette smoking by gender were observed in more than half (87) of the 151 sites where the GYTS was conducted from 2000 to 2007.[22] The potential increase in female youth smoking raises great concern for the future burden of tobacco use and tobacco-related disease among women.

Trends in Smoking Prevalence

Fortunately, tobacco consumption has fallen over the past several decades in many industrialized countries. Consumption among men peaked around 1970 in many countries, but patterns over time among women have been more variable. In the United States, the prevalence of smoking increased steadily between the 1930s and 1964, when more than 40% of all adult Americans smoked.[23] Since then, smoking prevalence has decreased, and it dropped below 20% in 2007 (22% in men, 17% in women).[24] In Japan, smoking prevalence was highest in 1966, when the proportions of adult male and female smokers reached 84% and 18%, respectively. By 1996, the proportions had declined to 59% and 15%.[25] In 2004, smoking prevalence in Japan was down to 39.9% among men and 10% among women.[1] In the United Kingdom, cigarette smoking prevalence fell from 51% in men and 41% in women in 1974 to 23% and 21%, respectively, in 2006.[20]

In contrast, cigarette consumption per capita increased in developing countries at a rate of about 3.7% per annum between 1970 and 2000, almost 10 times the

Table 3.2. Smoking Prevalence by Socioeconomic Status, Sex, and Number of Smokers Age 15 or Older, 2006[a]

Income Group	Smoking Prevalence (%)[b]			Total Smokers (millions)	% of All Smokers[b]
	Male	Female	Overall		
High	32	18	25	215	18
Middle	45	7	26	830	71
Low	28	4	16	119	10
Total	40	9	24	1 164	100

Source: Based on *WHO Report on the Global Tobacco Epidemic, 2009: Implementing Smoke-Free Environments*. Geneva, World Health Organization, 2009.

[a]   These estimates are not age-standardized (i.e. the effects of the underlying age structures across countries are not removed) and should be used with caution when making comparisons of smoking prevalence across regions. For this reason, these estimates differ to those published in WHO's *World Health Statistics Report, 2010*.

[b]   All estimates have been rounded off.

World Health Organization

Table 3.3. **Prevalence of Daily and Current Tobacco Smoking in Adult Men and Women in Selected Countries**

Country	Year	Daily smoking (%)			Current smoking (%)		
		Men	Women	Difference	Men	Women	Difference
African Region (AFR)							
Burkina Faso	2003	19	10.3	9.3	23.6	11.1	12.5
Chad	2003	13.2	2.1	11.1	17.4	2.9	14.5
Côte d'Ivoire	2003	14.5	1.2	13.3	19.3	2.3	17
Ethiopia	2003	5.3	0.4	4.9	6.3	0.5	5.8
Ghana	2003	6.2	0.4	5.8	9	1.2	7.8
Kenya	2004	21.2	0.9	20.3	26.2	1.9	24.3
Uganda[a]	2000–2001	25.2	3.3	—	—	—	—
South Africa	2003	31.7	9	22.7	35.1	10.2	24.9
Region of the Americas (AMR)							
Argentina[b]	2005	26.2	18.6	7.6	35.1	24.9	10.2
Brazil	2008	17.3	11	6.3	20.5	12.4	8.1
Chile	2006	29.7	26.3	3.4	42.7	39.2	3.5
Canada[b]	2007	16.4	14.3	2.1	20.4	18.1	2.3
Mexico[b]	2006	21.6	6.5	15.1	30.4	9.5	20.9
Paraguay	2003	23.5	6.5	17	41.6	13.3	28.3
United States	2007	—	—	—	22.3	17.4	4.9
Uruguay	2006	37.2	28.6	8.6	40.8	31.7	9.1
Venezuela (Bolivarian Republic of)	2005	20.9	13	7.9	22.6	13.6	9
Eastern Mediterranean Region (EMR)							
Egypt	2005	22.9	0.3	22.6	29.5	0.4	29.1
Iran (Islamic Republic of)	2005	20.9	2.9	18	24.1	4.3	19.8
Pakistan	2002–2003	27.3	4.4	22.9	32.4	5.7	26.7
Tunisia	2005–2006	53.1	6.6	46.5	—	—	—
United Arab Emirates	2003	17.6	1.4	16.2	28.1	2.4	25.7
European Region (EUR)							
Austria	2004	40.2	35.5	4.7	48	47	1
Bosnia and Herzegovina	2003	46.6	24.9	21.7	54.2	34.2	20
Czech Republic	2008	26.1	19.3	6.8	34.9	27.4	7.5
Denmark	2008	24	22	2	29	27	2
France	2005	28.2	21.7	6.5	33.3	26.5	6.8
Germany	2005	27.9	18.8	9.1	32.2	22.4	9.8
Hungary	2003	38.6	27.7	10.9	42.5	31.3	11.2
Kazakhstan	2003	38.7	5.8	32.9	52.2	9.6	42.6
Norway	2007	27	26	1	38	38	0
Poland	2007	34	23	11	—	—	—
Russian Federation[a]	2001	60.4	15.5	44.9	—	—	—
Spain	2006	32	22	10	36	24	12

World Health Organization

Table 3.3. *(continued)*

Country	Year	Daily smoking (%)			Current smoking (%)		
		Men	Women	Difference	Men	Women	Difference
Sweden	2007	12	16	-4	24	24	0
Switzerland	2007	23	16	7	33	24	9
Turkey	2006	—	—	—	50.6	16.6	34
Ukraine	2005	62.3	16.7	45.6	66.8	19.9	46.9
United Kingdom[a]	2007	—	—	—	22	20	2
South-East Asia Region (SEAR)							
Bangladesh	2004	—	—	—	41	1.8	39.2
India[c]	2005–2006	—	—	—	32.7	1.4	31.3
Indonesia	2007	46.8	3.1	43.7	56.8	4.5	52.3
Myanmar	2003	35.6	10.4	25.2	48.9	13.7	35.2
Sri Lanka	2003	24.5	1.6	22.9	39	2.6	36.4
Thailand	2007	36.6	1.6	35	41.8	2	39.8
Western Pacific Region (WPR)							
China[b]	2002	…	…	…	57.4	2.6	54.8
Japan	2006	…	…	…	39.9	10	38.9
Malaysia	2006	…	…	…	46.4	1.6	44.8
New Zealand	2007	19.3	17	2.3	21.1	18.8	2.3
Philippines	2003	40.3	7.1	33.2	57.5	12.3	45.2
Singapore[b]	2007	22.8	3.6	19.2	25.2	4.2	21
Viet Nam	2003	34.8	1.8	33	49.4	2.3	47.1

Note: All surveys were conducted among adults, but age groups and survey methodologies varied.
[a] The difference cannot be calculated, because the age range for males differs from that for females.
[b] Cigarette smoking.
[c] Cigarette or bidi smoking.
Source: Ref. 1. See Ref. 1 for more detail on data sources and smoking prevalence in other countries.

rate of increase in industrialized countries.[26] By 2005, developing countries accounted for approximately 70% of world cigarette consumption.[1] The ratio of average cigarette consumption per adult between industrialized and developing countries narrowed from 3.3 in the early 1970s to 1.8 in the early 1990s.[27]

Just as the gap in cigarette consumption has narrowed between industrialized and developing countries, it is clearly narrowing between men and women. The tobacco pandemic is reaching men and women equally as multinational tobacco companies expand their focus from men in high-income countries to men in developing countries and women in both industrialized and developing countries. At the same time, the divide between socioeconomic groups is broadening. In areas

where women have been smoking for several decades, the relationship between socioeconomic status (SES) and smoking in women is similar to that seen in men. In most high-income countries, there are significant differences in smoking prevalence between different socioeconomic groups. In the United Kingdom in 2006, for example, only 14% of women and 17% of men in the highest socioeconomic groups were smokers, in contrast to 28% and 32%, respectively, in the lowest socioeconomic groups.[20] In a sample of nine Western European countries, between 1985 and 2000, smoking prevalence and/or consumption decreased more rapidly, on average, among the more highly educated than among the less-educated. The gap was greatest among women.[28] In contrast, recent surveys in the Russian Federation and Ukraine have suggested that smoking prevalence

Table 3.4. Number of Cigarettes Smoked per Smoker per Day by Gender in Selected Countries

Country	Cigarettes smoked per day			Survey year
	Men	Women	Difference	
American Samoa[9]	14.2	12.4	-1.8	2004
Australia[10]	14.7	13.3	-1.4	2004
Brazil[11]	12.6	10.2	-2.4	2003
Cambodia[12]	14.2	11.1	-3.1	2004
Canada[13]	16.9	13.8	-3.1	2006
China[14]	15	10	-5	2002
Egypt[9]	19.6	18.2	-1.4	2005
Fiji[15]	7.3	5.4	-1.9	2002
India[9]	7.3	4.8	-2.5	2005
Côte d'Ivoire[9]	7	3.5	-3.5	2005
Maldives[9]	14.8	8.3	-6.5	2004
Mongolia[9]	12.6	7.5	-5.1	2006
Netherlands[16]	15.5	14.9	-0.6	2004
New Zealand[9]	14	11	-3	2002
Russian Federation[17]	16.9	11.2	-5.7	2004
Seychelles[9]	10.6	8.1	-2.5	2004
Sri Lanka[9]	7.1	6.8	-0.3	2003
United Republic of Tanzania[18]	6	3	-3	1998
Ukraine[19]	16	11	-5	2005
United Kingdom[20]	15	13	-2	2006
United States[21]	18.1	15.3	-2.8	2004

Note: Data compiled from varied sources, as noted by country. Survey methodologies and smoking definitions may vary by survey and are not necessarily nationally representative.

in women is highest among the highly educated, more urban, and least economically deprived.[17,19]

The historical trajectories of tobacco use among men and women reflect different sociocultural motivating and constraining forces, which have acted to determine tobacco use patterns among women. The constraints against smoking have weakened in many countries, and smoking prevalence among women has risen, often accelerated by marketing campaigns targeted directly at girls and women. In some countries, the prevalence of smoking among girls and women is still rising. In Spain, the prevalence of cigarette smoking among women remained low after the Second World War, because of traditional norms reinforced by the government. A dramatic increase was observed after the democratization of Spain in the 1970s, which allowed the entry of the multinational tobacco industry and large

increases in cigarette marketing expenditures.[29] Among 21- to 30-year-olds, the prevalence of cigarette smoking increased from 9.4% in 1970, to 31.9% in 1980, to 49.9% in 1990.[30] The rapid increase in cigarette smoking in Spain provides a warning about the impact of aggressive tobacco marketing in the context of increasing education, liberalization, and economic prosperity of women.[29] This pattern, which has been seen in many industrialized countries throughout the 20th century, seems likely to be repeated in developing countries during the present century unless effective tobacco control measures are implemented.

Case-Study: Tobacco Use in India

India provides a case-study of the challenges of controlling tobacco use in a population that uses

World Health Organization

Table 3.5. Prevalence of Tobacco Use by Boys and Girls by Gender and WHO Region

Region	% Currently smoked cigarettes [a]			% Currently used tobacco products other than cigarettes [b]		
	Boys	Girls	Difference	Boys	Girls	Difference
African Region (AFR)	13.5	5.2	−8.3[c]	11.9	10.6	−1.3
Region of the Americas (AMR)	13.5	15	1.5	12.3	6.8	−5.5[c]
Eastern Mediterranean Region (EMR)	7.3	2	−5.3[c]	14.3	9.1	−5.2[c]
European Region (EUR)	21	17.4	−3.6	12.1	7.5	−4.6[c]
South-East Asia Region (SEAR)	9.5	2	−7.5[c]	12.5	7.1	−5.4[c]
Western Pacific Region (WPR)	18.5	8.4	−10.1[c]	7.2	6.1	−1.1
Total	12.1	6.8	−5.3[c]	12.2	7.5	−4.7[c]

Note: These data are from a subset of countries in each region. For details concerning how the data were aggregated, see Ref. 22.
[a]   Smoked on at least one day during the month preceding the survey.
[b]   Used tobacco products other than cigarettes on at least one day during the month preceding the survey.
[c]   Significant differences.

numerous types of tobacco products. These products include smoked tobacco, such as bidi and chutta, and chewed tobacco, such as khaini, mawa, and betel quid. The prevalence of smoking and chewing differs widely by region of the country.[31,32] In general, men both smoke and chew tobacco, whereas women generally only chew tobacco, except in a few areas where the prevalence of smoking among women is high. In the coastal areas of Andhra Pradesh and Orissa, women smoke cheroots (cigars, also called chutta) in a reverse manner (i.e. with the burning end inside the mouth), and in some northern parts of the country, many women smoke hookah or hubble bubble.[32] Table 3.6 shows the prevalence of different forms of tobacco use among adult men and women in urban and rural areas of India. Rural men and women are more likely to smoke and chew tobacco than are their urban counterparts. Additionally, women are more likely to chew tobacco than to smoke cigarettes or bidis. The prevalence of tobacco use is only slightly lower among pregnant women than in the general population of reproductive age, suggesting a lack of awareness of the potential harm of tobacco use on the part of these women, their families, and their health-care providers.

The prevalence of tobacco use by women increases with age. In 2005–2006, the reported prevalence of tobacco use was 3.5% among 15- to 19-year-olds, 9.1% among 20-

to 34-year-olds, and 18.3% among 35- to 49-year-olds.[33] Results from the 2006 GYTS show that 1.6% of 13- to 15-year-old female students smoke cigarettes, and another 8.5% use other tobacco products. Further, among girls who were ever-smokers, more than half began before age 10.[34,35] It should be noted, however, that survey methodologies,

Figure 3.1. Tobacco Use Among Men and Women Ages 15–49 in India by Level of Wealth

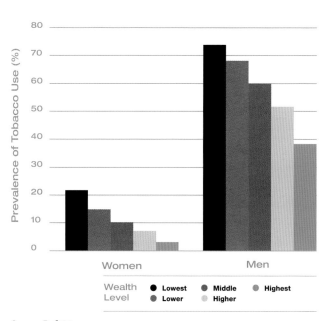

Source: Ref. 33.

Table 3.6. **Tobacco Use Among Men And Women Ages 15–49 in India, 2005–2006**

Tobacco Type	Women (%)			Men (%)		
	Urban	Rural	Total	Urban	Rural	Total
Cigarettes/bidis	0.5	1.8	1.4	28.7	35.0	32.7
Chewing tobacco (paan masala, gutkha, other)	5.5	9.8	8.4	31.1	39.6	36.5
Any tobacco use	6.7	12.9	10.9	49.9	61.1	57.0

Source: Adapted from Ref. 33.

smoking definitions, and target populations differ between studies, limiting the ability to make comparisons.

There is also a strong socioeconomic element in tobacco use in India. Figure 3.1 shows that among both men and women, there is a clear inverse relationship between level of wealth and prevalence of tobacco use. A similar relationship is observed when education is used as the measure of SES. These data indicate a need for targeted efforts with effective programmes and policies to reach the lowest-income and most-vulnerable populations. There is also considerable variation in tobacco use by members of different religions, with Sikhs and Jains reporting the lowest prevalence.[33]

The tobacco profile of women in rural India is varied. In general, female tobacco users in rural India are housewives or farmers working in the fields, and their literacy levels are low. The main reasons for starting to use tobacco in various forms include accepted sociocultural norms, beliefs, and use as a medicinal aid (e.g. to cure toothaches or during labour).[33] For example, women in Kerala tend to chew tobacco with betel leaf and areca nut. These women are full-time housewives who also work in the fields, growing, tending, and harvesting paddy. The literacy rate in Kerala is higher than in most parts of India, and in addition, the women are independent, have their private supplies of chewing tobacco, and indulge whenever they want to. Their counterparts in Andhra Pradesh are poorer and less literate, and those who do not chew tobacco smoke chutta.[33]

Although the prevalence of tobacco use among women in India is relatively low, there are many users given the country's large population. Further, there is concern about an increase in the prevalence of smoking among urban women, with increasing independence, modernization, and purchasing power and a decrease in the cultural pressures constraining tobacco use. In the past, the tobacco industry has aggressively exploited the image of the emancipated woman to increase sales.[31]

Because of the high prevalence of tobacco use and the manner in which it is used, tobacco poses a large burden of morbidity and mortality in India. It has been estimated that 20% of deaths among men and 5% of deaths among women between the ages of 30 and 69 are caused by smoking. Recent estimates indicate that by 2010, almost 1 million adult deaths per year of people between the ages of 30 and 69 in India will be caused by smoking.[36]

Case-Study: Tobacco Use in Singapore

Singapore offers a case-study of a country with a well-established tobacco control programme and a smoking prevalence that is relatively low among high-income countries.[1] Singapore has been a leader in tobacco control policy. It was the first country to implement a tobacco advertising ban, which it did as early as 1970. Legislation that followed included protection from exposure to tobacco smoke, rotating and graphic health warnings, cessation policies for youth, and public education campaigns.[1]

A recent national survey showed that since the start of Singapore's National Smoking Control Programme in 1986, there has been an overall decrease in smoking prevalence from 20% in 1984, to 15% in 1998, to 14% in 2007.[37,38] Of concern is the plateau in smoking prevalence among females and an increase in smoking by young

World Health Organization

women 20 to 24 years of age in recent years.[37] The decrease observed in overall smoking prevalence since 1986 is largely due to a decrease in male smoking, as female smoking prevalence increased from 3% in 1984 to 4% in 2007.[37,38] In particular, between 1992 and 1998, there was a significant increase in the prevalence of smoking among 20- to 24-year-old women, according to National Health Survey data: from 2.5% in 1992 to 6.7% in 1998.[37] Table 3.7 presents a summary of the trends in smoking prevalence among 18- to 69-year-olds in Singapore.

The reason for the increase in smoking prevalence among young women is unclear; however, the Ministry of Health has responded to it by targeting smoking cessation efforts at young women.[39] Recent GYTS data indicate that smoking prevalence among 13- to 15-year-old girls is 7.5%, and prevalence among boys is 10.5%.[22] Morrow and Barraclough[40] suggest that recent changes in smoking among young women and the small difference in smoking prevalence between young men and young women may be the result of shifting social dynamics in Singapore. The significance of gender is not recognized in tobacco control policies and programmes, since Singapore is a country where policies are gender-neutral. Increased attention is needed to trends among women to avoid the uptake of smoking seen in Western countries with the attainment of social and economic equality.

Another trend of concern in Singapore is the educational gradient reported in the most recent National Health Survey: as daily smoking prevalence has increased, the level of education has decreased for both men and women 18 to 69 years of age. Similar to trends in other countries, less-educated men are 12.6 times more likely to smoke daily than the most-educated cohort, and less-educated women are 8.8 times more likely.[41]

Despite Singapore's achievements in tobacco control policies and programmes, the changing prevalence among young women is cause for concern. The case-study of Singapore shows the need for continued monitoring of changing patterns of tobacco use, even after decades of success in tobacco control, and the need for responses to unfavourable trends.

Initiation of Tobacco Use

Most tobacco use begins in early adolescence—almost all first use occurs before the age of 18.[42] In most countries, few people start smoking after the age of 21; however, in some countries, such as China, prevalence is low during adolescence and increases during early adulthood. In a 1996 national survey in China, the average age at initiation of tobacco use was 19 for men and 25 for women.[43] Many factors have been reported to affect initiation. These factors differ between industrialized and developing countries and among various groups within a country. Most of the available evidence comes from the industrialized world, but where possible, we highlight representative studies from developing countries.

The development of tobacco use is influenced by a complex interplay of personal, social, and cultural factors which can vary over time and stage of development and may vary in impact on girls and boys.[44,45] Personal factors include personality type and characteristics that may predispose individuals to risk-taking behaviour. Social influences include the behaviour and attitudes of the individual's social support network, including friends, family, and peers. Cultural influences constitute the broader environmental context regarding social norms and acceptability in communities, neighbourhoods, and countries.[44,45] Here, we discuss some of the interpersonal and environmental determinants that may influence initiation of tobacco use among adolescents.

Personal Factors

Personal factors that have consistently been associated with tobacco use by young people include sociodemo-

Table 3.7. Prevalence of Daily Cigarette Smoking Among 18- to 69-Year-Olds in Singapore by Gender and Survey Year

Survey year	Female (%)	Male (%)
1992	3.0	33.2
1995	2.7	31.9
1998	3.1	26.9
2004	3.6	22.8

Source: National Health Survey.
Note: Cigarette smoking prevalence is defined as having smoked at least one cigarette per day.

graphic factors; socioeconomic factors; knowledge, attitudes, and beliefs; self-esteem; and self-image.

Sociodemographic factors. Sociodemographic factors include age, gender, ethnicity and acculturation, family size and structure, and SES. It is difficult to isolate effects of these factors because they interrelate and overlap. Initiation and prevalence of tobacco use among adolescents typically rises with increasing age and grade, peaking during late adolescence and the early twenties.[46] Adolescents who begin smoking at a younger age are more likely to become regular smokers[47] and are less likely to quit smoking.[48]

Price affects not only whether adolescents smoke, but also how much they smoke.

In the United States, Afro-American youths report significantly lower levels of initiation and current smoking than whites or Hispanics.[3,49–56] Recent data from the US National Youth Tobacco Survey show little difference in current tobacco use between Afro-American and white middle-school students,[57] but significant differences among high-school students. In 2006, 16% of Afro-American high-school students had smoked within the past 30 days, compared with 28% of white students. The reasons for these differences are not clear given the correlation between race and SES in the United States. However, the mechanisms contributing to initiation for Afro-Americans who do smoke may be different from those for whites; e.g. smoking may serve more of a social function for white adolescents, because they may be more strongly influenced by peer smoking.[56,58,59]

Studies of family structure have found that intact, two-parent families tend to be protective against smoking.[3,53,60–63] The effect of household size on risk of tobacco use is unclear: larger families have been associated with both lower[64,65] and higher levels of tobacco use,[60] and some studies do not associate family size with smoking.[66] Higher levels of parental SES, such as higher education and social class, are found in some studies to be inversely related to tobacco use among adolescents.[54,67–70]

Socioeconomic factors. Socioeconomic status has been implicated in the risk for onset of smoking among

adolescents.[44,71–73] Adolescents from lower socioeconomic backgrounds are more likely to smoke than are other adolescents.[73] This difference may reflect, in part, divergent beliefs and attitudes about tobacco use,[74] along with other interpersonal and environmental risk factors. Moreover, cigarette advertising has been shown to influence low-income youth beliefs and attitudes about tobacco use. A field study in Mumbai[75] found that the tobacco industry in India targeted both high- and low-SES youth, using minor variations on similar themes of Westernization and affluence in marketing campaigns. Such advertising associates cigarette smoking with financial success and may make it appear attractive.[31]

In a cross-sectional survey of approximately 12 000 sixth- and eighth-grade students in Delhi and Chennai, India, in 2004, Mathur et al.[76] compared government and private schools as a proxy for SES and found that students from government schools were more likely to be current (within the previous 30 days) and ever-smokers of bidis and cigarettes. They were also about four times as likely as private-school students to have ever used bidis. The survey found a higher prevalence of many psychosocial risk factors among students in government schools, suggesting greater susceptibility to tobacco use. Although this study was not representative of all schoolchildren, and many children do not attend school at all, it suggests that socioeconomic differences observed in Indian adults may hold for children as well.

Personal income of adolescents is also associated with adolescent tobacco use. Some studies indicate that young people with more spending money have higher levels of tobacco use.[21,23,77,78] In several countries, adolescents are even more sensitive than adults to the price of cigarettes: price affects not only whether adolescents smoke, but also how much they smoke.[78–80] Thus, a rise in the price of tobacco products can have a substantial impact on youth tobacco consumption.[78]

Knowledge, attitudes, and beliefs. There is a lack of consensus on the role of tobacco-related knowledge in smoking uptake.[3,72] Studies have shown that in industrialized countries, adolescents who smoke are usually less knowledgeable about the health risks involved, do not believe that smoking will affect them personally, or feel that the short-term benefits outweigh any health risks.[81] However, knowledge alone is not sufficient to prevent smoking among adolescents, since many misinterpret the risks involved. In developing countries, young girls' knowledge about smoking and its effects on health is likely to be particularly low because of cultural beliefs and lack of systematic health-education programmes.[34] Knowledge about the health consequences of smoking is limited in many low- and middle-income countries, but this may be changing in some. In China, for example, 61% of adult smokers surveyed in 1996 believed that cigarettes did them "little or no harm".[8] In a 1998 survey among youth, about 80% of the respondents were aware that smoking causes lung cancer and other negative health outcomes.[82] A cross-sectional survey in Egypt conducted in 2005 found that among females, knowledge of the immediate negative consequences of smoking reduced susceptibility to future tobacco use.[83]

In high-income countries, general awareness of the health effects of smoking has undoubtedly increased over the past four decades. Nevertheless, there is some debate about how accurately smokers perceive the risks of developing disease. Various studies conducted over the past several decades have produced mixed conclusions, in part because of differing methodologies and possibly the reluctance of respondents to answer interviewer-administered questions honestly.[84] Recent evidence suggests that most smokers in the United States are aware of their increased risk of disease, but they significantly underestimate the magnitude of this risk relative to that of non-smokers.[84] Young adult smokers, in particular, have been found to underestimate the risk of light smoking.[85] Moreover, even individuals with a reasonably accurate perception of the health risks faced by smokers minimize the personal relevance of this information, believing that other smokers' risks are greater than their own.[8,84]

Children and adolescents may know less about the health effects of smoking than adults do. In a study of smoker perceptions in the United States, the majority of youth smokers reported giving no thought to how long they would continue to smoke when they began smoking. The majority of those who had given it thought reported expecting to smoke for less than five years. Although many young smokers reported being addicted, they tended to believe that they were less addicted than the average smoker and would be able to quit more easily than other smokers. Young people's overestimation of their ability to quit may play a role in the initiation of regular smoking.[86] Even adolescents who know about the risks of tobacco use may have a limited capacity to use the information wisely.

Positive attitudes towards tobacco use and tobacco users tend to be related to an increased likelihood of tobacco use.[44,71,72,87,88] In a study in northern England, Charlton and Blair[89] found a significant relationship between positive attitudes towards smoking and initiation of smoking among females. Positive beliefs about smoking have also been associated with youth smoking.[44,84,85,89,90] In general, adolescent smokers have less knowledge about the negative consequences of smoking than their non-smoking counterparts, discount the addictive property of tobacco, and negate the risks of experimental smoking.[44] Data from the 2003 GYTS in Turkey found that having positive beliefs about smokers is cross-sectionally associated with youth susceptibility to smoking, ever-smoking, and established smoking behaviour.[91]

In a series of focus groups among a small sample (n = 27) of Chinese high-school girls in Beijing in 2006, about half of the respondents believed that smoking makes a woman look independent.

Self-esteem. The process of individuation and identity formation is inherent in adolescence. The adolescent's sense of self evolves as she or he interacts with parents, school, and peers and considers options for the future. Self-esteem, or qualitative self-evaluation, emerges from these contexts.[92] In some studies, lack of self-esteem has been implicated in tobacco use among adolescents.[44,71,93–98] In other research, however, no association was found between self-esteem and smoking initiation.[99,100] Different measures of self-esteem have been used in the literature, and this may have contributed to the inconsistent findings. The 2001 report of the Surgeon General of the United States concluded that adolescents who smoke are more likely to have low self-esteem and low expectations for future achievement.[44] In fact, they may regard smoking as a means of coping with the stress, anxiety, and depression associated with lack of self-confidence. Several studies have found that girls have lower self-esteem than boys.[96,97,101] One study of schoolchildren in Calgary, Canada, found that girls have lower self-esteem than boys, and a significant association was observed between low self-esteem and smoking behaviour in girls only.[96] Young and Werch[92] also found that young non-smokers and those with no intention of smoking in the future had higher self-esteem than frequent users or those who intended to use in the future.

Self-image. Some adolescents may smoke cigarettes to enhance their self-esteem by improving their external image, i.e. by appearing mature or "cool". Role models who smoke are frequently seen as tough, sociable, and sexually attractive.[102] Adolescents who believe that smoking bestows these attributes may see smoking as a powerful mechanism for self-enhancement. These adolescents may experiment with smoking in an attempt to adopt a perceived positive social image and thereby improve the way others, particularly peers, view them.[102] If peers respond favourably to this strategy, these new young smokers may continue to smoke, since the behaviour has proved functional for them. In a series of focus groups among a small sample (n = 27) of Chinese high-school girls in Beijing in 2006, about half of the respondents believed that smoking makes a woman look independent. These respondents also approved of smoking by celebrities.[103]

Smoking is portrayed in advertising as a means of attaining maturity and adulthood and, for women, of being sophisticated, sociable, feminine, and sexually attractive. In industrialized countries, where the media promote an image of female attractiveness that equates being thin with desirability, weight control and dieting are major obsessions among adolescent girls.[104] Being slim gives these girls self-confidence and seems fashionable. The expected benefits of smoking on body weight may play an important role in smoking uptake.[44] The association between dieting and smoking initiation among adolescents has been studied in high-income countries,[105–109] including the United States, where Austin et al.[106] found that girls who reported dieting at baseline were four times more likely to become smokers at the two-year follow-up than girls who were not dieting at baseline. In a prospective study of young girls in Massachusetts, putting a greater value on being thin was associated with becoming an "established" smoker (smoking at least 100 cigarettes in one's lifetime) later on in adolescence.[105]

In a survey of high-school students in an urban location in the United States, nearly 40% of white female cigarette smokers reported using smoking as a method to control their appetite and weight, in contrast to only 12% of white male smokers.[110] No such use of smoking for weight control was reported for Afro-American adolescent smokers. A larger survey of ninth- and twelfth-grade students in Minnesota found that close to 50% of adolescent female smokers and 28% of male smokers reported smoking cigarettes to lose weight or control weight in the previous 12 months. After controlling for grade level, Afro-American female smokers were found to be half as likely as white female smokers to use smoking for weight control. In addition, heavy smoking was shown to correlate with weight-control behaviour, as adolescent heavy smokers were more than three times as likely as light smokers to report smoking for weight control or weight loss.[111]

Socioenvironmental Factors

Environmental factors that influence initiation and maintenance of tobacco use by adolescents include parental influence, peer tobacco use, and marketing and advertising of tobacco products.

Parental influence. The impact of parental smoking has been studied in a wide range of contexts in a large number of studies, which have resulted in a variety of outcomes.[112] Most studies of the association between parent smoking and adolescent smoking have been conducted in industrialized countries. Some have found significant associations, and some have not.[3] Bauman et al.[113] found that smoking among adolescents is more strongly related to whether a parent has ever smoked than to whether a parent currently smokes. However, several other studies observed that adolescents with parents who are current smokers are more likely to smoke than adolescents with parents who are former smokers.[114,115] Further, the influence of parental smoking may be gender-specific, as young girls have been found to be more likely to smoke when their mother is a current smoker.[44,116–118] Ashley et al. found in a nationally representative sample of US adolescents in 2002 and 2003 that cigarette smoking among mothers was associated with a greater risk of cigarette smoking by daughters than by sons.[119] Data from a nationally representative sample in New Zealand did not show gender-specific associations of parental smoking with adolescent smoking for the same sex, although it found that parental smoking behaviour in combination with other factors under parental control (i.e. provision

World Health Organization

of pocket money and allowing smoking in the home) is a key determinant of daily smoking by adolescents.[120]

The relationship between parental smoking and adolescent smoking could be interpreted in a variety of ways. The most straightforward interpretation is that parents who smoke serve as models for the behaviour of their children.[44] Alternatively, being raised in a home where parents smoke exposes a young person to cigarette smoke, and such exposure may lead to greater perceived parental approval of smoking by adolescents.[121,122] Finally, parents who smoke may facilitate their children's smoking simply by giving children easier access to cigarettes or allowing smoking in the home.[123]

Studies comparing the associations between peer and adolescent smoking and between parent and adolescent smoking have generally found that peer smoking is a better predictor of adolescent smoking, although the study context and the stage of adolescent tobacco use affect this finding.[3,124] Bricker et al.[125] studied smoking by adolescents and determined that parental influence was substantial throughout the transition from non-use to experimentation and daily use, whereas peer influence was stronger for the transition from not smoking to experimentation. Other research found similar results, i.e. that parental influence on initiation and escalation to daily smoking remains constant or decreases over time, while smoking by friends is more predictive of initiation than of escalation.[3]

Some evidence indicates that adolescents are more likely to smoke if their older siblings smoke.[118,126] Presumably, this is partly because older siblings model, prompt, and reinforce smoking behaviour with their younger siblings. Households in which older siblings smoke may also be households in which parents do not clearly oppose youth smoking. Even if relationships between parents' current smoking or lifetime smoking status and their children's smoking are weak, parents may still play a role in preventing their children from becoming smokers.

Less information is available on the role of parents in developing countries. The few recent studies of parental influence produced mixed results, similar to studies in industrialized countries. Gender differences in the association between parent smoking and adolescent smoking were reported in Brazil, similar to those found in some studies in the United States.[44] A prospective birth-cohort study in Brazil found that parental smoking during pregnancy and childhood may be a more important determinant of smoking in adolescent girls than in boys.[127]

In China, parental current smoking status and parental monitoring of youth have been identified as risk factors for youth tobacco use in some studies, but not in others. A longitudinal study in seven Chinese cities found that parental monitoring was predictive of smoking within the previous 30 days by male and female adolescents.[128] Cross-sectional data from the same study sampled ninth-grade students in urban and rural areas and showed that adolescent smoking was not strongly associated with current parental smoking in either type of area.[129] A cross-sectional survey of students in Huangpu, Guangzhou, found a significant association between mothers' smoking and experimental smoking by females and males, although the association with female youth was greater.[130] In contrast, fathers' smoking was significantly associated only with smoking among males.

In a 2003 study of students in Alexandria, Egypt, parental and sibling smoking was associated with ever-smoking, smoking in the prior 30 days, and susceptibility to smoking.

Finally, findings on the importance of parental smoking relative to peer influence are inconsistent in recent literature. In a 2003 study of students in Alexandria, Egypt, parental and sibling smoking was associated with ever-smoking, smoking in the prior 30 days, and susceptibility to smoking (defined as the likelihood of smoking in the next year or when the child is older).[131] Other traditional risk factors, including peer smoking, positive beliefs about smoking, and perceived social norms, were also associated with smoking or smoking susceptibility. In general, the associations with parental and sibling smoking were found to be stronger than those with peer smoking, leading to the conclusion that in this more collective society, the family unit may have a stronger influence than it typically has in some Western countries. However, in a small study of female university smokers in Cairo, Labib et al.[132] reported

World Health Organization

that almost all the respondents had friends who smoked, and more than half of the water pipe smokers reported being introduced to water pipes by a female friend. Relatively few female smokers reported being introduced by a male or female relative. While the importance and predictive value of parental influence on adolescent tobacco use is inconsistent in the literature, the potential gender-specific and cultural differences indicate that parental influence is an important predictor of adolescent smoking, but it is one of many risk factors.

Peer tobacco use. Peers have been variously defined as classmates, friends, best friends, opposite- or same-sex friends, and boyfriends or girlfriends.[72] Regardless of the definition used, however, peer tobacco use is consistently related to adolescent tobacco use initiation, maintenance, and intentions.[3,133–135] Taylor et al.[136] found that adolescents in the United States who had one significant peer who smoked were almost four times more likely to smoke than those without a significant peer who smoked. In some settings, smoking may be a shared activity with important socializing functions for female youth,[137,138] and same-sex friends may be particularly influential in the smoking behaviour of female adolescents.[117,137,138]

From the findings of cross-sectional studies, it is difficult to determine whether female adolescents model their behaviour after friends or select peers with similar behaviour. To some extent, it is possible that an adolescent begins to smoke, then becomes friends with others who smoke.[139,140] However, evidence from longitudinal studies shows that adolescents who have friends who smoke but do not yet smoke themselves are more likely to become smokers in the future than those with non-smoking friends.[141,142]

Social influences appear to be important even after a young person begins smoking regularly. Peer smoking has been shown to predict continued smoking by young people.[141] Presumably, adolescents who begin to smoke and continue receive social reinforcement from peers. Christakis and Fowler[143] conducted a network analysis using prospective data from the United States and found that groups of individuals tended to quit smoking together and were heavily influenced by their social networks, including spouses, friends, and siblings.

Studies conducted in other countries, including Mexico and the Russian Federation, point to the strong influence of peer smoking on adolescent smoking behav-

iour.[94,144] Recent studies of the relationship between social factors and adolescent smoking behaviour among Chinese have also highlighted the importance of peer smoking influences.[128–130,145] In a study of college students in China, having friends who smoke, parental SES, depression, alienation, and other health risk behaviours were associated with women's intention to smoke.[146] In another study, nearly 40% of Chinese women smokers in China, Hong Kong Special Administrative Region reported the influence of friends or colleagues as a reason for beginning to smoke. Substantially fewer (9%) reported familial influence on smoking initiation.[147] These data suggest that many of the factors related to smoking uptake among youth in Western cultures—in particular, the role of peer smoking—may be applicable to Chinese youth as well.

Marketing and advertising of tobacco products. Tobacco advertising and promotion have a direct effect on the initiation of tobacco use among adolescents.[3,54,148] Tobacco companies deny marketing cigarettes to young people, but a great deal of evidence indicates that they are hard at work recruiting young people to smoke. In the United States, about 4000 adolescents start smoking cigarettes every day, and about 1140 adolescents become daily cigarette smokers. About 1100 smokers die every day from smoking-related illnesses in the United States, and more than 3000 quit smoking.[149,150] The majority of smokers begin smoking before age 18.[55] Thus, recruiting young people to smoke is vital to profit maintenance for the tobacco companies. A recent meta-analysis of tobacco marketing in various countries found that exposure to all pro-tobacco marketing and media doubles the odds of tobacco use initiation.[151]

Marketing to young people is not just a matter of ensuring future sales. Sales to minors are also a significant source of profit for the tobacco companies. Healton et al.[152] estimated that in 2002, the wholesale value of cigarettes sold annually to adolescents under age 18 in the United States was about US$ 1.2 billion (and virtually all these sales are illegal). This represents a substantial increase over the 1997 estimate of US$ 737 million and is primarily the result of increasing wholesale prices.

In addition to direct and indirect advertising and promotion, exposure to other external cues, such as smoking in movies, has been shown to increase the risk for subsequent initiation in children.[153–156] A recent study in Germany found that youths in the highest quartile of movie-smoking exposure were almost twice as likely to try smoking as those in the lowest quartile, after controlling for known determinants of initiation such as peer and parental smoking.[157] Wills et al.,[158] using longitudinal data from a representative sample in the United States, modelled movie-smoking exposure, mediators, and smoking onset and found a direct effect of movie-smoking exposure on smoking onset, as well as a larger effect on changing smoking expectancies among girls.[158] The relationship between movie-smoking exposure and adolescent smoking has also been studied in Mexico. Thrasher et al.[94] performed a cross-sectional study of 3876 schoolchildren in two cities in Mexico in 2006 and found a positive association between exposure to smoking in films and current and ever-smoking. Among ever-smokers, positive associations were observed between exposure to smoking in films and susceptibility to smoking, favourable attitudes towards smoking, and perceived peer smoking prevalence.

Maintenance of Tobacco Use

Women continue to smoke because of a complex interplay of factors, including physiological addiction to nicotine and psychological and social factors.

Physiological Dependence

It is well known that cigarettes and other forms of tobacco are addictive and that nicotine is the drug in tobacco that leads to addiction.[4,5] The American Psychiatric Association[159] and WHO[160] have classified nicotine dependence as a mental disorder. These organizations' definitions of dependence include a strong desire for a substance and difficulty controlling use; physiological withdrawal when use is stopped or reduced; evidence of tolerance; and persistent use despite knowledge of harms. Smokers who are deprived of cigarettes experience withdrawal and tend to compensate for periods of deprivation by increasing consumption when cigarettes become available; such compensatory activity regulates the nicotine level in the bloodstream.[161] Evidence indicates that use of smokeless tobacco produces the same effects,[162] with symptoms associated with withdrawal including nausea, headache, constipation, diarrhoea, increased appetite, drowsiness, fatigue, insomnia, inability to concentrate, irritability, hostility, anxiety, and craving for tobacco.[4,5]

The dependence-producing properties of nicotine are responsible for its reinforcing effects. Once a person has begun to use tobacco habitually, attempts to quit using it produce symptoms of withdrawal. These symptoms can be reduced or terminated by resuming smoking or chewing tobacco, which constitutes negative reinforcement. A tobacco user experiences numerous trials each day when the aversive effects of nicotine withdrawal are terminated by consuming tobacco. A person who tries to quit but fails experiences longer and more substantial aversive events, which are then reinforced by giving in to the urges. In unsuccessful efforts to quit, most tobacco users inadvertently shape powerful aversive reactions to nicotine withdrawal.[4]

> *Several studies have suggested that women may have a harder time quitting smoking than men, which may be due in part to the greater tendency for women to smoke in response to negative affect, stress, or depression, or to control weight.*

Several studies have suggested that women may have a harder time quitting smoking than men, which may be due in part to the greater tendency for women to smoke in response to negative affect, stress, or depression, or to control weight.[163–168] A recent study found that nicotine metabolism was faster among women than among men and faster among women taking oral contraceptives, which may have relevance for the efficacy of nicotine replacement medications for women.[169] Some studies have shown that women are less sensitive than men to the reinforcing effects of nicotine but more sensitive to non-nicotine smoking cues, such as social cues.[44,164–166,168,170] The evidence for differences between men and women in the extent of withdrawal symptoms is mixed. Most research suggests no differences;[164] however, the extent of women's symptoms may vary as a function of menstrual cycle stage.[164,171]

Psychosocial Factors

Stress. Many women smoke in response to negative life experiences.[44,72] Although both men and women may smoke to reduce stress, they experience different stresses. For example, in recent years, women have entered the workforce in large numbers, but they still shoulder the majority of child care, elder care, and household responsibilities. Women in the workforce also generally hold lower-level service or manufacturing jobs, which provide little sense of autonomy or control and may increase stress.

> *Because women may initiate smoking in order to lose or maintain weight and continue to smoke in fear of weight gain, weight control may represent an important motivational factor in their cigarette use.*

Women may smoke in response to other types of emotional distress as well, such as anger, resentment, or anxiety.[164,172] A recent survey in the United Kingdom found that women were more likely than men to report stress as a reason for smoking again after a failed quit attempt.[173]

Women may use smoking to temper negative emotions and to better fit the societal norm. Traditionally, in Western culture, women are praised and rewarded for their beauty, defined as being youthful and thin. Many women strive for this cultural ideal, regardless of the cost to their health, using smoking as a means of weight control.[44] The factors that contribute to women's maintenance of smoking may be indicative of women's lower status in the society and the inequality women often face.

Depression. Prevalence of cigarette smoking has been found to be higher for persons having psychiatric disorders[44] such as schizophrenia, mania, personality disorders;[174] depression;[175–180] or panic disorders.[178,180] Depressed smokers are more likely to be nicotine dependent[164,181] and less likely to quit smoking.[164,175,177,182,183] Smokers with a history of depression also have a greater risk of relapse after a cessation attempt.[181,184] It has been reported that smoking cessation causes more-intense depressed moods in smokers with a history of depression, resulting in lower success rates for cessation.[61] A study of patients hospitalized for cardiovascular disease suggests that recent quitters exhibiting depressive symptoms during hospitalization are more likely to relapse, and their depression may be exacerbated by stronger withdrawal symptoms.[185] The prevalence of depression among women is twice that among men,[159] and women may be more likely to smoke in response to negative affect,[164,186] indicating that the associations between smoking and depression may be particularly important for women.

Several longitudinal studies have shown an association between smoking and depression among adolescents.[139,183,187,188] In a longitudinal study in the United States, Kandel and Davies[139] reported that depressed adolescents were more likely than non-depressed adolescents to report daily smoking nine years after initiation of smoking. Patton et al.[187] studied adolescents in Australia and showed that depressive symptoms increased the risks for experimental smoking in the presence of peer smoking. Goodman and Capitman[189] found that, after controlling for other determinants of smoking, smoking among adolescents was a predictor of subsequent depressive symptoms rather than vice versa. This finding suggests a complex and dynamic process between depressive symptoms and smoking uptake and maintenance.[164,181]

Body weight. Body weight is an important concern in the initiation and maintenance of smoking by women. Several studies of female adolescents and adults have found relationships between smoking and body image, body weight, and dieting behaviour.[44,105–109,190,191] Women's concerns about weight may encourage smoking initiation, be a barrier to smoking cessation, and increase relapse rates among women who stop smoking.[110,192–197] Women who smoke to control weight report greater dietary restraints[191] and more eating-disorder symptoms.[192] In addition, restrained eaters endorse the use of smoking for weight-control purposes significantly more than unrestrained eaters do.[197]

Much research has also investigated whether fear of gaining weight discourages attempts to quit.[192,198–200] The findings suggest that concerns about weight gain often hinder smoking cessation, especially among women,[191] although some results have not supported this.[192] Additionally, women tend to gain more weight than men do after quitting.[200] Because women may initiate smoking in order to lose or maintain weight and continue to smoke for fear of weight gain, weight control may represent an important motivational factor in their cigarette use. Gerend et al.[201] found that a minority of women reported using smokeless tobacco for weight management, but its use for this reason may not be a predominant mediator, as cigarette smoking is.

Summary and Recommendations

Summary

Over the past several decades, the tobacco pandemic has been shifting from industrialized to developing nations to increasingly involve women. The increase in tobacco use among women has typically followed weakening social, cultural, and political constraints, which have been exploited by multinational tobacco companies. Global estimates show wide variation in the prevalence of smoking among women. In some regions, prevalence is comparable among men and women, while in others, there are very large differences by sex and gender. Recent estimates of tobacco use among youth show similar patterns among boys and girls in many areas of the world, suggesting that these differences may be narrowing. Although effective tobacco control policies are available, they could be optimized by understanding the factors that influence uptake and maintenance of tobacco use and how these factors may differ between boys and girls. Evidence suggests that girls and women may be more influenced by beliefs about weight control and self-image and by female friends or role models, and that women smoke to cope with stress and negative feelings more than men do. However, most of the literature on smoking initiation comes from industrialized countries, where the mix of social, environmental, and cultural influences may be quite different from that in developing countries. Further research is needed to understand the extent to which these well-established factors relate to smoking initiation and maintenance in a variety of settings.

Recommendations

- Develop culturally sensitive and gender-specific community programmes to prevent initiation and maintenance of tobacco use.

- In developing tobacco control strategies, incorporate the changing cultural, psychosocial, and environmental factors that influence initiation and maintenance of tobacco use among girls and women of all ages as well as boys and men.

- Monitor patterns of tobacco use specific to girls and women through the life-course.

- Ensure that sex-disaggregated data and a gender analysis are included in surveillance systems, research, monitoring, and evaluation of tobacco control programmes.

References

1. *WHO report on the global tobacco epidemic, 2009: implementing smoke-free environments.* Geneva, World Health Organization, 2009.
2. Lopez AD, Collishaw NE, Piha T. A descriptive model of the cigarette epidemic in industrialized countries. *Tobacco Control,* 1994, 3:242–247.
3. US Department of Health and Human Services, Public Health Service, Centers for Disease Control and Prevention. *Preventing tobacco use among young people: a report of the Surgeon General.* Washington, DC, US Government Printing Office, 1994.
4. Institute of Medicine. *Ending the tobacco problem: a blueprint for the nation.* Washington, DC, National Academies Press, 2007.
5. *Harm reduction in nicotine addiction: helping people who can't quit. A report by the Tobacco Advisory Group of the Royal College of Physicians.* London, Royal College of Physicians, 2007.
6. Shafey O et al. *The tobacco atlas,* 3rd ed. Atlanta, GA, American Cancer Society, 2009.
7. Asma S, Gupta PC. *Bidi smoking and public health.* Mumbai, India Ministry of Health, 2008.
8. *Curbing the epidemic: governments and the economics of tobacco control.* Washington, DC, The World Bank, 1999.
9. *STEPwise approach to surveillance (STEPS).* Geneva, World Health Organization, 2008. (http://www.who.int/chp/steps/en/).
10. *2004 National Drug Strategy Household Survey: first results.* (http://www.aihwgovau/publications/phe/ndshs04/ndshs04-c00 pdf).
11. Monteiro CA et al. Population-based evidence of a strong decline in the prevalence of smokers in Brazil (1989–2003). *Bulletin of the World Health Organization,* 2007, 85:527–534.
12. *WHO Global InfoBASE: data for saving lives.* Geneva, World Health Organization, 2008 (http://www.who.int/infobase/report.aspx?rid=115&dm=8&iso=KHM).
13. *Statistics Canada: Canadian Tobacco Use Monitoring Survey.* Ottawa, Government of Canada, 2008 (http://www.statcan.ca/english/Dli/Data/Ftp/ctums.htm).
14. Yang GH et al. Smoking and passive smoking in China, 2002 [in Chinese]. *Zhonghua Liu Xing Bing Xue Za Zhi,* 2005, 26:77–83.
15. *Fiji non-communicable diseases (NCD) STEPS survey 2002.* Fiji, Ministry of Health, 2002 (http://www.who.int/chp/steps/FijiSTEPSReport pdf).
16. The Netherlands National Drug Monitor. *Annual report 2005.* Utrecht, Trimbos Institute, Netherlands Institute of Mental Health and Addiction, 2006.

 World Health Organization

17. Bobak M et al. Changes in smoking prevalence in Russia, 1996–2004. *Tobacco Control*, 2006, 15:131–135.

18. Jagoe Ket al. Tobacco smoking in Tanzania, East Africa: population based smoking prevalence using expired alveolar carbon monoxide as a validation tool. *Tobacco Control*, 2002, 11:210–214.

19. Andreeva TI, Krasovsky KS. Changes in smoking prevalence in Ukraine in 2001–5. *Tobacco Control*, 2007, 16:202–206.

20. Goddard E. *General Household Survey 2006: smoking and drinking among adults*. Newport, United Kingdom Office for National Statistics, 2008.

21. Centers for Disease Control and Prevention. *Cigarette smoking among adults —United States, 2004*. November 2005 (http://www cdc gov/ mmwr/preview/mmwrhtml/mm5444a2 htm).

22. Warren CW et al. Global youth tobacco surveillance, 2000–2007. *MMWR Surveillance Summary*, 2008, 57:1–28.

23. Gajalakshmi CK et al. Patterns of tobacco use, and health consequences. In: Jha P, Chaloupka F, eds. *Tobacco control policies in developing countries*. New York, NY, Oxford University Press, 2000.

24. *Early release of selected estimates based on data from the 2007 National Health Interview Survey*. Atlanta, GA, National Center for Health Statistics, Centers for Disease Control and Prevention, 2008 (http:// www.cdc.gov/nchs/about/major/nhis/released200806.htm#8).

25. Japanese Public Welfare Ministry. *Smoking problems and health II*. Tokyo, Health and Medical Foundation, 1993.

26. *Projections of tobacco production, consumption and trade to the year 2010*. Rome, Food and Agriculture Organization of the United Nations, 2003.

27. Gajalakshmi CK et al. Global patterns of smoking and smoking attributable mortality. In: Jha P, Chaloupka F, eds. *Tobacco control policies in developing countries*. New York, NY, Oxford University Press, 2000.

28. Giskes K et al. Trends in smoking behaviour between 1985 and 2000 in nine European countries by education. *Journal of Epidemiology and Community Health*, 2005, 59:395–401.

29. Shafey O et al. Cigarette advertising and female smoking prevalence in Spain, 1982–1997: case-studies in international tobacco surveillance. *Cancer*, 2004, 100:1744–1749.

30. Fernandez E et al. Prevalence of cigarette smoking by birth cohort among males and females in Spain, 1910–1990. *European Journal of Cancer Prevention*, 2003, 12:57–62.

31. Reddy KS, Gupta PC, eds. *Report on tobacco control in India*. Mumbai, Ministry of Health & Family Welfare, Government of India, 2004.

32. Rani M et al. Tobacco use in India: prevalence and predictors of smoking and chewing in a national cross sectional household survey. *Tobacco Control*, 2003, 12:e4.

33. *2005–06 National Family Health Survey (NFHS-3)*. Mumbai, Ministry of Health & Family Welfare, Government of India, 2007.

34. Sinha DN et al. Tobacco control in schools of India: review from India Global School Personnel Survey 2006. *Indian Journal of Public Health*, 2007, 51:101–106.

35. Sinha DN et al. Linking Global Youth Tobacco Survey 2003 and 2006 data to tobacco control policy in India. *Journal of School Health*, 2008, 78:368–373.

36. Jha P et al. A nationally representative case-control study of smoking and death in India. *New England Journal of Medicine*, 2008, 358:1137–1147.

37. *National Health Survey 1998*. Singapore, Ministry of Health, 1999.

38. *National Health Survey 2007*. Singapore, Ministry of Health, 2007. (http://www.moh.gov.sg/mohcorp/publicationsreports.aspx?id=22520

39. Lim TK. Singapore and the tobacco pandemic. *Annals Academy of Medicine Singapore*, 2008, 37:363–364.

40. Morrow M, Barraclough S. Tobacco control and gender in South-East Asia. Part II: Singapore and Viet Nam. *Health Promotion International*, 2003, 18:373–380.

41. Fong C et al. Educational inequalities associated with health-related behaviours in the adult population of Singapore. *Singapore Medical Journal*, 2007, 48:1091–1099.

42. US Department of Health and Human Services. *The health effects of active smoking: a report of the Surgeon General*. Washington, DC, US Government Printing Office, 2004.

43. Yang G et al. Smoking in China: findings of the 1996 National Prevalence Survey. *Journal of the American Medical Association*, 1999, 282:1247–1253.

44. *Women and smoking: a report of the Surgeon General*. Rockville, MD, US Department of Health and Human Services, 2001.

45. Flay BR. Understanding environmental, situational and intrapersonal risk and protective factors for youth tobacco use: the theory of triadic influence. *Nicotine & Tobacco Research*, 1999, 1 (Suppl. 2):S111–S114.

46. Centers for Disease Control and Prevention. *Reducing tobacco use: a report of the Surgeon General*. Washington, DC, US Department of Health and Human Services, 200 (Report No. English (US) S/N 017-001-00544-4).

47. Escobedo LG et al. Sociodemographic characteristics of cigarette smoking initiation in the United States: implications for smoking prevention policy. *Journal of the American Medical Association*, 1990, 264:1550–1555.

48. Breslau N, Peterson EL. Smoking cessation in young adults: age at initiation of cigarette smoking and other suspected influences. *American Journal of Public Health*, 1996, 86:214–220.

49. Bachman JG et al. Racial/ethnic differences in smoking, drinking, and illicit drug use among American high school seniors, 1976–89. *American Journal of Public Health*, 1991, 91:372–377.

50. McDermott RJ et al. Multiple correlates of cigarette use among high school students. *Journal of School Health*, 1992, 62:146–150.

51. Flint AJ, Yamada EG, Novotny TE. Black-white differences in cigarette smoking uptake: progression from adolescent experimentation to regular use. *Preventive Medicine*, 1998, 27:358–364.

52. Harrell JS et al. Smoking initiation in youth: the roles of gender, race, socioeconomics, and developmental status. *Journal of Adolescent Health*, 1998, 23:271–279.

53. Kandel DB et al. Racial/ethnic differences in cigarette smoking initiation and progression to daily smoking: a multilevel analysis. *American Journal of Public Health*, 2004, 94:128–135.

54. National Cancer Institute. *Changing adolescent smoking prevalence: where it is and why*. Bethesda, MD, US Department of Health and Human Services, National Institutes of Health, 2001 (Smoking and tobacco control monograph 14. NIH Pub. No. 02-5086).

55. Substance Abuse and Mental Health Services Administration. *Results from the 2005 national survey on drug use and health: national findings*. Rockville, MD, US Department of Health and Human Services, 2006 (DHHS Publication SMA 06-4194).

56. Hu MC, Davies M, Kandel DB. Epidemiology and correlates of daily smoking and nicotine dependence among young adults in the United States. *American Journal of Public Health*, 2006, 96:299–308.

57. *National youth tobacco survey: 2006 NYTS data and documentation*. Atlanta, GA, Centers for Disease Control and Prevention, 2008. (http://www.cdc.gv/tobacco/data_statistics/surveys/nyts/index. htm#NYTS2006).

58. Headen SW et al. Are the correlates of cigarette smoking initiation different for black and white adolescents? *American Journal of Public Health*, 1991, 81:854–858.

59. Ellickson PL et al. From adolescence to young adulthood: racial/ ethnic disparities in smoking. *American Journal of Public Health*, 2004, 94:293–299.

60. Isohanni M, Moilanen I, Rantakallio P. Determinants of teenage smoking, with special reference to non-standard family background. *British Journal of Addiction*, 1991, 86:391–398.

61. Covey LS, Tam D. Depressive mood, the single-parent home, and adolescent cigarette smoking. *American Journal of Public Health*, 1990, 80:1330–1333.

62. Botvin GJ et al. Factors promoting cigarette smoking among black youth: a causal modeling approach. *Addictive Behaviors*, 1993, 18:397–405.

63. Griesbach D, Amos A, Currie C. Adolescent smoking and family structure in Europe. *Social Science & Medicine*, 2003, 56:41–52.

64. Boyle MH et al. *Substance abuse among adolescents and young adults: prevalence, sociodemographic correlates, associated problems and familial aggregation*. Toronto, Ontario Ministry of Health, 1993, (Ontario Health Survey, Working Paper No. 2).

65. Burchfiel CM et al. Initiation of cigarette smoking in children and adolescents of Tecumseh, Michigan. *American Journal of Epidemiology*, 1989, 130:410–415.

66. Stanton WR, Oei TP, Silva PA. Sociodemographic characteristics of adolescent smokers. *International Journal of Addiction*, 1994, 29:913–925.

67. Droomers M et al. Father's occupational group and daily smoking during adolescence: patterns and predictors. *American Journal of Public Health*, 2005, 95:681–688.

68. Huurre T, Aro H, Rahkonen O. Well-being and health behaviour by parental socioeconomic status: a follow-up study of adolescents aged 16 until age 32 years. *Social Psychiatry and Psychiatric Epidemiology*, 2003, 38:249–255.

69. Jefferis BJ et al. Effects of childhood socioeconomic circumstances on persistent smoking. *American Journal of Public Health*, 2004, 94:279–285.

70. Jefferis B et al. Cigarette consumption and socio-economic circumstances in adolescence as predictors of adult smoking. *Addiction*, 2003, 98:1765–1772.

71. Conrad KM, Flay BR, Hill D. Why children start smoking cigarettes: predictors of onset. *British Journal of Addiction*, 1992, 87:1711–1724.

72. Tyas SL, Pederson LL. Psychosocial factors related to adolescent smoking: a critical review of the literature. *Tobacco Control*, 1998, 7:409–420.

73. Hanson MD, Chen E. Socioeconomic status and health behaviors in adolescence: a review of the literature. *Journal of Behavioral Medicine*, 2007, 30:263–285.

74. Siahpush M et al. Socio-economic variations in tobacco consumption, intention to quit and self-efficacy to quit among male smokers in Thailand and Malaysia: results from the International Tobacco Control-South-East Asia (ITC-SEA) survey. *Addiction*, 2008, 103:502–508.

75. Bansal R, John S, Ling PM. Cigarette advertising in Mumbai, India: targeting different socioeconomic groups, women, and youth. *Tobacco Control*, 2005, 14:201–206.

76. Mathur C et al. Differences in prevalence of tobacco use among Indian urban youth: the role of socioeconomic status. *Nicotine & Tobacco Research*, 2008, 10:109–116.

77. Scragg R, Laugesen M, Robinson E. Cigarette smoking, pocket money and socioeconomic status: results from a national survey of 4th form students in 2000. *New Zealand Medical Journal*, 2002, 115(1158):U108.

78. Slater SJ et al. The impact of retail cigarette marketing practices on youth smoking uptake. *Archives of Pediatric Adolescent Medicine*, 2007, 161:440–445.

79. Chaloupka FJ. Explaining recent trends in smoking prevalence. *Addiction*, 2005, 100:1394–1395.

80. Ross H, Chaloupka FJ. The effect of cigarette prices on youth smoking. *Health Economics*, 2003, 12:217–230.

81. Cohn LD et al. Risk-perception: differences between adolescents and adults. *Health Psychology*, 1995, 14:217–222.

82. Yang G et al. Smoking among adolescents in China: 1998 survey findings. *International Journal of Epidemiology*, 2004, 33:1103–1110.

83. Islam SM, Johnson CA. Influence of known psychosocial smoking risk factors on Egyptian adolescents' cigarette smoking behavior. *Health Promotion International*, 2005, 20:135–145.

84. Weinstein ND, Marcus SE, Moser RP. Smokers' unrealistic optimism about their risk. *Tobacco Control*, 2005, 14:55–59.

85. Murphy-Hoefer R et al. A review of interventions to reduce tobacco use in colleges and universities. *American Journal of Preventive Medicine*, 2005, 28:188–200.

86. Weinstein ND, Slovic P, Gibson G. Accuracy and optimism in smokers' beliefs about quitting. *Nicotine & Tobacco Research*, 2004, 6 (Suppl. 3):S375–S380.

87. Wang MQ et al. Attitudes and beliefs of adolescent experimental smokers: a smoking prevention perspective. *Journal of Alcohol and Drug Education*, 1996, 41:1–12.

88. Hill AJ et al. Predicting the stages of smoking acquisition according to the theory of planned behavior. *Journal of Adolescent Health*, 1997, 21:107–115.

89. Charlton A, Blair V. Absence from school related to children's and parental smoking habits. *British Medical Journal*, 1989, 298:90–92.

90. Gilchrist LD, Schinke SP, Nurius P. Reducing onset of habitual smoking among women. *Preventive Medicine*, 1989, 18:235–248.

91. Ertas N. Factors associated with stages of cigarette smoking among Turkish youth. *European Journal of Public Health*, 2007, 17:155–161.

92. Young M, Werch CE. Relationship between self-esteem and substance use among students in fourth through twelfth grade. *Wellness Perspectives: Research, Theory and Practice*, 1990, 7:31–44.

93. Murphy NT, Price CJ. The influence of self-esteem, parental smoking, and living in a tobacco production region on adolescent smoking behaviors. *Journal of School Health*, 1988, 58:401–405.

94. Thrasher JF et al. Exposure to smoking imagery in popular films and adolescent smoking in Mexico. *American Journal of Preventive Medicine*, 2008, 35:95–102.

95. Simon TR et al. Prospective correlates of exclusive or combined adolescent use of cigarettes and smokeless tobacco: a replication-extension. *Addictive Behaviors*, 1995, 20:517–524.

96. Abernathy TJ, Massad L, Romano-Dwyer L. The relationship between smoking and self-esteem. *Adolescence*, 1995, 30:899–907.

97. Kawabata T et al. Relationship between self-esteem and smoking behavior among Japanese early adolescents: initial results from a three-year study. *Journal of School Health*, 1999, 69:280–284.

98. Byrne D, Davenport S, Mazanov J. Profiles of adolescent stress: the development of the adolescent stress questionnaire (ASQ). *Journal of Adolescence*, 2007, 30:393.

99. Brunswick AF, Messeri P. Causal factors in onset of adolescents' cigarette smoking: a prospective study of urban black youth. *Advances in Alcohol & Substance Abuse*, 1983, 3:35–52.

100. Winefield HR, Winefield AH, Tiggemann M. Psychological attributes of young adult smokers. *Psychological Reports*, 1992, 70:675–681.

101. Croghan IT et al. Is smoking related to body image satisfaction, stress, and self-esteem in young adults? *American Journal of Health Behavior*, 2006, 30:322–333.

102. Chassin L et al. The natural history of cigarette smoking from adolescence to adulthood: demographic predictors of continuity and change. *Health Psychology*, 1996, 15:478–484.

103. Ho MG et al. Perceptions of tobacco advertising and marketing that might lead to smoking initiation among Chinese high school girls. *Tobacco Control*, 2007, 16:359–360.

104. Tomeo CA et al. Weight concerns, weight control behaviors, and smoking initiation. *Pediatrics*, 1999, 104:918–924.

105. Honjo K, Siegel M. Perceived importance of being thin and smoking initiation among young girls. *Tobacco Control*, 2003, 12:289–295.

106. Austin SB, Gortmaker SL. Dieting and smoking initiation in early adolescent girls and boys: a prospective study. *American Journal of Public Health*, 2001, 91:446–450.

107. Voorhees CC et al. Early predictors of daily smoking in young women: the National Heart, Lung, and Blood Institute Growth and Health Study. *Preventive Medicine*, 2002, 34:616–624.

108. Leatherdale ST et al. Susceptibility to smoking and its association with physical activity, BMI, and weight concerns among youth. *Nicotine & Tobacco Research*, 2008, 10:499–505.

109. Kaufman AR, Augustson EM. Predictors of regular cigarette smoking among adolescent females: does body image matter? *Nicotine & Tobacco Research*, 2008, 10:1301–1309.

110. Camp DE, Klesges RC, Relyea G. The relationship between body weight concerns and adolescent smoking. *Health Psychology*, 1993, 12:24–32.

111. Fulkerson JA, French SA. Cigarette smoking for weight loss or control among adolescents: gender and racial/ethnic differences. *Journal of Adolescent Health*, 2003, 32:306–313.

112. Vitaro F et al. Differential contribution of parents and friends to smoking trajectories during adolescence. *Addictive Behaviors*, 2004, 29:831–835.

113. Bauman KE et al. Effect of parental smoking classification on the association between parental and adolescent smoking. *Addictive Behaviors*, 1990, 15:413–422.

114. Farkas AJ et al. The effects of household and workplace smoking restrictions on quitting behaviours. *Tobacco Control*, 1999, 8:261–265.

115. Jackson C, Henriksen L. Do as I say: parent smoking, antismoking socialization, and smoking onset among children. *Addictive Behaviors*, 1997, 22:107–114.

116. Elkind AK. The social definition of women's smoking behaviour. *Social Science & Medicine*, 1985, 20:1269–1278.

117. Gottlieb NH. The effects of peer and parental smoking and age on the smoking careers of college women: a sex-related phenomenon. *Social Science & Medicine*, 1982, 16:595–600.

118. Nofziger S, Lee HR. Differential associations and daily smoking of adolescents: the importance of same-sex models. *Youth & Society*, 2006, 37:453–478.

119. Ashley OS et al. Moderation of the association between parent and adolescent cigarette smoking by selected sociodemographic variables. *Addictive Behaviors*, 2008, 33:1227–1230.

World Health Organization

120. Scragg R, Laugesen M. Influence of smoking by family and best friend on adolescent tobacco smoking: results from the 2002 New Zealand national survey of year 10 students. *Australian and New Zealand Journal of Public Health*, 2007, 31:217–223.

121. Harakeh Z et al. Parental factors and adolescents' smoking behavior: an extension of the theory of planned behavior. *Preventive Medicine*, 2004, 39:951–961.

122. Roberts KH et al. Longitudinal analysis of the effect of prenatal nicotine exposure on subsequent smoking behavior of offspring. *Nicotine & Tobacco Research*, 2005, 7:801–808.

123. Scragg R, Laugesen M, Robinson E. Parental smoking and related behaviours influence adolescent tobacco smoking: results from the 2001 New Zealand national survey of 4th form students. *New Zealand Medical Journal*, 2003, 116(1187):U707.

124. Krosnick JS, Judd CM. Transitions in social influence at adolescence: who induces cigarette smoking? *Developmental Psychology*, 1982, 18:359–368.

125. Bricker JB et al. Changes in the influence of parents' and close friends' smoking on adolescent smoking transitions. *Addictive Behaviors*, 2007, 32:740–757.

126. Slomkowski C et al. Sibling effects on smoking in adolescence: evidence for social influence from a genetically informative design. *Addiction*, 2005, 100:430–438.

127. Menezes AM, Hallal PC, Horta BL. Early determinants of smoking in adolescence: a prospective birth cohort study. *Cademos Saúde Pública*, 2007, 23:347–354.

128. Grenard JL et al. Influences affecting adolescent smoking behavior in China. *Nicotine & Tobacco Research*, 2006, 8:245–255.

129. Ma H et al. Risk factors for adolescent smoking in urban and rural China: findings from the China seven cities study. *Addictive Behaviors*, 2008, 33:1081–1085.

130. Wen X et al. Modifiable family and school environmental factors associated with smoking status among adolescents in Guangzhou, China. *Preventive Medicine*, 2007, 45:189–197.

131. Islam SM, Johnson CA. Correlates of smoking behavior among Muslim Arab-American adolescents. *Ethnicity & Health*, 2003, 8:319–337.

132. Labib N et al. Comparison of cigarette and water pipe smoking among female university students in Egypt. *Nicotine & Tobacco Research*, 2007, 9:591–596.

133. Biglan A et al. Peer and parental influences on adolescent tobacco use. *Journal of Behavioral Medicine*, 1995, 18:315–330.

134. Spear SF, Akers RL. Social learning variables and the risk of habitual smoking among adolescents: the Muscatine Study. *American Journal of Preventive Medicine*, 4:336–342.

135. Krohn MD et al. Social bonding theory and adolescent cigarette smoking: a longitudinal analysis. *Journal of Health and Social Behavior*, 1983, 24:337–349.

136. Taylor JE et al. Saturation of tobacco smoking models and risk of alcohol and tobacco use among adolescents. *Journal of Adolescent Health*, 2004, 35:190–196.

137. Barton J et al. Social image factors as motivators of smoking initiation in early and middle adolescence. *Child Development*, 1982, 53:1499–1511.

138. McGraw SA et al. Sociocultural factors associated with smoking behavior by Puerto Rican adolescents in Boston. *Social Science & Medicine*, 1991, 33:1355–1364.

139. Kandel DB, Davies M. Adult sequelae of adolescent depressive symptoms. *Archives of General Psychiatry*, 1986, 43:255–262.

140. de Vries H et al. Challenges to the peer influence paradigm: results for 12-13 year olds from six European countries from the European Smoking Prevention Framework Approach study. *Tobacco Control*, 2006, 15:83–89.

141. Ary DV, Biglan A. Longitudinal changes in adolescent cigarette smoking behavior: onset and cessation. *Journal of Behavioral Medicine*, 1988, 11:361–382.

142. Bricker JB et al. Childhood friends who smoke: do they influence adolescents to make smoking transitions? *Addictive Behaviors*, 2006, 31:889–900.

143. Christakis NA, Fowler JH. The collective dynamics of smoking in a large social network. *New England Journal of Medicine*, 2008, 358:2249–2258.

144. Rogacheva A et al. Smoking and related factors of the social environment among adolescents in the Republic of Karelia, Russia in 1995 and 2004. *European Journal of Public Health*, 18:630–636, published online 27 September 2008.

145. Chen X et al. Perceived smoking norms, socioenvironmental factors, personal attitudes and adolescent smoking in China: a mediation analysis with longitudinal data. *Journal of Adolescent Health*, 2006, 38:359–368.

146. Mao R et al. Psychosocial correlates of cigarette smoking among college students in China. *Health Education Research*, 2009, 24:105–118, published online 16 February 2008.

147. Lau EM et al. The epidemiology of cigarette smoking in Hong Kong Chinese women. *Preventive Medicine*, 2003, 37:383–388.

148. DiFranza JR et al. Tobacco promotion and the initiation of tobacco use: assessing the evidence for causality. *Pediatrics*, 2006, 117:e1237-e1248.

149. *Youth and tobacco use: current estimates*. Atlanta, GA, Centers for Disease Control and Prevention, 2006 (http://www.cdc.gov/tobacco/data_statistics/fact_sheets/youth_data/youth_tobacco.htm).

150. US Department of Health and Human Services. *The health benefits of smoking cessation: a report of the Surgeon General*. Washington, DC, US Government Printing Office, 1990.

151. Wellman RJ et al. The extent to which tobacco marketing and tobacco use in films contribute to children's use of tobacco: a meta-analysis. *Archives of Pediatric Adolescent Medicine*, 2006, 160:1285–1296.

152. Healton C et al. Youth smoking prevention and tobacco industry revenue. *Tobacco Control*, 2006, 15:103–106.

153. Dalton MA et al. Effect of viewing smoking in movies on adolescent smoking initiation: a cohort study. *The Lancet*, 2003, 362:281–285.

154. Charlesworth A, Glantz SA. Smoking in the movies increases adolescent smoking: a review. *Pediatrics*, 2005, 116:1516–1528.

155. Titus-Ernstoff L et al. Longitudinal study of viewing smoking in movies and initiation of smoking by children. *Pediatrics*, 2008, 121:15–21.

156. Sargent JD et al. Exposure to movie smoking: its relation to smoking initiation among US adolescents. *Pediatrics*, 2005, 116:1183–1191.

157. Hanewinkel R et al. Longitudinal study of parental movie restriction on teen smoking and drinking in Germany. *Addiction*, 2008, 103:1722–1730.

158. Wills TA et al. Movie smoking exposure and smoking onset: a longitudinal study of mediation processes in a representative sample of US adolescents. *Psychology of Addictive Behaviors*, 2008, 22:269–277.

159. *Diagnostic and statistical manual of mental disorders DSM-IV*, 4th ed. Arlington, VA, American Psychiatric Association, 2000.

160. ICD 10: International classification of disease and related health problems. In: *Manual of the international classification of diseases, injuries, and causes of death*, 10th ed. Geneva, World Health Organization, 1992.

161. US Department of Health and Human Services. *A report of the Advisory Committee to the Surgeon General: the health consequences of using smokeless tobacco*. Washington, DC, US Government Printing Office, 1986.

162. Holm H et al. Nicotine intake and dependence in Swedish snuff takers. *Psychopharmacology (Berl)*, 1992, 108:507–511.

163. Schnoll RA, Patterson F, Lerman C. Treating tobacco dependence in women. *Journal of Women's Health (Larchmont)*, 2007, 16:1211–1218.

164. Benowitz NL, Hatsukami D. Gender differences in the pharmacology of nicotine addiction. *Addiction Biology*, 1998, 3:383–404.

165. Perkins KA, Donny E, Caggiula AR. Sex differences in nicotine effects and self-administration: review of human and animal evidence. *Nicotine & Tobacco Research*, 1999, 1:301–315.

166. Pomerleau OF et al. Nicotine dependence, depression, and gender: characterizing phenotypes based on withdrawal discomfort, response to smoking, and ability to abstain. *Nicotine & Tobacco Research*, 2005, 7:91–102.

167. Leventhal AM et al. Gender differences in acute tobacco withdrawal: effects on subjective, cognitive, and physiological measures. *Experimental and Clinical Psychopharmacology*, 2007, 15:21–36.

168. Pauly JR. Gender differences in tobacco smoking dynamics and the neuropharmacological actions of nicotine. *Frontiers in Bioscience*, 2008, 13:505–516.

169. Benowitz NL et al. Female sex and oral contraceptive use accelerate nicotine metabolism. *Clinical Pharmacology & Therapeutics*, 2006, 79:480–488.

170. Field M, Duka T. Cue reactivity in smokers: the effects of perceived cigarette availability and gender. *Pharmacology Biochemistry and Behavior*, 2004, 78:647–652.

171. Carpenter MJ et al. Menstrual cycle phase effects on nicotine withdrawal and cigarette craving: a review. *Nicotine & Tobacco Research*, 2006, 8:627–638.

172. McDermott LJ, Dobson AJ, Owen N. From partying to parenthood: young women's perceptions of cigarette smoking across life transitions. *Health Education Research*, 2006, 21:428–439.

173. West R, McEwen M, Bates C. *Sex and smoking: comparisons between male and female smokers*. London, No Smoking Day, 1999 (http://www.rjwest.co.uk/resources/sexandsmoking.pdf.

174. Hughes JR, Hatsukami D. Signs and symptoms of tobacco withdrawal. *Archives of General Psychiatry*, 1986, 43:289–294.

175. Hall SM et al. Nicotine, negative affect, and depression. *Journal of Consulting and Clinical Psychology*, 1993, 61:761–767.

176. Anda RF et al. Depression and the dynamics of smoking: a national perspective. *Journal of the American Medical Association*, 1990, 264:1541–1545.

177. Glassman AH et al. Smoking, smoking cessation, and major depression. *Journal of the American Medical Association*, 1990, 264:1546–1549.

178. Breslau N, Kilbey M, Andreski P. Nicotine dependence, major depression, and anxiety in young adults. *Archives of General Psychiatry*, 1991, 48:1069–1074.

179. Kendler KS et al. Smoking and major depression: a causal analysis. *Archives of General Psychiatry*, 1993, 50:36–43.

180. Pohl R et al. Smoking in patients with panic disorder. *Psychiatry Research*, 1992, 43:253–262.

181. Wilhelm K et al. Smoking cessation and depression: current knowledge and future directions. *Drug and Alcohol Review*, 2006, 25:97–107.

182. Borrelli B et al. The impact of depression on smoking cessation in women. *American Journal of Preventive Medicine*, 1996, 12:378–387.

183. Lam TH et al. Depressive symptoms and smoking among Hong Kong Chinese adolescents. *Addiction*, 2005, 100:1003–1011.

184. Weissman MM et al. Affective disorders. In: Robins LN, Regier DA, eds. *Psychiatric disorders in America: the epidemiologic catchment area study*. Toronto, Free Press, 1991:53–80.

185. Thorndike AN et al. Depressive symptoms and smoking cessation after hospitalization for cardiovascular disease. *Archives of Internal Medicine*, 2008, 168:186–191.

186. National Cancer Institute. *Women, tobacco, and cancer: an agenda for the 21st century*. Bethesda, MD, US Department of Health and Human Services, 2004.

187. Patton GC et al. Depression, anxiety, and smoking initiation: a prospective study over 3 years. *American Journal of Public Health*, 1998, 88:1518–1522.

188. Escobedo LG, Reddy M, Giovino GA. The relationship between depressive symptoms and cigarette smoking in US adolescents. *Addiction*, 1998, 93:433–440.

189. Goodman E, Capitman J. Depressive symptoms and cigarette smoking among teens. *Pediatrics,* 2000, 106:748–755.

190. US Department of Health and Human Services. *The health consequences of smoking: nicotine addiction. a report of the Surgeon General*. Washington, DC, US Government Printing Office, 1988.

191. Weekley CK III, Klesges RC, Reylea G. Smoking as a weight-control strategy and its relationship to smoking status. *Addictive Behaviors*, 1992, 17:259–271.

192. French SA et al. Do weight concerns hinder smoking cessation efforts? *Addictive Behaviors*, 1992, 17:219–226.

193. Klesges RC et al. Smoking, body weight, and their effects on smoking behavior: a comprehensive review of the literature. *Psychological Bulletin*, 1989, 106:204–230.

194. Gritz ER et al. Ethnic variations in the prevalence of smoking among registered nurses. *Cancer Nursing*, 1989, 12:16–20.

195. Pirie PL, Murray DM, Luepker RV. Gender differences in cigarette smoking and quitting in a cohort of young adults. *American Journal of Public Health*, 1991, 81:324–327.

196. Gritz ER et al. National working conference on smoking and body weight. Task Force 3: implications with respect to intervention and prevention. *Health Psychology*, 1992, 11(Suppl.):17–25.

197. Ogden J, Fox P. Examination of the use of smoking for weight control in restrained and unrestrained eaters. *International Journal of Eating Disorders*, 1994, 16:177–185.

198. Pirie PL et al. Smoking cessation in women concerned about weight. *American Journal of Public Health*, 1992, 82:1238–1243.

199. Talcott GW et al. Is weight gain after smoking cessation inevitable? *Journal of Consulting and Clinical Psychology*, 1995, 63:313–316.

200. Williamson DF et al. Smoking cessation and severity of weight gain in a national cohort. *New England Journal of Medicine*, 1991, 324:739–745.

201. Gerend MA et al. Eating behavior and weight control among women using smokeless tobacco, cigarettes, and normal controls. *Addictive Behaviors*, 1998, 23:171–178.

Pin-up
The Smoker's Body

Every 6.5 seconds someone dies from tobacco use, says the World Health Organization. Research suggests that people who start smoking in their teens (as more than 70 percent do) and continue for two decades or more will die 20 to 25 years earlier than those who never light up. It is not just lung cancer or heart disease that cause serious health problems and death. Below, some of smoking's less publicized side effects – from head to toe.

1. Hair loss
Smoking weakens the immune system, leaving the body more vulnerable to diseases such as lupus erythematosus, which can cause hair loss, ulcerations in the mouth and rashes on the face, scalp and hands.

2. Cataracts
Smoking is believed to cause or worsen several eye conditions. Smokers have a 40 percent higher rate of cataracts, a clouding of the eye's lens that blocks light and may lead to blindness. Smoke causes cataracts in two ways: by irritating the eyes and by releasing chemicals into the lungs that then travel up the bloodstream to the eyes. Smoking is also associated with age-related macular degeneration, an incurable eye disease caused by the deterioration of the central portion of the retina, known as the macula. The macula is responsible for focusing central vision in the eye and controls our ability to read, drive a car, recognize faces or colours, and see objects in fine detail.

3. Wrinkling
Smoking prematurely ages skin by wearing away proteins that give it elasticity, depleting it of vitamin A and restricting blood flow. Smokers' skin is dry, leathery and etched with tiny lines, especially around the lips and eyes.

4. Hearing loss
Because smoking creates plaque on blood vessel walls, decreasing blood flow to the inner ear, smokers can lose their hearing earlier than non-smokers and are more susceptible to hearing loss caused by ear infections or loud noise. Smokers are also three times more likely than non-smokers to get middle ear infections that can lead to further complications such as meningitis and facial paralysis.

5. Cancer
More than 40 chemicals in tobacco smoke have been shown to cause cancer. Smokers are 20 times more likely to develop lung cancer than non-smokers. And according to many studies, the longer one smokes, the greater the risk of developing cancers at several sites, including a two-fold risk of developing cancer of the nasal and paranasal cavities 5b; cancer of the oral cavity 5a (4 to 5 times); two-fold risk of developing cancer of nasopharynx; six and hypopharynx (4 to 5 times); larynx (10 times); oesophagus 5c (2 to 5 times); stomach 5d (2 times) and pancreas 5e (2 to 4 times). Some recent studies have also suggested a link between heavy smoking and breast cancer 5f, and smoking cessation substantially reduces the risk for most of the above mentioned smoking-related cancers.

6. Tooth decay
Smoking interferes with the mouth's chemistry, creating excess plaque, yellowing teeth and contributing to tooth decay. Smokers are one and half times more likely to lose their teeth.

7. Emphysema
In addition to lung cancer, smoking causes emphysema, a swelling and rupturing of the lung's air sacs that reduces the lungs' capacity to take in oxygen and expel carbon dioxide. In extreme cases, a tracheotomy allows patients to breathe. An opening is cut in the windpipe and a ventilator to force air into the lungs (see image). Chronic bronchitis (not shown) creates a build-up of pus-filled mucus, resulting in a painful cough and breathing difficulties.

8. Osteoporosis
Carbon monoxide, the main poisonous gas in car exhaust fumes and cigarette smoke, binds to blood much more readily than oxygen, cutting the oxygen-carrying power of heavy smokers' blood by as much as 15 percent. As a result, smokers' bones lose density. Fracture more easily and take up to 80 percent longer to heal. Smokers may also be more susceptible to back problems: one study shows that industrial workers who smoke are five times as likely to experience back pain after an injury.

9. Heart disease
One out of three deaths in the world is due to cardiovascular diseases. Smoking is one of the biggest risk factors for developing cardiovascular diseases. These diseases kill more than a million people a year in industrialized countries. Smoking-related cardiovascular diseases kill more than 600 000 people each year in developed countries. Smoking makes the heart beat faster, raises blood pressure and increases the risk of hypertension and clogged arteries and eventually causes heart attacks and strokes.

10. Stomach ulcers
Smoking reduces resistance to the bacteria that cause stomach ulcers. It also impairs the stomach's ability to neutralize acid after a meal, leaving the acid to eat away the stomach lining. Smokers' ulcers are harder to treat and more likely to recur.

11. Discoloured fingers
The tar in cigarette smoke collects on the fingers and fingernails, staining them a yellowish-brown.

12. Uterine cancer and miscarriage
Besides increasing the risk of cervical and uterine cancer, smoking creates fertility problems for women and complications during pregnancy and childbirth. Smoking during pregnancy increases the risk of low weight babies and future ill health consequences. Miscarriage is 2 to 3 times more common in smokers, as are stillbirths due to fetal oxygen deprivation and placental abnormalities induced by carbon monoxide and nicotine in cigarette smoke. Sudden infant death syndrome is also associated with smoking. In addition, smoking can lower estrogen levels causing premature menopause.

13. Deformed sperm
Smoking can deform sperm and damage its DNA, which could cause miscarriage or birth defects. Some studies have found that men who smoke have an increased risk of fathering a child who contracts cancer. Smoking also diminishes sperm count and reduces the blood flow to the penis, which can cause impotence. Infertility is more common among smokers.

14. Psoriasis
Smokers are two to three times as likely to develop psoriasis, a noncontagious inflammatory skin condition that leaves itchy, oozing red patches all over the body.

15. Buerger's disease
Buerger's disease, also known as thromboangiitis obliterans, is an inflammation of arteries, veins, and nerves in the legs, principally, leading to restricted blood flow. Left untreated, Buerger's disease can lead to gangrene (death of body tissue) and amputation of the affected areas.

The original image has been adapted for the Arabic-English version.

This poster is an updated reproduction of 'The smoker's body' originally produced by COLORS magazine, issue 21, July-August 1997.

Tobacco Free Initiative
http://www.who.int/tobacco

A product of M&H Communications.
Creating space for public health.
© World Health Organization, Geneva, 2002

ملصق
جسم المدخِّن

تقول منظمة الصحة العالمية إن شخصا ما يموت نتيجة لتعاطي التبغ كل ٦٫٥ ثوان، وتوحي الدراسات أن من يبدأ التدخين في العقد الثاني من عمره (وهؤلاء يشكلون أكثر من سبعين بالمئة من المدخنين) ويستمر على التدخين مدة عقدين أو أكثر سيموتون في الفترة الباكرة قبل ٢٠-٢٥ سنة من أقرانه الذين لم يدخنوا. ولا تقتصر المشكلات الخطيرة التي قد تؤدي للوفاة على سرطان الرئة وأمراض القلب. فهناك الكثير من الأمراض التي تصيب أي من البدن، من قمة الرأس إلى أخمص القدم. ولكنها غير مشهورة بين الناس.

(١) سقوط الشعر

(٢) الساد (الكتاراكت العيني)

(٣) التجاعيد الجلدية

(٤) فقد السمع

(٥) السرطان

(٦) تسوس الأسنان

(٧) النفاخ الرئوي

(٨) تخلخل العظام

(٩) أمراض القلب

(١٠) القرحات المعدية

(١١) اصطباغ الأصابع

(١٢) سرطان الرحم والإجهاض

(١٣) تشوه النطاف

(١٤) الصُّدَفية

(١٥) داء برغر

4. Impact of Tobacco Use on Women's Health

Introduction

Cigarette smoking was initially adopted by men in industrialized countries and was later taken up by women in those countries and men in developing countries. With the recent decline in smoking in industrialized countries, the multinational tobacco companies have moved aggressively into the developing nations. Consequently, there is a risk of an epidemic of tobacco-related diseases in the developing world, where tobacco use is increasingly becoming a major health issue for women as well as men.[1] The high percentage of non-smoking women in those countries makes them an attractive target for the industry.

The health effects of smoking in a population become fully pronounced only about a half-century after the habit is adopted by a sizeable percentage of young adults. Thus, most of what is known about the health effects of tobacco use among women comes from studies in industrialized countries, where women began smoking cigarettes decades ago and there has been adequate time to monitor the consequences. Despite the relative paucity of epidemiological data on women in developing countries, there is no reason to think that female smokers there will be spared the serious health effects of smoking. In those countries where female smoking is increasing, it may be several decades before the full health impact is felt, but devastating health consequences are inevitable unless action is taken today. Data from industrialized countries show that mortality of women who smoke is elevated by 90% or more compared with mortality among those who do not smoke,[2–4] with evidence that risk increases as the number of cigarettes smoked and the duration of smoking increase. Thus, the risk of premature death for tens of millions of women worldwide is nearly doubled by a single factor—tobacco use—that is entirely preventable.

It is well established that lung cancer is generally rare in populations where smoking prevalence is low and that its occurrence tends to increase following increases in smoking prevalence. Given this relationship, lung cancer mortality rates—which are available for most countries of the world, even though accuracy and completeness of reporting vary

considerably—can serve as an indicator of the "maturity" of the tobacco epidemic across populations. Although this review focuses much more on lung cancer than on other smoking-related diseases, lung cancer is only one of myriad adverse health consequences of smoking for women. Lung cancer accounted for approximately 13% of all smoking-attributable deaths among women in high-income countries in 2004;[5] the remaining 87% of tobacco's toll on women in high-income countries was due to other diseases. Moreover, lung cancer rates are a reflection of smoking patterns two to three decades earlier, so they inadequately reflect the more immediate health effects of women's smoking, such as adverse reproductive outcomes.

Most of what is known about the health effects of tobacco is based on the smoking of manufactured cigarettes, although in some areas of the world, other forms of tobacco use among women are common (e.g. smoking of traditional hand-rolled flavoured cigarettes (bidis), use of water pipes to smoke tobacco, use of snuff and other types of smokeless tobacco, and reverse cigarette smoking). Further studies of the health effects of these forms of tobacco use are needed, although no form can be considered safe.[6] Moreover, many women throughout the world are involved in tobacco agriculture and factory work. Although the literature contains descriptions of some of the toxic effects of handling tobacco,[7,8] there has been little study of the health effects of employment in tobacco production on women; for example, effects of such employment on pregnancy outcomes should be investigated. However, this chapter focuses on the health consequences of active smoking. The effects of exposure to second-hand smoke (SHS) are reviewed elsewhere in this monograph.

Effects of Smoking on Women's Health

Effects of Smoking on the Health of Infants and Children

The infants of mothers who smoke during pregnancy have birth weights approximately 200 g to 250 g lower, on average, than those of infants born to non-smoking women,[9–11] and they are more likely to be small for gestational age.[12–15] Risks of stillbirth,[16–19] neonatal death,[16,17,20] and sudden infant death syndrome (SIDS)[21–24] are also greater among the offspring of women who smoke. In addition, it appears that breastfeeding is less common or of shorter duration among women who smoke than among non-smokers and that smokers who breastfeed may produce less breast milk than non-smokers do.[25–29]

> *Women who smoke are more likely than non-smokers to experience primary and secondary infertility and delays in conceiving.*

Exposure to SHS has numerous effects on the health of children, particularly relating to respiratory illnesses and ear infections, lung function, and asthma; these are reviewed elsewhere in this monograph in the chapter on SHS, women, and children. Older children and adolescents who are active smokers have increased risks of respiratory illness, cough, and phlegm production; slower rates of lung growth; reduced lung function; and poorer lipid profiles than their non-smoking counterparts.[30]

Effects of Smoking on Reproduction and Menstrual Function

Women who smoke are more likely than non-smokers to experience primary and secondary infertility[31,32] and delays in conceiving.[33–36] Women smokers who become pregnant are also at increased risk of premature rupture of membranes, abruptio placentae (premature separation of the implanted placenta from the uterine wall), placenta previa (partial or total obstruction by the placenta of the cervical os), and pre-term delivery.[18,37–53] As noted above, their infants have lower average birth weights, are more likely to be small for gestational age, and are at increased risk of stillbirth and perinatal mortality than are the infants of non-smoking women. The proportion of pregnant women who smoke exceeds 30% in some populations, such as the poor and the less educated,[54–64] and in light of the serious health consequences and the strong motivation of pregnant women to ensure the health of their newborns, efforts to help pregnant women quit smoking (and to prevent postpartum relapse) should be a high priority in public health programmes focusing on women and children.

Additional studies of the effects of smoking on menstrual function, including menstrual regularity, are needed. From the evidence to date, it appears that women who smoke are more likely to experience dysmenorrhoea (painful menstruation)[65–68] and more severe and more frequent menopausal symptoms.[68] Early menopause is also more common among women who smoke. On average, women who are current smokers go through menopause about one to two years earlier than non-smoking women.[68–72]

Effects of Smoking on Cardiovascular Disease

In both industrialized and developing countries, cardiovascular diseases are the major causes of death among women, as well as among men.[73,74] Women who smoke have an increased risk of cardiovascular disease, including coronary heart disease (CHD), ischaemic stroke, and subarachnoid haemorrhage. Numerous prospective and case–control studies document the finding that smoking is one of the major causes of CHD in women.[2,75–81] Relative risks of CHD associated with smoking are greater for younger women than for older women. Data from the American Cancer Society's Cancer Prevention Study II (CPS II) for 1982–1986 indicate that age-adjusted relative risks of CHD were 3.0 (95% confidence interval (CI) = 2.5, 3.6) in women 35 to 64 years of age and 1.6 (95% CI = 1.4, 1.8) in women 65 years of age or older.[82] In the 1980s, evidence suggested that smoking may account for a majority of cases of CHD among women in the United States under the age of 50.[83] Risk of CHD increases with the number of cigarettes smoked daily and with the duration of smoking.[77,78] In the Nurses' Health Study, current smokers who began to smoke before the age of 15 years had an estimated relative risk of 9.3 (95% CI = 5.3, 16.2) in comparison with non-smokers.[78]

Women who use oral contraceptives and also smoke have a particularly elevated risk of CHD.[83,84] Earlier studies found that use of oral contraceptives alone was associated with a moderate increase in CHD risk and that the risk was 20- to 40-fold greater among oral contraceptive users who also smoked heavily, compared with women who neither used oral contraceptives nor smoked.[85,86] Recent studies based on lower-dose formulations show the overall risk of CHD associated with oral contraceptive use to be less than was observed with the first-generation formulations; however, the relative risk among smokers—

especially heavy smokers—who use oral contraceptives is still markedly higher than that among non-smokers who do not use them.[87–89] It is important that all women who wish to use oral contraceptives be informed of these risks and encouraged not to smoke.

Women who smoke also have elevated risks of ischaemic stroke and subarachnoid haemorrhage.[2,76,90–93] In a meta-analysis published in 1989 that was based on 31 studies, risk of stroke among female smokers was 1.72 (95% CI = 1.59, 1.86) times that of women who had never smoked.[94] More recent studies have reported a twofold to threefold excess risk for ischaemic stroke and subarachnoid haemorrhage among women who smoked over that for women who never smoked.[29] In CPS II, 55% (95% CI = 45, 65) of cerebrovascular deaths among women younger than 65 years of age were attributed to smoking.[82] Women who smoke also have significantly increased risks of carotid atherosclerosis,[95–97] peripheral vascular atherosclerosis,[98,99] and death from ruptured abdominal aortic aneurysm.[80,100–102]

Effects of Smoking on Chronic Obstructive Pulmonary Disease

Women who smoke have markedly increased risks of developing and dying of chronic obstructive pulmonary disease (COPD), which includes chronic bronchitis and emphysema with airflow obstruction.[103,104] In CPS II, the relative risk of COPD was 12.8 (95% CI = 10.4, 15.9) in current smokers, compared with non-smokers.[105] Risk increases with the number of cigarettes smoked per day.[2] At the population level, increases in smoking prevalence rates have been followed by steep increases in COPD mortality in countries around the world. In industrialized countries, prevalence of COPD is now almost the same in women and men.[106] Approximately 90% of COPD among women in CPS II was attributed to smoking.[105] Consistent with these findings, longitudinal studies have shown that lung function (as measured by forced expiratory volume in 1 sec (FEV1)) declines more steeply with age in women who smoke than it does in non-smokers.[107–110]

Effects of Smoking on Cancer

An estimated one fifth of all cancer deaths worldwide are attributable to smoking.[5] Women who smoke have higher risks for many cancers, including cancers of the lung, mouth, pharynx, oesophagus, larynx, bladder, pancreas, kidney, cervix, and possibly other sites, along with acute myelogenous leukaemia. In 2004, approximately 6% of new cases of cancer among women in low- and middle-income countries and 11% of new cases among women in high-income countries were attributable to tobacco.[5]

Age-adjusted lung cancer mortality rates among women in the United States have increased approximately 800% since 1950; by 1987, lung cancer had surpassed breast cancer to become the leading cause of cancer death among women in that country.

Lung cancer. Lung cancer was a rare disease among both men and women in the early decades of the 20th century. By the 1950s, however, it had become the leading cause of cancer death among men in many industrialized countries. By the 1970s and 1980s, lung cancer mortality rates were increasing among men in developing countries, as well as among women in many industrialized regions where female cigarette smoking was already well established (e.g. in North America, Northern Europe, and Australia/New Zealand). In 1950, lung cancer accounted for only about 3% of all cancer deaths of women in the United States, but today it accounts for 25%.[111] In 1955–1959, the lung cancer death rate among women aged 35 to 64 years in the 15 countries of the European Union combined was 7.7 per 100 000;[112] in 2006, the estimated age-standardized rate for all women was 18.4 per 100 000 in the 25 countries of the European Union.[113]

Age-adjusted lung cancer mortality rates among women in the United States have increased approximately 800% since 1950 (see Figure 4.1); by 1987, lung cancer had surpassed breast cancer to become the leading cause of cancer death among women in that country. However, mortality rates for female lung cancer appear to have recently levelled off for the first time, after increasing for several decades.[111] In countries where smoking among women became common relatively early in the 20th century, the vast majority of lung cancer deaths (about 90% in the United States[2]) are caused by smoking.[114,115] Worldwide, an estimated 53% of lung cancer in women is attributable to smoking.[5]

Current lung cancer rates among women vary dramatically between countries (Figure 4.2), reflecting historical differences in cigarette smoking across populations. Thus, lung cancer rates are intermediate or remain low in populations of women in which smoking was adopted later or is still relatively uncommon. Even within countries, there can be dramatic differences in subgroups of the population. For example, in the United States, the lung cancer death rate in the state of Utah is less than half the national average (13.9 per 100 000 vs 33.2 per 100 000);[117] the prevalence of smoking is low in Utah because of the predominance there of the Mormon religion, which proscribes smoking. In California, Asian women have much lower lung cancer death rates (24.9 per 100 000 in 1992–1996) than Caucasian women (48.9 per 100 000),[118] reflecting historical differences in smoking prevalence in the two racial groups.

Epidemiological studies consistently demonstrate that smoking is strongly associated with an increased risk of lung cancer in women and that risk increases with duration and amount of smoking and decreases with time since smoking cessation.[119-121] For example, in CPS II, which included more than 676 000 women 30 years of age or older, during follow-up from 1982 through 1988, those who were current smokers at the time of enrolment were approximately 12 times more likely than non-smokers to die of lung cancer.[2] The relative risk increased from 3.9 for women who smoked from one to nine cigarettes per day to 19.3 for women who smoked 40 cigarettes per day.[2]

Among women in industrialized countries, lung cancer ranks third (after cancers of the breast and colon/rectum) among all cancers in the number of new cases, and second (after cancer of the breast) among all cancers in the number of deaths. Among women in developing countries, lung cancer ranks fourth among cancers, after cancers of the cervix, breast, and stomach, in both number of new cases and deaths.[122] An estimated 379 000 women worldwide died from lung cancer in 2004 (compared with 940 000 men), accounting for 12% of all female cancer

Figure 4.1. **Annual Age-Adjusted Death Rates from Selected Cancer Types Among Females in the United States, 1930–2001 (age-adjusted to the US standard population)**

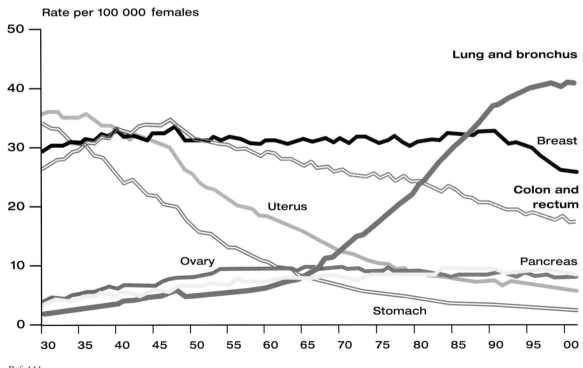

Source: Ref. 111.

World Health Organization

deaths (compared with 23% for men).[5] These numbers are expected to increase dramatically in the future, paralleling increases in female smoking prevalence in most countries of the world.

Not only is active smoking a well-established cause of lung cancer in women, many studies now document causal association of exposure to SHS with lung cancer in non-smoking women.

Other cancers. Women who smoke have markedly increased risk of cancers of the mouth and pharynx (oral cancers), oesophagus, larynx, bladder, pancreas, and kidney.[119,123–136] Risk of cervical cancer also has been shown in many studies to be higher in smokers than in non-smokers. While human papilloma virus (HPV) is now considered to be a cause of cervical cancer, the rate of development of cervical cancer is increased in HPV-infected women who smoke. The 2004 report of the US Surgeon General concluded that smoking should be considered a cause of cervical cancer.[137] Although the extent to which this relationship is independent of HPV infection is uncertain,[138] at least two prospective cohort studies have found smoking to be significantly associated with cervical cancer neoplasia in HPV-infected women.[139,140] An accumulating body of evidence indicates a possible link between active smoking and breast cancer, particularly premenopausal breast cancer.[141–146] Available data also show increased risks of acute myeloid leukaemia[147,148] in women who smoke, compared with non-smokers. Both the International Agency for Research on Cancer (IARC) and the Surgeon General of the United States have found that smoking is a cause of acute myeloid leukaemia.[149] In the United States, the majority of deaths due to several cancers in addition to lung cancer, including cancers of the larynx, pharynx, and oesophagus, among both men and women are attributable to smoking.[150]

Effects of Smoking on Bone Density and Fractures

Although smoking has not been consistently shown to have an effect on bone density in premenopausal or perimenopausal women, many studies have found that postmenopausal women who smoke have lower bone densities than non-smokers have.[29,151–156] Three recent meta-analyses examined the risk of hip fracture associated with

smoking and found reported increases in risk ranging from 31% to 84% among predominantly female study samples. The relative risk of hip fracture in smokers, compared with non-smokers, appears to be strongly associated with age. There is also evidence of an association between smoking and risk of fractures at other sites, but the highest observed risk is for fractures of the hip.[157]

Other Health Effects of Smoking

Cigarette smoking and depression are strongly associated, although it is difficult to determine whether the association reflects an effect of smoking on the etiology of depression, results from the use of smoking for self-medication by depressed individuals, or is due to common genetic or other factors that predispose people to both smoking and depression.[158–165] Because depression is a major cause of morbidity worldwide and is more prevalent in women than in men, the association between smoking and depression is important for women's health and needs further study.

Risk of a number of other conditions is higher among women who smoke than among non-smokers. These conditions include, but are not limited to, periodontal disease,[137,166] gall bladder disease,[167–171] peptic ulcer,[29,137,170–172] some forms of cataract,[137,173,174] and facial wrinkling.[100,175,176] While not necessarily life-threatening, these conditions can have considerable impact on the quality of women's lives.

Figure 4.2. Age-Standardized Lung Cancer Incidence Rates per 100 000 Women, by World Region, 2000 (standardized to the world population)

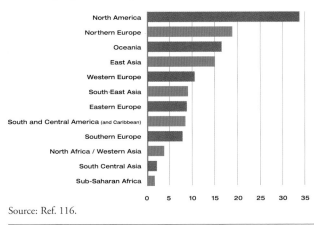

Source: Ref. 116.

Effects of Smoking on Total Mortality Worldwide: Narrowing of the Gender Gap

Peto et al.[114] estimated mortality from smoking during 1955–1995 for the major populations of the world that are classified by the United Nations as "developed". The proportion of all deaths attributed to smoking in these populations increased over time among persons of both sexes. In 1955, the proportion of all deaths resulting from smoking by persons 35 to 69 years of age in industrialized countries was 2% among women and 20% among men.[114] A more recent WHO report estimated global mortality caused by smoking in 2004.[5] In the 30-to-69-year age group, the proportion of all deaths due to smoking in industrialized countries was 12% among women and 33% among men. While these figures of estimated mortality from smoking are drawn from different studies with some of the changes attributable to methodological changes, nevertheless they demonstrate the narrowing of the gender gap in deaths due to smoking, as the increase was relatively greater among women. According to Peto,[114] each smoker in this age group who died (men and women combined) lost an average of 22 years of life expectancy.

Risk of CHD is markedly reduced (by 25% to 50%) within one to two years of smoking cessation.

Most of the deaths attributable to smoking worldwide have occurred in industrialized countries, but the situation is changing dramatically as the impact of the rising prevalence of smoking among women in the developing world is felt. It has been estimated that during the 1990s, about 2 million smoking-attributable deaths among men and women combined occurred annually in industrialized countries, and 1 million occurred in developing countries.[114] In 2004, the estimated numbers of smoking-attributable deaths in industrialized and developing countries were approximately equal: 2.43 million in industrialized countries and 2.41 million in developing countries.[5] However, by 2025, there will be an estimated 0.6 million such deaths among women every year in industrialized countries, compared with 1.98 million among women in developing countries.

In 2004, 3.8 million deaths among men worldwide were attributable to smoking (2.0 million in developing countries and 1.8 million in industrialized countries), and 1.0 million among women were attributable to smoking (0.4 million in developing countries and 0.6 million in industrialized countries).[5] However, women will account for an increasing proportion of all smoking-attributable deaths in the future. Recent estimates and projections from a WHO report[5] indicate that mortality from tobacco use at the global level will increase by 80% among women between 2004 and 2030; the increase in men will be 60% over the same time period. The gender gap is closing as smoking prevalence in women approximates that of men.

It is instructive to compare the experience of the United States, where smoking among women became common in the 1930s and 1940s and peaked (at about 33%) in the 1960s, with that of Japan, where female smoking prevalence has been low. The estimated proportion of deaths attributable to smoking among women in the United States 35 to 69 years of age increased from 0.6% in 1955 to 15% in 1975 to 31% in 1995; the increase in Japanese women was much less: from 0% in 1955 to 3% in 1975 to 4% in 1995.[114,115]

Reports from CPS II (conducted during 1982–1988) suggest that perhaps as many as half (47.9%) of the deaths among women who were smokers at the time of enrolment in the study were attributable to smoking.[105] In other words, about half of the persistent smokers in that study were eventually killed by their smoking. This proportion was higher than that for female smokers in the American Cancer Society's earlier CPS I study (1959–1965) (18.7%), reflecting the fact that female smokers in CPS I had started smoking later in life and had smoked fewer cigarettes per day than women in CPS II had.[105]

Based on a recent analysis of data from three large Danish population-based studies, it is estimated that among female smokers who inhaled, those who smoked 15 or more cigarettes per day lost 9.4 years of life expectancy, and lighter smokers lost 7.4 years, compared with women who had never smoked.[177]

World Health Organization

The Benefits of Smoking Cessation

Women who quit smoking experience marked reductions in disease risks. Some of the most extensively documented effects are discussed here, but the benefits are not limited to these examples.

Many studies suggest that the infants of women who stop smoking by the first trimester of pregnancy have weight and body measurements similar to those of infants born to non-smoking women.[11,13,51,178–186]

Risk of CHD is markedly reduced (by 25% to 50%) within one to two years of smoking cessation. There is a continued but more gradual reduction to the level of risk of non-smokers by approximately 10 to 15 years following cessation.[78,182–185] Stroke risk among smokers also decreases with smoking cessation; the estimated amount of time needed for risks to approximate those of individuals who have never smoked ranges from less than five years of abstinence to 15 or more years of abstinence.[90,100,183,186]

Individuals who quit smoking experience a slowing in the decline of pulmonary function,[100] a benefit that is considerably greater when cessation occurs at younger ages,[109,187] presumably because the cumulative adverse effects of smoking are less in young people than they are in older smokers who quit. A small improvement in lung function decline occurs during the first year following cessation, and the rate of decline slows in comparison with that of continuing smokers.[188] A number of years after quitting, former smokers have lower relative risks of COPD than continuing smokers, but in most studies their risks are still elevated, compared with those of non-smokers.[103] An analysis based on a large cohort of women in the United States suggests that former smokers' risk of developing chronic bronchitis approached that of individuals who had never smoked approximately 5 years after quitting.[104]

Risk of lung cancer and other cancers also declines with duration of smoking cessation. In CPS II, female former smokers who smoked up to 19 cigarettes per day had a relative risk of lung cancer of 9.1 (compared with women who had never smoked) after 1 to 2 years of not smoking. The risk declined to 2.9 after only 3 to 5 years of not smoking. Among former smokers of 20 or more cigarettes per day, the relative risk was 9.1 for women who had quit 6 to 10 years previously (compared with women

who had never smoked) and declined to 2.6 with 16 or more years of smoking abstinence.[100] Although risk of lung cancer in former smokers declines dramatically, compared with that of continuing smokers, it may never reach the low risk level of individuals who never smoked. Benefits of reduced tobacco consumption are now becoming apparent at the national level in some areas. Among adult women in the United States, smoking prevalence has declined since the mid-1970s, and lung cancer incidence is now declining in all age groups under 60 years of age; in fact, overall age-adjusted lung cancer incidence rates appear to have peaked in the 1990s.

Existing evidence suggests that the health effects of smoking tobacco with a water pipe – including lung cancer, cardiovascular disease, and harm to the fetus in the case of pregnant women – are similar to those of smoking cigarettes.

China: Hope for Women

Large-scale epidemiological studies of smoking in relation to all-cause and cause-specific mortality among Chinese adults confirm the significant increases in overall risk associated with smoking previously seen in North America and Europe,[189–191] although, at least in men, the principal causes of tobacco-related death are proportionately very different from those in Western countries. Approximately two thirds of Chinese males begin to smoke in early adulthood, and it appears that about half of them will eventually die prematurely as a result of their smoking. The proportion of deaths attributed to smoking has been estimated to increase from 12% in 1990 to 33% in 2030.[192] However, smoking prevalence among young Chinese women is low and may even be declining;[193–195] if the decline continues, the proportion of smoking-attributable deaths among Chinese women will drop from 3% in 1990 to 1% in 2030.[194] Preventing an epidemic of tobacco-related diseases among women in China and other countries where female smoking prevalence is still low is a tremendous public health opportunity.

Effects of Using Forms of Tobacco Other Than Cigarettes

Few epidemiological studies have addressed the health effects in women of using forms of tobacco other than modern cigarettes. This is an area that definitely requires further study given that large numbers of women, especially in developing countries, use oral snuff, practise reverse smoking, smoke hand-rolled herbal or other traditional cigarettes, or use other forms of tobacco. Existing evidence suggests that the health effects of smoking tobacco with a water pipe—including higher risks of lung cancer, cardiovascular disease, and harm to the fetus in the case of pregnant women—are similar to those of smoking cigarettes.[196,197] There is some evidence that smokeless tobacco is associated with poor health outcomes at different stages of life; such outcomes include low birth weight of infants, modest cardiovascular disease risk, pancreatic cancer, and oral cancer.[112,198–203] Research in this area is continuing.

Research Gaps

Additional research on women and smoking is needed in several areas:

- A life-course approach is essential to fully comprehend the health of girls and women of all ages.[204] However, little is known concerning the implications of tobacco smoke exposure from childhood, through adolescence, during the reproductive years, and beyond to old age. More investigation is needed of the later consequences of early life exposures to tobacco smoke. Further research is also needed on how the age of starting to smoke regularly might affect children's growth, risks associated with pregnancy, and subsequent risk for diseases caused by smoking.

- Much better population-level data on smoking prevalence among women are needed, especially prevalence in the developing world. Data collection should occur at regular time intervals, and standardized measures should be used to define various aspects of active and passive smoking, so

that comparisons can be made over time and across populations. A step towards such data collection is being made with the launch of the Global Adult Tobacco Survey (GATS) in 15 high-burden countries.

- High-quality, population-based cancer-incidence data are needed to monitor changes in tobacco-related cancers and to enable compilation of data across countries for better estimation of the worldwide impact of tobacco use on women's health. Cause-specific mortality data would also be useful. The data should be sex- and age-disaggregated as appropriate.

- Studies of the possible modifying effects of lifestyle and environmental exposure on the disease risks associated with smoking are needed. This is especially true for women in the developing world whose dietary, occupational, and other exposures may differ from those of women in the industrialized world, on whom most of the research to date has been conducted.

- Studies are needed to determine whether there are sex differences in susceptibility to nicotine addiction and whether women and men with similar smoking patterns experience different disease risks.

- Studies are needed on girls' and women's understanding of the disease risks associated with tobacco use and on effective means of tobacco-use prevention and cessation among various subgroups of women and girls.

- Studies are needed on the health effects unique to women of using forms of tobacco other than cigarettes, such as smokeless tobacco and pipes.

- Studies are needed to determine whether women who work in tobacco production experience increased disease risks, including effects on the children of those who work in tobacco production while pregnant.

Conclusions

Smoking by women is causally associated with an increased risk of developing and dying from myriad diseases, including many cancers, cardiovascular disease, and COPD, as well as increased risk of adverse reproductive outcomes. During the latter half of the 20th century, tobacco-related diseases became epidemic among women in the industrialized world, following women's adoption of cigarette smoking earlier in the century. Tobacco-caused diseases will threaten women in developing countries in the 21st century unless sustained efforts are undertaken to curb tobacco use. Preventing an epidemic of tobacco-related diseases among women in the developing world presents one of the greatest public health opportunities of our time.

References

1. *Fact sheet on gender, health and tobacco.* Geneva, World Health Organization, 2003.
2. Thun MJ et al. Age and the exposure-response relationships between cigarette smoking and premature death in Cancer Prevention Study II. In: Shopland DR et al., eds. *Changes in cigarette-related disease risks and their implication for prevention and control.* Rockville, MD, National Cancer Institute, 1997:383–475.
3. Prescott E et al. Mortality in women and men in relation to smoking. *International Journal of Epidemiology*, 1998, 27:27–32.
4. Vogt MT et al. Smoking and mortality among older women: the study of osteoporotic fractures. *Archives of Internal Medicine*, 1996, 156:630–636.
5. *Global health risks: mortality and burden of disease attributable to selected major risks.* Geneva, World Health Organization, 2009 (http://www.who.int/healthinfo/global_burden_disease/global_health_risks/en/index.html, accessed November 2009).
6. Mackay J, Eriksen M, Shafey O. *The tobacco atlas.* 2nd ed. Atlanta, GA, American Cancer Society, 2006.
7. McBride JS et al. Green tobacco sickness. *Tobacco Control,* 1998, 7:294–298.
8. Ballard T et al. Green tobacco sickness: occupational nicotine poisoning in tobacco workers. *Archives of Environmental Health*, 1995, 50:384–389.
9. Murphy NJ et al. Tobacco erases 30 years of progress: preliminary analysis of the effect of tobacco smoking on Alaska Native birth weight. *Alaska Medicine*, 1996, 38:31–33.
10. Wilcox AJ. Birth weight and perinatal mortality: the effect of maternal smoking. *American Journal of Epidemiology,* 1993, 137:1098–1104.
11. Zaren B, Lindmark G, Gebre-Medhin M. Maternal smoking and body composition of the newborn. *Acta Paediatrica*, 1996, 85:213–219.
12. Cnattingius S. Maternal age modifies the effect of maternal smoking on intrauterine growth retardation but not on late fetal death and placental abruption. *American Journal of Epidemiology*, 1997, 145:319–323.
13. Lieberman E et al. Low birthweight at term and the timing of fetal exposure to maternal smoking. *American Journal of Public Health,* 1994, 84:1127–1131.
14. Nordentoft M et al. Intrauterine growth retardation and premature delivery: the influence of maternal smoking and psychosocial factors. *American Journal of Public Health,* 1996, 86:347–354.
15. Wen SW et al. Smoking, maternal age, fetal growth, and gestational age at delivery. *American Journal of Obstetrics & Gynecology,* 1990, 162:53–58.
16. Cnattingius S, Haglund B, Meirik O. Cigarette smoking as a risk factor for late fetal and early neonatal death. *British Medical Journal*, 1988, 297:258–261.
17. Cnattingius S et al. Delayed childbearing and risk of adverse perinatal outcome: a population-based study. *Journal of the American Medical Association,* 1992, 268:886–890.
18. Raymond EG, Mills JL. Placental abruption: maternal risk factors and associated conditions. *Acta Obstetricia et Gynecologica Scandinavica*, 1993, 72:633–639.
19. Schramm WF. Smoking during pregnancy: Missouri longitudinal study. *Paediatric and Perinatal Epidemiology*, 1997, 11:73–83.
20. Malloy M et al. The association of maternal smoking with age and cause of infant death. *American Journal of Epidemiology*, 1988, 128:46–55.
21. Dwyer T, Ponsonby AL, Couper D. Tobacco smoke exposure at one month of age and subsequent risk of SIDS: a prospective study. *American Journal of Epidemiology*, 1999, 149:593–602.
22. Kohlendorfer U, Kiechl S, Sperl W. Sudden infant death syndrome: risk factor profiles for distinct subgroups. *American Journal of Epidemiology*, 1998, 147:960–968.
23. Alm B et al. A case-control study of smoking and sudden infant death syndrome in the Scandinavian countries, 1992–1995. The Nordic Epidemiological SIDS Study. *Archives of Disease in Childhood*, 1998, 78:329–334.
24. Cooke RW. Smoking, intra-uterine growth retardation and sudden infant death syndrome. *International Journal of Epidemiology*, 1998, 27:238–241.
25. Horta BL et al. Environmental tobacco smoking and breastfeeding duration. *American Journal of Epidemiology,* 1997, 146:128–133.
26. Hopkinson JM. Milk production by mothers of premature infants. *Pediatrics*, 1992, 90:934–938.
27. Vio F, Salazar G, Infante C. Smoking during pregnancy and lactation and its effects on breast-milk volume. *American Journal of Clinical Nutrition*, 1991, 54:1011–1016.
28. Yeung DL, Leung M, Hall J. Breastfeeding: prevalence and influencing factors. *Canadian Journal of Public Health*, 1981, 72:323–330.
29. *Women and smoking: a report of the Surgeon General.* Rockville, MD, US Department of Health and Human Services, 2001.
30. *Preventing tobacco use among young people: a report of the Surgeon General.* Atlanta, GA, Centers for Disease Control and Prevention, National Center for Chronic Disease Prevention and Health Promotion, 1994.
31. Daling J et al. Cigarette smoking and primary tubal infertility. In: Rosenberg MJ, ed. *Smoking and reproductive health.* Littleton, MA, PSG Publishing Company, 1987, 40–46.
32. Joesoef MR et al. Fertility and use of cigarettes, alcohol, marijuana, and cocaine. *Annals of Epidemiology*, 1993, 3:592–594.
33. Baird DD, Wilcox AJ. Cigarette smoking associated with delayed conception. *Journal of the American Medical Association,* 1985, 253:2979–2983.
34. Curtis KM, Savitz DA, Arbuckle TE. Effects of cigarette smoking, caffeine consumption, and alcohol intake on fecundability. *American Journal of Epidemiology*, 1997, 146:32–41.
35. Howe G et al. Effects of age, cigarette smoking, and other factors on fertility: findings in a large prospective study. *British Medical Journal*, 1985, 290:1697–1700.
36. Spinelli A, Figa-Talamanca I, Osborn J. Time to pregnancy and occupation in a group of Italian women. *International Journal of Epidemiology*, 1997, 26:601–609.
37. Hadley CB, Main DM, Gabbe SG. Risk factors for pre-term premature rupture of the fetal membranes. *American Journal of Perinatology*, 1990, 7:374–379.
38. Harger JH et al. Risk factors for pre-term premature rupture of fetal membranes: a multicenter case-control study. *Annals of the Rheumatic Diseases*, 1990, 57:451–455.
39. Ekwo EE et al. Risks for premature rupture of amniotic membranes. *International Journal of Epidemiology*, 1993, 22:495–503.
40. Spinillo A et al. Factors associated with abruptio placentae in pre-term deliveries. *Acta Obstetricia et Gynecologica Scandinavica*, 1994, 73:307–312.
41. Williams MA et al. Cigarettes, coffee, and pre-term premature rupture of the membranes. *American Journal of Epidemiology*, 1992, 135:895–903.
42. Ananth CV, Savitz DA, Luther ER. Maternal cigarette smoking as a risk factor for placental abruption, placenta previa, and uterine bleeding in pregnancy. *American Journal of Epidemiology*, 1996, 144:881–889.
43. Handler AS et al. The relationship between exposure during pregnancy to cigarette smoking and cocaine use and placenta previa. *American Journal of Obstetrics & Gynecology*, 1994, 170:884–889.
44. Monica G, Lilja C. Placenta previa, maternal smoking and recurrence risk. *Acta Obstetricia et Gynecologica Scandinavica*, 1995, 74:341–345.
45. Chelmow D, Andrew DE, Baker ER. Maternal cigarette smoking and placenta previa. *Obstetrics & Gynecology*, 1996, 87:703–706.
46. Zhang J, Fried DB. Relationship of maternal smoking during pregnancy to placenta previa. *American Journal of Preventive Medicine*, 1992, 8:278–282.
47. Heffner LJ et al. Clinical and environmental predictors of pre-term labor. *Obstetrics & Gynecology*, 1993, 81:750–757.

48. Olsen P et al. Epidemiology of pre-term delivery in two birth cohorts with an interval of 20 years. *American Journal of Epidemiology*, 1995, 142:1184–1193.

49. Wen SW et al. Intrauterine growth retardation and pre-term delivery: prenatal risk factors in an indigent population. *American Journal of Obstetrics & Gynecology,* 1990, 162:213–218.

50. Cnattingius S et al. Effect of age, parity, and smoking on pregnancy outcome: a population-based study. *American Journal of Obstetrics & Gynecology*, 1993, 168:16–21.

51. McDonald AD, Armstrong BG, Sloan M. Cigarette, alcohol, and coffee consumption and prematurity. *American Journal of Public Health*, 1992, 82:91–93.

52. Meis PJ et al. Factors associated with pre-term birth in Cardiff, Wales. I. Indicated and spontaneous pre-term birth. *American Journal of Obstetrics & Gynecology*, 1995, 173:597–602.

53. Wisborg K et al. Smoking during pregnancy and pre-term birth. *British Journal of Obstetrics and Gynaecology*, 1996, 103:800–805.

54. Wisborg K et al. Smoking habits among Danish pregnant women from 1989 to 1996 in relation to sociodemographic and lifestyle factors. *Acta Obstetricia Gynecologica Scandinavica*, 1998, 77:836–840.

55. Eriksson KM et al. Smoking habits among pregnant women in Norway 1994–95. *Acta Obstetricia Gynecologica Scandinavica,* 1998, 77:159–164.

56. Horta BL et al. Tobacco smoking among pregnant women in an urban area in southern Brazil, 1982–93. *Revista de Saúde Pública,* 1997, 31:247–253.

57. Steyn K et al. Smoking in urban pregnant women in South Africa. *South African Medical Journal*, 1997, 87:460–463.

58. Dejin-Kaarlsson E et al. Psychosocial resources and persistent smoking in early pregnancy: a population study of women in their first pregnancy in Sweden. *Journal of Epidemiology and Community Health*, 1996, 50:33–39.

59. Dodds L. Prevalence of smoking among pregnant women in Nova Scotia from 1988 to 1992. *Canadian Medical Association Journal*, 1995, 152:185–190.

60. Stewart PJ et al. Change in smoking prevalence among pregnant women 1982–93. *Canadian Journal of Public Health*, 1995, 86:37–41.

61. Centers for Disease Control and Prevention. Cigarette smoking during the last 3 months of pregnancy among women who gave birth to live infants – Maine, 1988–1997. *Morbidity and Mortality Weekly Report*, 1999, 48:421–425.

62. Heaman MI, Chalmers K. Prevalence and correlates of smoking during pregnancy: a comparison of Aboriginal and non-Aboriginal women in Manitoba. *Birth*, 2005, 32:4.

63. Ward C, Lewis S, Coleman T. Prevalence of maternal smoking and environmental tobacco smoke exposure during pregnancy and impact on birth weight: retrospective study using millennium cohort. *BMC Public Health*, 2007, 7:81.

64. Chaaya M et al. Demographic and psychosocial profile of smoking among pregnant women in Lebanon: public health implications. *Maternal and Child Health Journal*, 2003, 7.

65. Wood C, Larsen L, Williams R. Social and psychological factors in relation to premenstrual tension and menstrual pain. *Australian and New Zealand Journal of Obstetrics and Gynaecology*, 1979, 19:111–115.

66. Pullon S, Reinken J, Sparrow M. Prevalence of dysmenorrhoea in Wellington women. *New Zealand Medical Journal*, 1988, 101:52–54.

67. Sundell G, Milsom I, Andersch B. Factors influencing the prevalence and severity of dysmenorrhoea in young women. *British Journal of Obstetrics and Gynaecology*, 1990, 97:588–594.

68. *Smoking and reproductive life: the impact of smoking on sexual, reproductive and child health*. London, British Medical Association, 2004 (www.bma. org.uk).

69. Willett W et al. Cigarette smoking, relative weight, and menopause. *American Journal of Epidemiology,* 1983, 117:651–658.

70. McKinlay SM, Bifano NL, McKinlay JB. Smoking and age at menopause in women. *Annals of Internal Medicine*, 1985, 103:350–356.

71. Hiatt RA, Fireman BH. Smoking, menopause, and breast cancer. *Journal of the National Cancer Institute*, 1986, 76:833–838.

72. Midgette AS, Baron JA. Cigarette smoking and the risk of natural menopause. *Epidemiology*, 1990, 1:474–480.

73. Gaziano TA Reducing the growing burden of cardiovascular disease in the developing world. *Health Affairs*, 2007, 26:13–24.

74. *Cardiovascular diseases*. Geneva, World Health Organization, 2007 (www.who.int/mediacentre/factsheets/fs317/en/index.html, accessed 7 December 2007).

75. Prescott E et al. Smoking and risk of myocardial infarction in women and men: longitudinal population study. *British Medical Journal*, 1998, 316:1043–1047.

76. Burns DM et al. The American Cancer Society Cancer Prevention Study I: 12-year follow-up of 1 million men and women. In: Shopland DR et al., eds. *Changes in cigarette-related disease risks and their implication for prevention and control*. Rockville, MD, National Cancer Institute, 1997: 13–42.

77. Njolstad I, Arnesen E, Lund-Larsen PG. Smoking, serum lipids, blood pressure, and sex differences in myocardial infarction: a 12-year follow-up of the Finnmark Study. *Circulation*, 1996, 93:450–456.

78. Kawachi I et al. Smoking cessation and time course of decreased risks of coronary heart disease in middle-aged women. *Archives of Internal Medicine*, 1994, 154:169–175.

79. Paganini-Hill A, Hsu G. Smoking and mortality among residents of a California retirement community. *American Journal of Public Health*, 1994, 84:992–995.

80. Doll R et al. Mortality in relation to smoking: 22 years' observations on female British doctors. *British Medical Journal*, 1980, 280:967–971.

81. Friedman GD et al. Smoking and mortality: the Kaiser Permanente experience. In: Shopland DR et al, eds. *Changes in cigarette-related disease risks and their implication for prevention and control*. Rockville, MD, National Cancer Institute, 1997, 477–499.

82. *Reducing the health consequences of smoking: 25 years of progress. A report of the Surgeon General*. Rockville, MD, Centers for Disease Control, Center for Chronic Disease Prevention and Health Promotion, 1989.

83. Rosenberg L et al. Myocardial infarction and cigarette smoking in women younger than 50 years of age. *Journal of the American Medical Association*, 1985, 253:2965–2969.

84. Owen-Smith V et al. Effects of changes in smoking status on risk estimates for myocardial infarction among women recruited for the Royal College of General Practitioners' Oral Contraception Study in the UK. *Journal of Epidemiology and Community Health*, 1998, 52:420–424.

85. Shapiro S et al. Oral contraceptive use in relation to myocardial infarction. *The Lancet*, 1979, 1:743–747.

86. Croft P, Hannaford PC. Risk factors for acute myocardial infarction in women: evidence from the Royal College of General Practitioners' Oral Contraception Study. *British Medical Journal*, 1989, 298:165–168.

87. D'Avanzo B et al. Oral contraceptive use and risk of myocardial infarction: an Italian case-control study. *Journal of Epidemiology and Community Health*, 1994, 48:324–325.

88. Lewis MA et al. Third generation oral contraceptives and risk of myocardial infarction: an international case-control study. *British Medical Journal*, 1996, 312:88–90.

89. WHO Collaborative Study of Cardiovascular Disease and Steroid Hormone Contraception. Acute myocardial infarction and combined oral contraceptives: results of an international multicentre case-control study. *The Lancet*, 1997, 349:1202–1209.

90. Kawachi I et al. Smoking cessation and decreased risk of stroke in women. *Journal of the American Medical Association,* 1993, 269:232–236.

91. Pedersen AT et al. Hormone replacement therapy and risk of non-fatal stroke. *The Lancet*, 1997, 350:1277–1283.

92. Hannaford PC, Croft PR, Kay CR. Oral contraception and stroke: evidence from the Royal College of General Practitioners' Oral Contraception Study. *Stroke*, 1994, 25:935–942.

93. Juvela S et al. Cigarette smoking and alcohol consumption as risk factors for aneurysmal subarachnoid hemorrhage. *Stroke*, 1993, 24:639–646.

94. Shinton R, Beevers G. Meta-analysis of relation between cigarette smoking and stroke. *British Medical Journal*, 1989, 298:789–794.

95. *The health consequences of smoking: cardiovascular disease: a report of the Surgeon General*. Rockville, MD, US Public Health Service, Office on Smoking and Health, 1983.

96. Ingall TJ et al. Predictors of intracranial carotid artery atherosclerosis: duration of cigarette smoking and hypertension are more powerful than serum lipid levels. *Archives of Neurology*, 1991, 48:687–691.

97. Tell GS et al. Relation of smoking with carotid artery wall thickness and stenosis in older adults: the Cardiovascular Health Study. *Circulation*, 1994, 90:2905–2908.

98. Fowkes FG et al. Sex differences in susceptibility to etiologic factors for peripheral atherosclerosis: importance of plasma fibrinogen and blood viscosity. *Arteriosclerosis, Thrombosis, and Vascular Biology*, 1994, 14:862–868.

99. Freund KM et al. The health risks of smoking. The Framingham Study: 34 years of follow-up. *Annals of Epidemiology*, 1993, 3:417–424.

100. US Department of Health and Human Services. *The health benefits of smoking cessation: a report of the Surgeon General*. Washington, DC, US Government Printing Office, 1990.

101. Hirayama T. *A large-scale census-based cohort study in Japan: contributions to epidemiology and biostatistics*. New York, NY, Karger, 1990.

102. Witteman JC et al. Cigarette smoking and the development and progression of aortic atherosclerosis: a 9-year population-based follow-up study in women. *Circulation*, 1993, 88:2156–2162.

103. *The health consequences of smoking: chronic obstructive lung disease. A report of the Surgeon General*. Rockville, MD, Office on Smoking and Health, US Public Health Service, 1984.

104. Troisi RJ et al. Cigarette smoking and incidence of chronic bronchitis and asthma in women. *Chest*, 1995, 108:1557–1561.

105. Thun MJ et al. Trends in tobacco smoking and mortality from cigarette use in Cancer Prevention Studies I (1959 through 1965) and II (1982 through 1988). In: Shopland DR et al., eds. *Changes in cigarette-related disease risks and their implication for prevention and control*. Rockville, MD, National Cancer Institute, 1997:3305–3382.

106. Rabe KF et al. Global strategy for the diagnosis, management, and prevention of chronic obstructive pulmonary disease: GOLD executive summary. *American Journal of Respiratory and Critical Care Medicine*, 2007, 176:532–555.

107. Xu X et al. Effects of cigarette smoking on rate of loss of pulmonary function in adults: a longitudinal assessment. *American Review of Respiratory Diseases*, 1992, 146:1345–1348.

108. Tashkin DP et al. The UCLA population studies of chronic obstructive respiratory disease. VIII. Effects of smoking cessation on lung function: a prospective study of a free-living population. *American Review of Respiratory Diseases*, 1984, 130:707–715.

109. Frette C, Barrett-Connor E, Clausen JL. Effect of active and passive smoking on ventilatory function in elderly men and women. *American Journal of Epidemiology*, 1996, 143:757–765.

110. Lange P et al. Decline of the lung function related to the type of tobacco smoked and inhalation. *Thorax*, 1990, 45:22–26.

111. Jemal A et al. Cancer statistics, 2005. *CA Cancer Journal for Clinicians*, 2005, 55:10–30.

112. Levi F et al. Trends in mortality from cancer in the European Union, 1955–94. *The Lancet*, 1999, 354:742–743.

113. Ferlay J et al. Estimates of the cancer incidence and mortality in Europe in 2006. *Annals of Oncology*, 2007, 18:581–592.

114. Peto R et al. *Mortality from smoking in industrialized countries 1950–2000: indirect estimates from national vital statistics*. New York, NY, Oxford University Press, 1994.

115. *The health consequences of smoking for women. a report of the Surgeon General*. Rockville, MD, US Public Health Service, Office on Smoking and Health, 1980.

116. Stewart B.W, Kleihues P, eds. *World cancer report*. Lyon, IARCPress. 2003 (http://www.iarc.fr/IARCPress/pdfs/wcr/).

117. Wingo PA et al. Annual report to the nation on the status of cancer, 1973–1996, with a special section on lung cancer and tobacco smoking. *Journal of the National Cancer Institute*, 1999, 91:675–690.

118. Lum R et al. *Cancer incidence and mortality in the San Francisco Bay Area, 1988–1996*. Union City, CA, Northern California Cancer Center, 1999.

119. *The health consequences of smoking: cancer. A report of the Surgeon General*. Rockville, MD, Office on Smoking and Health, 1982 (DHHS Publication (PHS) 82–50179).

120. Engeland A et al. The impact of smoking habits on lung cancer risk: 28 years' observation of 26 000 Norwegian men and women. *Cancer Causes & Control*, 1996, 7:366–376.

121. Ernster VL. Female lung cancer. *Annual Review of Public Health*, 1996, 276:33–38.

122. Parkin DM et al. Global cancer statistics, 2002. *CA Cancer Journal for Clinicians*, 2005, 55:74–108

123. Blot WJ et al. Smoking and drinking in relation to oral and pharyngeal cancer. *Cancer Research*, 1988, 48:3282–3287.

124. Negri E et al. Attributable risks for oral cancer in northern Italy. *Cancer Epidemiology Biomarkers & Prevention*, 1993, 2:189–193.

125. Tavani A et al. Attributable risk for laryngeal cancer in northern Italy. *Cancer Epidemiology Biomarkers & Prevention*, 1994, 3:121–125.

126. Negri E et al. Attributable risks for oesophageal cancer in northern Italy. *European Journal of Cancer*, 1992, 28A:1167–1171.

127. Tavani A et al. Risk factors for esophageal cancer in women in northern Italy. *Cancer*, 1993, 72:2531–2536.

128. Nordlund LA, Carstensen JM, Pershagen G. Cancer incidence in female smokers: a 26-year follow-up. *International Journal of Cancer*, 1997, 73:625–628.

129. McLaughlin JK et al. International Renal-Cell Cancer Study. I. Tobacco use. *International Journal of Cancer*, 1995, 60:194–198.

130. Hartge P et al. Smoking and bladder cancer risk in blacks and whites in the United States. *Cancer Causes & Control*, 1993, 4:391–394.

131. Fuchs CS et al. A prospective study of cigarette smoking and the risk of pancreatic cancer. *Archives of Internal Medicine*, 1996, 156:2255–2260.

132. Engeland A et al. Smoking habits and risks of cancers other than lung cancer: 28 years' follow-up of 26 000 Norwegian men and women. *Cancer Causes & Control*, 1996, 7:497–506.

133. Silverman DT et al. Cigarette smoking and pancreas cancer: a case-control study based on direct interviews. *Journal of the National Cancer Institute*, 1994, 86:1510–1516.

134. Sanderson RJ et al. The influence of alcohol and smoking on the incidence of oral and oropharyngeal cancer in women. *Clinical Otolaryngology*, 1997, 22:444–448.

135. Harnack LJ et al. Smoking, alcohol, coffee, and tea intake and incidence of cancer of the exocrine pancreas: the Iowa Women's Health Study. *Cancer Epidemiology Biomarkers & Prevention*, 1997, 6:1081–1086.

136. Muscat JE et al. Smoking and pancreatic cancer in men and women. *Cancer Epidemiology Biomarkers & Prevention*, 1997, 6:15–19.

137. US Department of Health and Human Services. *2004 Surgeon General's report—the health consequences of smoking*. Atlanta, GA, Centers for Disease Control and Prevention, 2004 (http://www.cdc.gov/tobacco/data_statistics/sgr/sgr_2004/chapters.htm).

138. Phillips AN, Smith GD. Cigarette smoking as a potential cause of cervical cancer: has confounding been controlled? *International Journal of Epidemiology*, 1994, 23:42–49.

139. Daling JR et al. The relationship of human papillomavirus-related cervical tumors to cigarette smoking, oral contraceptive use, and prior herpes simplex virus type 2 infection. *Cancer Epidemiology Biomarkers & Prevention*, 1996, 5:541–548.

140. Ylitalo N et al. Smoking and oral contraceptives as risk factors for cervical carcinoma in situ. *International Journal of Cancer*, 1999, 81:357–365.

141. Johnson KC. Accumulating evidence on passive and active smoking and breast cancer risk. *International Journal of Cancer*, 2005, 117:619–628.

142. Hanaoka T et al. Active and passive smoking and breast cancer risk in middle-aged Japanese women. *International Journal of Cancer*, 2005, 114:317–322.

143. Reynolds P et al. Active smoking, household passive smoking, and breast cancer: evidence from the California Teachers Study. *Journal of the National Cancer Institute*, 2004, 96:29–37.

144. Johnson KC, Hu J, Mao Y. Canadian Cancer Registries Epidemiology Research Group. Passive and active smoking and breast cancer risk in Canada, 1994–97. *Cancer Causes & Control*, 2000, 11:211–221.

145. Kropp S, Chang-Claude J. Active and passive smoking and risk of breast cancer by age 50 years among German women. *American Journal of Epidemiology*, 2002, 156:616–626.

146. Egan KM et al. Active and passive smoking in breast cancer: prospective results from the Nurses' Health Study. *Epidemiology*, 2002, 13:138–145.

147. Brownson RC, Novotny TE, Perry MC. Cigarette smoking and adult leukaemia: a meta-analysis. *Archives of Internal Medicine*, 1993, 153:469–475.

148. Siegel M. Smoking and leukaemia: evaluation of a causal hypothesis. *American Journal of Epidemiology*, 1993, 138:1–9.

149. *Tobacco smoke and involuntary smoking. Summary of data reported and evaluation*. IARC Monographs on the Evaluation of Carcinogenic Risks to Humans, Vol. 83 (http://monographs.iarc.fr/ENG/Monographs/vol83/volume83.pdf, accessed 7 January 2008).

150. Shopland DR. Tobacco use and its contribution to early cancer mortality with a special emphasis on cigarette smoking. *Environmental Health Perspectives*, 1995, 103 (Suppl. 8):131–141.

151. Orwoll ES et al. Axial bone mass in older women. *Annals of Internal Medicine*, 1996, 124:187–196.

152. Hollenback KA et al. Cigarette smoking and bone mineral density in older men and women. *American Journal of Public Health*, 1993, 83:1265–1270.

153. Nguyen TV et al. Lifestyle factors and bone density in the elderly: implications for osteoporosis prevention. *Journal of Bone and Mineral Research*, 1994, 9:1339–1346.

154. Kiel DP et al. The effect of smoking at different life stages on bone mineral density in elderly men and women. *Osteoporosis International,* 1996, 6:240–248.

155. Writing Group for the PEPI Trial. Effects of hormone therapy on bone mineral density: results from the Postmenopausal Estrogen/Progestin Interventions (PEPI) trial. *Journal of the American Medical Association*, 1996, 77:53–56.

156. Burger H et al. Risk factors for increased bone loss in an elderly population: the Rotterdam Study. *American Journal of Epidemiology,* 1998, 147:871–879.

157. Wong PKK, Christie JJ, Wark JD. The effects of smoking on bone health (review). *Clinical Science*, 2007, 113:233–241.

158. Borelli B et al. The impact of depression on smoking cessation in women. *American Journal of Preventive Medicine*, 1996, 12:378–387.

159. Breslau N, Kilbey MM, Andreski P. Nicotine withdrawal symptoms and psychiatric disorders: findings from an epidemiologic study of young adults. *American Journal of Psychiatry*, 1992, 149:464–469.

160. Breslau N. Psychiatric comorbidity of smoking and nicotine dependence. *Behavior Genetics*, 1995, 25:95–101.

161. Breslau N et al. Major depression and stages of smoking: a longitudinal investigation. *Archives of General Psychiatry*, 1998, 55:161–166.

162. Anda RF et al. Depression and the dynamics of smoking: a national perspective. *Journal of the American Medical Association*, 1990, 264:1541–1545.

163. Glassman AH et al. Smoking, smoking cessation, and major depression. *Journal of the American Medical Association*, 1990, 264:1546–1549.

164. Escobedo LG, Reddy M, Giovino GA. The relationship between depressive symptoms and cigarette smoking in US adolescents. *Addiction*, 1998, 93:433–440.

165. Kendler KS et al. Smoking and major depression. *Archives of General Psychiatry*, 1993, 50:36–43.

166. Sham ASK et al. The effects of tobacco use on oral health (review). *Hong Kong Medical Journal*, 2003, 9:271–277.

167. Murray FE et al. Cigarette smoking and parity as risk factors for the development of symptomatic gallbladder disease in women: results of the Royal College of General Practitioners' oral contraception study. *Gut*, 1994, 35:107–111.

168. Vessey M, Painter R. Oral contraceptive use and benign gallbladder disease revisited. *Contraception*, 1994, 50:167–173.

169. Grodstein F et al. A prospective study of symptomatic gallstones in women: relation with oral contraceptives and other risk factors. *Obstetrics & Gynecology*, 1994, 84:207–214.

170. Anda RF et al. Smoking and the risk of peptic ulcer disease among women in the United States. *Archives of Internal Medicine*, 1990, 150:1437–1441.

171. Schoon I-M et al. Peptic ulcer disease in older age groups in Gothenburg in 1985: the association with smoking. *Age and Ageing*, 1991, 20:371–376.

172. Kurata JH, Nogawa AN. Meta-analysis of risk factors for peptic ulcer: nonsteroidal anti-inflammatory drugs, *Helicobacter pylori*, and smoking. *Journal of Clinical Gastroenterology*, 1997, 24:2–17.

173. Hankinson SE et al. A prospective study of cigarette smoking and risk of cataract surgery in women. *Journal of the American Medical Association*, 1992, 268:994–998.

174. Klein BE et al. Cigarette smoking and lens opacities: the Beaver Dam Eye Study. *American Journal of Preventive Medicine*, 1993, 9:27–30.

175. Ernster VL et al. Facial wrinkling in men and women by smoking status. *American Journal of Public Health*, 1995, 85:78–82.

176. Castelo-Branco C et al. Facial wrinkling in postmenopausal women: effects of smoking status and hormone replacement therapy. *Maturitas*, 1998, 29:75–86.

177. Prescott EI et al. Smoking and life expectancy among Danish men and women. *Ugeskr Laeger*, 1999, 161:1261–1263.

178. MacArthur C, Knox EG. Smoking in pregnancy: effects of stopping at different stages. *British Journal of Obstetrics and Gynaecology*, 1988, 95:551–555.

179. Frank P et al. Effect of changes in maternal smoking habits in early pregnancy on infant birthweight. *British Journal of General Practice*, 1994, 44:57–59.

180. Mainous AG III, Hueston WJ. The effect of smoking cessation during pregnancy on pre-term delivery and low birthweight. *Journal of Family Practice,* 1994, 38:262–266.

181. Dolan-Mullen P, Ramirez G, Groff JY. A meta-analysis of randomized trials of prenatal smoking cessation interventions. *American Journal of Obstetrics & Gynecology*, 1994, 171:1328–1334.

182. Omenn GS et al. The temporal pattern of reduction of mortality risk after smoking cessation. *American Journal of Preventive Medicine*, 1990, 6:251–257.

183. Thompson SG, Greenberg G, Meade TW. Risk factors for stroke and myocardial infarction in women in the United Kingdom as assessed in general practice: a case-control study. *British Heart Journal*, 1989, 61:403–409.

184. Dobson AJ et al. How soon after quitting smoking does risk of heart attack decline? *Journal of Clinical Epidemiology*, 1991, 44:1247–1253.

185. Negri E et al. Acute myocardial infarction: association with time since stopping smoking in Italy. *Journal of Epidemiology and Community Health*, 1994, 48:129–133.

186. Wolf PA et al. Cigarette smoking as a risk factor for stroke: the Framingham Study. *Journal of the American Medical Association*, 1988, 259:1025–1029.

187. Xu X et al. Smoking, changes in smoking habits, and rate of decline in FEV1: new insights into gender differences. *European Respiratory Journal*, 1994, 7:1056–1061.

188. Anthonisen NR et al. Effects of smoking intervention and the use of an inhaled anticholinergic bronchodilator on the rate of decline of FEV1. *Journal of the American Medical Association*, 1994, 272:1497–1505.

189. Liu B-Q et al. Emerging tobacco hazards in China: 1. Retrospective proportional mortality study of one million deaths. *British Medical Journal*, 1998, 317:1411–1422.

190. Chen Z-M et al. Early health effects of the emerging tobacco epidemic in China: a 16-year prospective study. *Journal of the American Medical Association*, 1997, 278:1500–1504.

191. Yuan JM et al. Morbidity and mortality in relation to cigarette smoking in Shanghai, China. *Journal of the American Medical Association*, 1996, 275:1646–1650.

192. Peto R, Chen Z-M, Boreham J. Tobacco–the growing epidemic. *Nature Medicine*, 1999, 5:15–17.

193. Yang GH et al. Smoking and passive smoking in Chinese, 2002. *Zhonghua Liu Xing Bing Xue Za Zhi [Chinese Journal of Epidemiology]*, 2005, 26:77–83 [in Chinese].

194. Weng XZ, Hong ZG, Chen DY. Smoking prevalence in Chinese aged 15 and above. *Chinese Medical Journal*, 1987, 100:886–892.

195. Chinese Academy of Preventive Medicine, Chinese Association of Smoking or Health. *Smoking and health in China: 1996 national prevalence survey of smoking patterns.* Beijing, China Science and Technology Press, 1996.

196. Maziak W et al. Tobacco smoking using a waterpipe: a re-emerging strain in a global epidemic. *Tobacco Control*, 2004, 13:327–333.

197. World Health Organization Study Group on Tobacco Product Regulation. *Waterpipe tobacco smoking: health effects, research needs and recommended actions by regulators.* Geneva, World Health Organization, 2005 (www.who.int/tobacco/global_interaction/tobreg/Waterpipe%20 recommendation_Final.pdf).

198. Arabi Z. Metabolic and cardiovascular effects of smokeless tobacco (review). *Journal of the CardioMetabolic Syndrome*, 2006, 1:345–350.

199. Gupta R, Gurm H, Bartholomew JR. Smokeless tobacco and cardiovascular risk (review). *Archives of Internal Medicine*, 2004, 164:1845–1849.

200. Critchley JA, Unal B. Is smokeless tobacco a risk factor for coronary heart disease? A systematic review of epidemiological studies. *European Journal Cardiovascular Prevention & Rehabilitation*, 2004, 11:101–112.

201. Gupta PC, Ray CS. Smokeless tobacco and health in India and South Asia (review), *Respirology*, 2003, 8:419–431.

202. Critchley JA, Unal B. Health effects associated with smokeless tobacco: a systematic review (review). *Thorax*, 2003, 58:435–443.

203. Boffetta P et al. Smokeless tobacco use and risk of cancer of the pancreas and other organs. *International Journal of Cancer,* 2005, 114:992–995.

204. *Women and health—today's evidence, tomorrow's agenda.* Geneva, World Health Organization, 2009.

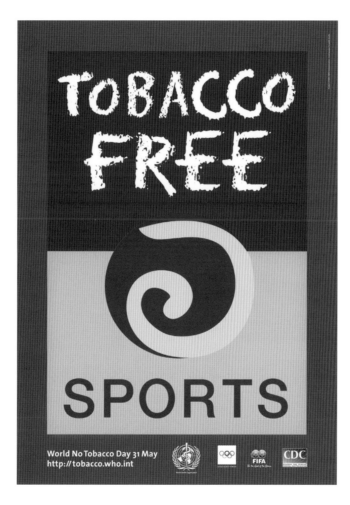

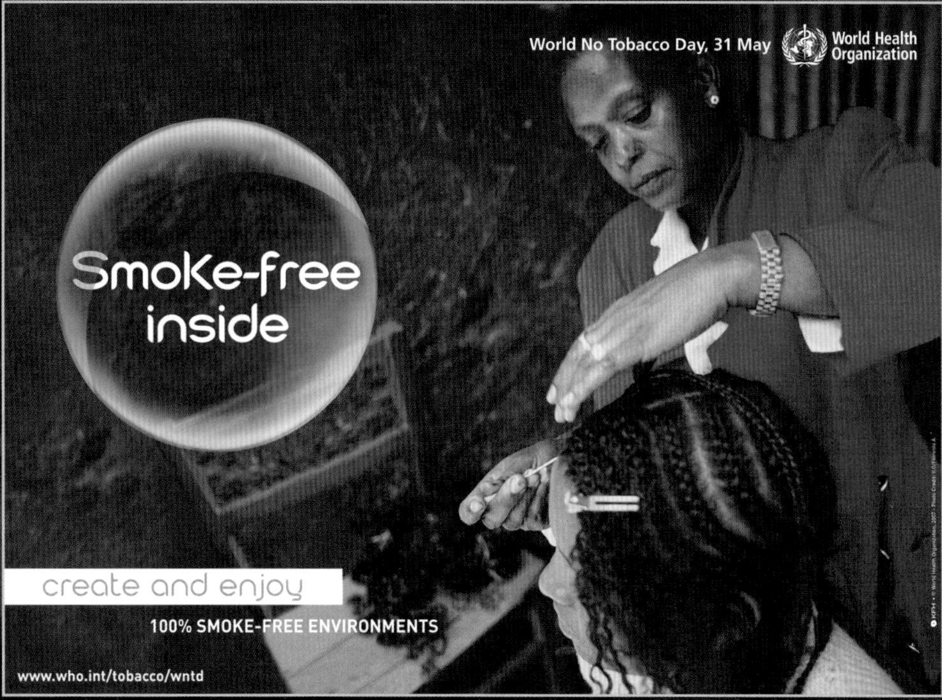
World No Tobacco Day, 31 May
World Health Organization
Smoke-free inside
create and enjoy
100% SMOKE-FREE ENVIRONMENTS
www.who.int/tobacco/wntd

5. Second-Hand Smoke, Women, and Children

Introduction and Definitions

Tobacco smoking, now and in the past, has been a custom and addiction primarily of men, leaving women and children as the majority of the world's passive, or involuntary, smokers. In 2004, second-hand smoke (SHS) is estimated to have caused about 600 000 premature deaths (28% among children). Of the 430 000 adult deaths, about 64% were among women. Although by 2008, 160 million people worldwide had been covered by comprehensive smoke-free laws, nearly 90% of the world's population is not protected, and laws do not limit exposure to SHS in homes where women and children are exposed through the smoking of male family members.[1] Globally, more than 1 billon people—almost one quarter of all adults worldwide—smoke,[1] leaving much of the world's non-smoking population vulnerable to SHS exposure. More than 80% of adult smokers live in low- and middle-income countries.[1] Rates of smoking prevalence, however, vary by gender and by country. Worldwide, about 40% of all men and about 9% of women smoke.[2] In high-income countries, smoking prevalence rates for men and women are similar, 32% and 18%, respectively. In middle-income countries, however, men smoke substantially more than women, 45% vs 7%. In low-income countries, smoking prevalence rates in men and in women are 28% and 4%, respectively.[1] These prevalence rates indicate that women, especially in developing countries, constitute a substantial portion of the population at risk of SHS exposure.

Exposure to SHS, also known as environmental tobacco smoke (ETS), is strongly associated with a number of adverse effects on children, involving, in particular, the respiratory tract. In a 1999 report on SHS and children's health, WHO stated, "The vast majority of children exposed to tobacco smoke do not choose to be exposed. Children's exposure is involuntary, arising from smoking, mainly by adults, in places where children live, work, and play. Given that more than 1 billion adults smoke, WHO estimates that approximately 700 million, or almost half, of the world's children are exposed to SHS. This high exposure, coupled with the evidence that SHS causes illness in children, suggests that SHS constitutes a substantial public health threat for children".[3]

Because the home is the predominant location for smoking, many women and children are exposed to tobacco smoke in their daily lives—while doing tasks such as eating, entertaining, and even sleeping. In addition to being exposed to tobacco smoke at home, women and children may be subjected to exposure at work, at school, and in transport. This may be particularly true in Asia and the Pacific region, where the majority of the men are smokers, while only a small percentage of the women smoke regularly.[2]

Tobacco smoking, now and in the past, has been a custom and addiction primarily of men, leaving women and children as the majority of the world's passive, or involuntary, smokers.

Cigarette smoke contains particles and gases generated by the combustion of tobacco, paper, and additives at high temperature. That smoke, which is involuntarily inhaled by non-smokers, contaminates indoor spaces as well as outdoor environments. It is a mixture of sidestream smoke released by smouldering cigarettes and the mainstream smoke that is exhaled by smokers. Sidestream smoke, generated at lower temperatures than mainstream smoke, tends to have higher concentrations of many of the toxins in cigarette smoke.[10,11] However, it is rapidly diluted as it travels away from the burning cigarette.

Second-hand smoke is an inherently dynamic mixture that changes in characteristics and concentration depending on when it is formed and how far it has travelled. The smoke particles change in size and composition as gaseous components are volatilized and moisture content changes; gaseous elements of SHS may be adsorbed onto materials, and particle concentrations drop with both dilution and impaction on surfaces. Because of its dynamic nature, SHS cannot be quantitatively defined, although such a definition is not needed for either research or public health purposes. A variety of indicators of smoking as the source of SHS and of SHS itself can be measured.

This chapter originated with the WHO Conference on Tobacco and Health, Making a Difference to Tobacco and Health: Avoiding the Tobacco Epidemic in Women and Youth, held in Kobe, Japan, in November 1999. A 1999 WHO consultation also focused on SHS and youth.[3] In 2001, WHO published a report on women and the tobacco epidemic,[4] and since that time, the evidence on SHS and disease risk and on control strategy has continued to mount. This chapter updates a paper prepared nearly a decade ago for the 1999 Conference. It covers the full spectrum of

issues related to SHS and women and children: indicators of exposure and prevalence of exposure, health effects of SHS, intervention strategies, policy recommendations, and research gaps.

We draw on the substantial literature on SHS worldwide, but we emphasize evidence from Asia and the Pacific region. This topic has been reviewed repeatedly,[5-8] most recently in 2006 by the US Surgeon General's Office.[9] We do not attempt to cover this extensive literature comprehensively; rather, we offer a synthesis of the evidence that targets areas in which the findings support intervention and identify research needs in areas in which the evidence is not yet conclusive.

Table 5.1. Indicators of SHS Exposure

Measure	Indicator
Surrogate measures	Prevalence of smoking in men and women
Indirect measures	Report of SHS exposures in the home and workplace
	Smoking in the household • Number of smokers • Parent smoking • Number of cigarettes smoked
	Smoking in the workplace • Presence of SHS • Number of smokers
Direct measures	Concentration of SHS components • Nicotine • Respirable particles • Other markers
	Biomarker concentrations • Cotinine • Carboxyhaemoglobin

Indicators of SHS Exposure

Exposure to SHS can take place in any environment where time is spent. A useful conceptual framework for considering exposure to SHS is offered by the micro-environmental model that describes personal exposure to SHS as the weighted sum of the concentrations of SHS in the micro-environments where time is spent and the weights supplied by the time spent in each.[12] A micro-environment is a space, e.g. a room in a residence or an office area, with a relatively uniform concentration of SHS during the time spent in it. For research purposes and for considering health risks, personal exposure is the most relevant measure for evaluating and projecting risk. Within the framework of the micro-environmental model, we consider the contributions of various micro-environments to personal exposures of women and children to SHS.

For children, the micro-environmental model makes clear the dominance of exposures in the home, where they spend the majority of their time. Other micro-environments where children spend time—transportation environments, public places, and even schools—are also potentially associated with exposure to SHS. The home is a key micro-environment for women, as well, and employed women may also experience significant exposures in work environments and in transportation micro-environments, public places, and other sites where leisure time is spent. Although it has not been well characterized, the interplay of family members within the home may heighten exposure because of the frequency of physical proximity of parents and children and of spouses.

World Health Organization

Within the framework set by the micro-environmental model, there are a number of useful indicators of exposure to SHS, ranging from surrogate indicators to direct measurements of exposure and of biomarkers, which are reflective of dose (Table 5.1). One useful surrogate—and the only indicator available for many countries—is the rate of smoking prevalence among men and women. Among adults, smoking tends to aggregate within couples, so the proportion of non-smoking women married to smokers is not necessarily estimable under the independent assumption of smoking among husbands and wives. Nonetheless, the rates of smoking prevalence provide at least a measure of the likelihood of exposure. For the countries of Asia, for example, where men have very high smoking rates and women have low smoking rates, the prevalence data for men imply that the majority of women are exposed to tobacco smoke at home.

The indirect measures listed in Table 5.1 are usually ascertained by questionnaire. These measures include self-reported exposure and descriptions of the source of SHS (i.e. smoking) in relevant micro-environments, most often the home and the workplace. The components of SHS include a number of irritating and odiferous gaseous components, such as aldehydes. Non-smokers typically describe the odour of SHS as annoying, and the threshold for detecting SHS is at low concentrations.[9] Self-reported exposure to SHS is thus a useful indicator of exposure, although the validity of questionnaire reports of intensity of exposure is uncertain. Questionnaires are also used to ascertain the prevalence of SHS and for research on smoking in home and work environments.

A simple mass-balance model obtains the concentration of SHS from the rate of its generation, i.e. the numbers of smokers and of cigarettes smoked, the volume into which the smoke is released, and the rate of removal of SHS by either air exchange or air cleaning.[13] Information on smoking can be collected readily from parents and other adults within the household, although reports of numbers of cigarettes smoked in the home are not easy to measure precisely. Smoking in workplace environments can be reported by co-workers, although the complexity of workplace environments may preclude the determination of the numbers of smokers in the work area or the numbers of cigarettes smoked. The other determinants of SHS concentration—room volume, air exchange, and removal—are not readily determined by questionnaire and are assessed only for research purposes.

The direct measures of SHS exposure include measurement of concentrations of SHS components in the air and of SHS biomarker levels in biological specimens. Using the micro-environmental model, researchers can estimate SHS exposure by measuring the concentration of SHS in the home, workplace, or other environments and then combining the concentration data with information on the time spent in the micro-environments where exposure took place. For example, to estimate SHS exposure in the home, the concentration of a marker in the air, e.g. nicotine, would be measured and the time spent in the home would be tracked, possibly with a time-activity diary that collects information on all locations where time is spent.

Biomarkers of exposure are compounds that can be measured in biological materials such as blood, urine, or saliva. Cotinine, a metabolite of nicotine, is a highly specific indicator of exposure to SHS in non-smokers.

The selection of a particular SHS component for monitoring is based largely on technological feasibility. Air can be sampled either actively, using a pump that passes air through a filter or a sorbent, or passively, using a badge that operates on the principle of diffusion. A number of SHS components have been proposed as potential indicators, including small particles in the respirable size range, nicotine, and carbon monoxide; other proposed indicators include more specific measures of particles and other gaseous components.[11,14] The most widely studied components are respirable particles, which are sampled actively with a pump and filter, and nicotine, which is present in the gas phase in SHS and is collectible with both active and passive sampling methods. The respirable particles in indoor air may come from sources other than active smoking and are nonspecific indicators of SHS; nicotine in air, by contrast, is highly specific, because smoking is its only source. Nicotine concentration can be readily measured using a passive filter badge, which is small enough to be worn by a child or can be placed in a room.[15]

Biomarkers of exposure are compounds that can be measured in biological materials such as blood, urine, or saliva. Cotinine, a metabolite of nicotine, is a highly specific indicator of exposure to SHS in non-smokers,[16] although some foods also contain small amounts of nicotine.[16] In non-smokers, the half-life of cotinine is about 20 hours, so cotinine level can indicate exposure to SHS over several days. It is an integrative measure, reflective of exposure to SHS in all environments where time has been spent. Cotinine can be readily measured in blood, urine, and even saliva, with either radioimmunoassay or chromatography. Newer methods for analysis extend the sensitivity of measurement to extremely low levels.[16] Nicotine can also be measured in hair, where it is incorporated. The first several centimetres of hair adjacent to the scalp give an integrated measure of exposure over the previous several weeks.[17] Carboxyhaemoglobin is a far less sensitive and specific measure that is of little utility for measuring involuntary exposure, although it is a fairly valid indicator of active smoking.

Prevalence of Exposure

Overview

We cannot readily estimate how much of the world's population is exposed to SHS, because few countries routinely collect relevant data. In fact, national estimates based on surveys are available for only a few countries, including the United States and China. The surveys of SHS exposure that have been conducted, however, have used a variety of methods and definitions; most of them have been carried out as part of specific research projects and were not intended to provide national estimates. In the following sections, we present estimates of the prevalence of SHS exposure based on the available information. First, we estimate the global prevalence of smoking, assuming that the prevalence of SHS exposure tracks with that of smoking. We then estimate the prevalence of SHS, using data on both active and passive smoking from several countries. We also address the prevalence of exposure to SHS in women and children. Finally, we use data from some small-scale surveys to further characterize the severity of SHS exposure in women and children.

Table 5.2. Age-Standardized Current Tobacco-Smoking Prevalence Among Adult (15 Years and Older) Males and Females of WHO Member States in the South-East Asia and Western Pacific Regions

Country	Adult Smoking Prevalence	
	Men (%)	Women (%)
South-East Asia Region		
Bangladesh	47	4
Bhutan	-	-
Democratic People's Republic of Korea	58	-
India	33	4
Indonesia	62	5
Maldives	45	12
Myanmar	43	15
Nepal	36	28
Sri Lanka	32	2
Thailand	43	2
Timor-Leste	-	-
Western Pacific Region		
Australia	22	19
Brunei Darussalam	-	-
Cambodia	49	7
China	59	4
Cook Islands	42	34
Fiji	22	4
Japan	42	13
Kiribati	-	-
Lao People's Democratic Republic	64	15
Malaysia	53	3
Marshall Islands	36	6
Micronesia, Federated States of	30	18
Mongolia	46	6
Nauru	47	54
New Zealand	22	20
Niue	-	-
Palau	38	9
Papua New Guinea	-	-
Philippines	53	12
Republic of Korea	53	6
Samoa	58	23
Singapore	36	6
Solomon Islands	-	-
Tonga	62	15
Tuvalu	54	21
Vanuatu	50	7
Viet Nam	44	2

Note: All surveys were conducted among adults, but age groups and survey methodologies varied.
Source: Ref. 1.

 World Health Organization

Prevalence of Smoking as an Indicator of SHS Exposure

Data for global trends have been cited above. Table 5.2 lists age-standardized smoking prevalence rates for the countries of the South-East Asia and Western Pacific Regions, highlighting differences in smoking prevalence between men and women. In general, smoking prevalence in these countries is lower among women than among men. In the South-East Asia Region, smoking prevalence ranges from 2% to 28% for women and 32% to 62% for men. In the Western Pacific Region, smoking prevalence ranges from 2% to 54% for women and from 22% to 64% for men. In the country of Nauru in the Western Pacific Region, smoking prevalence is higher among women than among men, 54% vs 47%.[1] In all regions, much more data are needed on how these patterns may change throughout the life-course of men and women.[18]

Prevalence Estimates of SHS Exposure

Various methods have been used to estimate the extent of exposure to SHS among non-smokers. These range from simple questionnaire reports to measurements of tobacco combustion products in the air of indoor environments and of biomarkers of tobacco smoke in human fluids and tissues. Studies comparing questionnaire indexes of SHS exposure with levels of biomarkers have shown that they are correlated, although their results are not perfectly concordant. Consequently, there is variation in the findings of studies that have used different approaches, and true differences in exposure may not be separable from methodological differences.

Table 5.3 presents data from a number of population-based studies that used questionnaires to determine SHS exposure. Some of these studies were national in scope, e.g. the national samples in China, Australia, and the United States, while others were from states or specific localities. Several studies incorporated cotinine as a biomarker. Unfortunately, data from developing countries are quite limited.

In spite of the limitations of the data, it is clear that involuntary exposure to SHS is widespread throughout the world (see Table 5.3). In industrialized countries, nearly half of the children and adolescents surveyed were exposed, primarily at home. As predicted by the

micro-environmental model of SHS exposure, smoking by household members was a prominent contributor to exposures of children. The workplace also contributed substantially to exposures of adults, both men and women.

The data from the national surveys are particularly informative. In a 1996 national survey in China,[30] 54% of all current non-smokers reported exposure to SHS, defined as being in the presence of passive smoke at least 15 minutes per day on more than one day per week. The prevalence of SHS exposure was higher in women (57%) than in men (45%). The highest prevalence of exposure to SHS was in women of reproductive age (up to 60%), with exposure in the younger age groups higher than that in older groups. The majority of passive smokers were exposed to SHS every day, with 71.2% reporting exposure at home, 25.0% reporting exposure in their work environments, and 32.5% reporting exposure in public places.

The 2006 US Surgeon General's report estimated that in 2000, 126 million US residents over 3 years of age were exposed to SHS.[9] National estimates are also available from several other surveys in the United States, including the National Health Interview Survey in 1988,[22] the National Health and Nutrition Examination Survey III,[31] and the Hispanic Health and Nutrition Survey.[29] These surveys indicate that SHS exposure was common in the United States through the 1990s.

More-detailed information comes from a number of different states and for specific populations in the United States. A population-based cross-sectional study carried out in 1985 by Coultas et al.[19] found that 39% of 1360 Hispanic adults in New Mexico were exposed to SHS. Cummings et al.,[44] using a questionnaire-based cross-sectional study, interviewed 663 non-smokers and ex-smokers who attended the Roswell Park Memorial Institute cancer screening clinic in Buffalo, New York, in 1986. They found that 28% of those interviewed reported exposure to SHS at work, 27% reported exposure at home, 16% reported exposure at restaurants, and 11% reported exposure at social gatherings.

Further information on SHS exposure can be found in the results of more-focused epidemiological studies, some of which were conducted to assess the effects of SHS exposure (Table 5.4). The studies listed in Table 5.4 were selected to provide data from countries throughout the world and to include both children and adults. In general,

Table 5.3. **Prevalence of Exposure to SHS: Population-Based Studies**

Reference	Study Design and Population	Results
Coultas et al., 1987[19]	Cross-sectional study, 2029 Hispanic children and adults in New Mexico (1360 non-smokers and ex-smokers also had salivary cotinine measured)	Prevalence=39% 18 years+, 48% 13–17 years, 45% 6–12 years, and 54% <5 years and infants; Mean salivary concentrations=0 to 6 ng/ml; 35% prevalence of cotinine in non-smoking households
Somerville et al., 1988[20]	Cross-sectional study, 4337 children aged 5 to 11 years in England and 766 in Scotland, from the 1982 National Health Interview Survey on Child Health in the United Kingdom	Prevalence=42% in England and 60% in Scotland
Chilmonczyk et al., 1990[21]	Cross-sectional study, 518 infants aged 6 to 8 weeks receiving routine well-child care in private physicians' offices in greater Portland, Maine	41% infants lived in a smoking household with urinary cotinine levels > 10 µg/L ; 8% had urinary cotinine levels >10 µg/L among those with no smoking reported
Overpeck and Moss, 1991[22]	Cross-sectional study, sample of 5356 children < 5 years of age from the National Health Interview Survey in 1988	Approximately 50% of all US children < 5 years of age exposed to prenatal maternal smoking and/or SHS from household members after birth; 28% had prenatal and postnatal exposure, 21% only after birth, 1.2% prenatally
Borland et al., 1992[23]	Cross-sectional study, sample of 7301 non-smokers from the larger study of Burns and Pierce, 1992	31.3% non-smoking workers reported exposure at work >1 time in the preceding 2 weeks, 35.8% males vs 22.9% females, 41.9% < 25 years vs 26.4% for older workers, 43.1% with <12 years of education vs 18.6% with a college education
Burns and Pierce, 1992[24]	Cross-sectional study, head of household in 32 135 homes in California, contacted via stratified random-digit dialing from June 1990 to July 1991	32.2% children aged 5 to 11 years and 36.5% adolescents aged 12 to 17 years exposed at home
Jaakkola et al., 1994[25]	Population-based cross-sectional study, random sample of 1003 children, aged 1 to 6 years in Espoo, Finland	25.2% children reported SHS exposure at home, 74.8% did not, assessed by parent-completed questionnaire
Jenkins, 1992[26]	Cross-sectional study, telephone interviews with 1579 English-speaking adults and 183 adolescents (12 to 17 years of age) with telephones in California	46% male adult non-smokers exposed at work, 15–23% exposed at other locations, 35% female adult non-smokers exposed at work, 31% at other indoor locations, 20% at home and 13% at outdoor locations; 42% adolescents exposed at home and other indoor locations, 13% at outdoor locations and 4.5% at school, 54% children aged 6 to 11 years and 62% < 5 years exposed at home
Jenkins et al., 1992[26] **and Lum et al., 1994**[27]	Cross-sectional study, same population as described above and another interview of 1200 children aged <11 years (< 8 years old with a parent or guardian) from April 1989 to February 1990 in California	Prevalence for non-smokers=43% for adults and 64% for adolescents (self-report); among smokers and non-smokers=61% for adults and 70% for adolescents during the day; children, infants, and preschoolers reported 35% to 45% exposure, average duration=3.5 hours
Pierce et al., 1994[28]	Cross-sectional study using the California Adult Tobacco Surveys in 1990, 1992, 1993 with 8224 to 30 716 adults 18 years and older and 1789 to 5040 adolescents 12 to 17 years of age sampled	15.1% smoked prior to pregnancy, and of these, 37.5% quit during the pregnancy (9.4% of California women smoke during pregnancy); 17.7% of those < 5 years of age exposed in their homes and 19.6% of those <17 years
Pletch, 1994[29]	Cross-sectional study, 4256 Hispanic women aged 12 to 49 years who participated in the Hispanic Health and Nutrition Examination Survey (HHANES) from 1982 to 1984	Age-specific household exposure for non-smokers=31% to 62% for Mexican-Americans, 22% to 59% for Puerto Ricans, and 40% to 53% for Cuban-Americans; 59% of Puerto Rican and 62% of Cuban-American adolescents had high exposures
Yang et al., 1996[30]	Cross-sectional study, 122 700 records (65 000 males and 57 000 females) of persons 15 years and older from the 1996 National Prevalence Survey of Smoking Patterns in China	Prevalence for males=45.5%, females=57%

World Health Organization

Table 5.3. *(continued)*

Reference	Study Design and Population	Results
Pirkle et al., 1996[31]	Cross-sectional study, 9744 adults aged 17 years or older from the NHANES III Study, 1988 to 1991	Prevalence for males=43.5%, females=32.9%; 87.9% had detectable serum cotinine levels
Lister and Jorn, 1998[32]	Cross-sectional study, data from the ABS 1989–1990 National Health Survey of parents and their children (n=4281), aged 0 to 4 years, Australia	45% of children lived in households with > 1 current smoker, 29% had a mother who smoked; odds ratio (OR)=1.52, 95% CI=1.19, 1.94 for maternal smoking significantly associated with parent-reported asthma and OR=1.51, 95% CI=1.26, 1.80 asthma wheezing
CDC, 2003[33]	Cross-sectional study, data from the 2001 Texas Youth Tobacco Survey, 8696 students in grades 6–12 from 192 schools in Texas	50.6% of middle school students reported SHS exposure (95% CI=+/-3.1%) and 65.8% of high school students reported SHS exposure (95% CI=+/-2.2%); 80.1% of students who lived with a smoker reported SHS exposure (95% CI=+/- 2.2%)
Gu et al., 2004[34]	Cross-sectional study, 15 540 adults aged 35 to 74 years in China, surveyed between 2000 and 2001	Among non-smokers surveyed, 12.1% of men and 51.3% of women reported SHS exposure at home, and 26.7% of men and 26.2% of women reported SHS exposure at work
Nebot et al., 2004[35]	Cross-sectional study, data from Barcelona Health Interview Survey 2000, 10 000 people aged 15 to 64 years in Barcelona, Spain	69.7% of the population reported SHS exposure, 22.6% reported SHS exposure at work and home, 29.7% reported exposure only at work, and 17.5% reported exposure only at home; by sex, 23.5% of women and 12.6% of men reported SHS at home only, and 34.2% of men and 24.2% women reported SHS at work only
Martinez-Donate et al., 2005[36]	Cross-sectional household survey, population-based sample of 400 adult residents of Tijuana, Baja California, Mexico, during 2003–2004	53.9% of Tijuana adults reported chronic exposure to SHS (95% CI=48.8%, 58.9%); 44.4% of Tijuana adults reported their workplace had a non-smoking policy, and 65.8% reported their households were smoke-free
Maziak et al., 2006[37]	Cross-sectional population-based survey, 2038 participants aged 18 to 65 years residing in Aleppo, Syrian Arab Republic	Among non-smokers (n=419), 97.6% had detectable saliva cotinine levels (mean +/- SD 1.7 +/- 1.5 ng/ml)
Pickett et al., 2006[38]	Cross-sectional study, data from 1999–2002 National Health and Nutrition Examination Survey; 5866 non-smoking adults from 57 survey locations in the United States	12.5% of non-smoking adults living in counties with extensive smoke-free law coverage were exposed to SHS; 35.1% of non-smoking adults living in counties with limited smoke-free law coverage were exposed to SHS; 45.9% of non-smoking adults living in counties with no laws were exposed to SHS
GTSS Collaborative Group, 2006[39]	Global Youth Tobacco Survey of youth aged 13 to 15 years from 132 countries between 1999 and 2005	43.9% of students were exposed to SHS at home, 55.8% of students were exposed to SHS in public places, and 46.5% of students had parents who smoke
CDC, 2007[40]	Cross-sectional study, data from students aged 13 to 15 years from 137 jurisdictions worldwide surveyed during 2000–2007 in the Global Youth Tobacco Survey	46.8% of never-smokers were exposed to SHS at home, 47.8% of never-smokers were exposed to SHS in places other than the home
Perez-Rios et al., 2007[41]	Cross-sectional study, 6492 individuals aged 16 to 74 years living in Galicia, Spain, and enrolled in the regional health-care system	74.6% of the Galician population was exposed to SHS (95% CI=73.2, 75.9); 80.5% (95% CI=79, 82.1) of males were exposed to SHS, and 68.2% (95% CI=66.1, 70.4) of females were exposed to SHS
Rudatsikira et al., 2007[42]	Cross-sectional study within the framework of the Global Youth Tobacco Survey in 2003 in Mongolia	73.9% of males and 71.7% of females reported SHS exposure in their home or elsewhere; OR=5.85 (95% CI 3.83, 8.92) for SHS exposure when both parents were smokers, OR=3.65 (95% CI=3.10, 4.30) for SHS exposure when only the father smoked, OR=6.54 (95% CI=3.48, 12.32) for SHS exposure when only the mother smoked
Twose et al., 2007[43]	Cohort study, follow-up interview of 1608 participants in the Cornella Health Interview Survey Follow-up Study from Cornella de Llobregat, Barcelona, Catalonia	Self-reported prevalence of SHS exposure was 69.5% (95% CI=64.5%, 74.4%) in men and 62.9% (95% CI=58.1%, 67.6%) in women; 25.9% (95%CI=21.8%, 30.1%) of men and 34.1% (95% CI=29.8%, 38.5%) reported passive smoking at home; 55.1% (95% CI=50.8%, 59.4%) of men and 44.3% (95% CI=40.5%, 48.2%) of women reported SHS exposure during leisure time; 34.0% (95% CI=23.5%, 45.6%) of men and 30.1% (95% CI=18.9%, 41.3%) of women reported SHS exposure in the workplace

Table 5.4. **Prevalence of Exposure to SHS: Selected Epidemiological Studies**

Reference	Study Design and Population	Results
Kauffmann et al., 1983[48]	Cross-sectional study, data from the French Cooperative Study PAARC with spirometric measurements for 95% of participants, 7818 adult residents (3915 men and 3903 women) aged 25 to 49 years, living in seven cities of France, 1975	Prevalence for males=4.2%, females=49.7%; non-smoking participants with spouses who smoked at least 10 g. of tobacco a day had significantly lowered forced expiratory volume in 25 to 75 seconds (FEF_{25-75}); women also had a significant difference in forced expiratory volume in 1 second (FEV_1) and a dose-response relationship with amount of smoking from their husbands
Ware et al., 1984[49]	Cohort study, 10 106 schoolchildren with respiratory illness in six US communities, aged 6 to 9 years	Prevalence=68%; maternal smoking associated with 20 to 35% increase in childhood respiratory illness rates; FEV_1 lower for children living with current smokers and lowest for those living with ex-smokers
Greenberg et al., 1989[50]	Questionnaire-based cross-sectional study, mothers of 433 infants from a representative population of healthy neonates from 1986–1987 in North Carolina	55% of infants lived in a household with at least one smoker; 42% were exposed during the week preceding data collection; cotinine was detected in 60% of urine samples (median=121 ng/mg creatinine)
Cummings et al., 1990[44]	Questionnaire-based cross-sectional study, interview of 663 non-smokers and ex-smokers who attended the Roswell Park Memorial Institute cancer screening clinic in 1986 in Buffalo, New York	28% reported exposure at work, 27% at home, 16% at restaurants, 11% at social gatherings, 10% in car or airplane, and 8% in public buildings; cotinine levels for self-reported non-smokers ranged from 0 to 85 ng/ml (average 8.84 ng/ml)
Dijkstra et al., 1990[51]	Cohort study, non-smoking children aged 6 to 12 years over a 2-year period, The Netherlands	Prevalence=66%; association between exposure to SHS in the home and development of wheeze, based on lung function tests and questionnaire for respiratory symptoms
Masjedi et al., 1990[45]	Cross-sectional study, 288 adults (167 men and 108 women) aged 18 to 65 years living in Tehran, Islamic Republic of Iran	Men=47%, women=50%; significant reductions in FEV_1 (5.7%), FVC (4.6%), FEV_{25-75} (9.9%) for men
Butz and Rosenstein, 1992[52]	Questionnaire-based cross-sectional study, 102 children with asthma, 103 with cystic fibrosis, 50 with rheumatoid arthritis, and 105 well children from June 1989 to October 1989	30% reported $\geq$ 1 smoker(s) in the household, reported more often by cystic fibrosis and rheumatoid arthritis respondents (C^2=9.24, P=0.03); 12% reported $\geq$ 2 smokers in household; cystic fibrosis and rheumatoid arthritis subjects reported higher rates of exposure in low socioeconomic groups (C^2=9.68, P=0.02)
Sherrill et al., 1992[53]	Longitudinal cohort study, 634 children aged 9 to 15 years, New Zealand	Overall prevalence=40%; parental smoking associated with mild reduction in FEV_1/VC (forced expiratory volume in 1 second/vital capacity) in males; children with asthma had more serious and progressive reduction with parental smoking (mean=3.9% for males and 2.3% for females) by age 15 years, based on self-report asthma/wheeze and pulmonary function tests
Cummings, 1994[54]	Cross-sectional study, 339 currently employed non-smokers who were exposed at home (n=122) and non-smokers who were not exposed at home (n=217), using the same population as in Cummings, 1990[44]	81% employed non-smokers were exposed at work and home, 76% were exposed only at work; SHS exposure at home was not predictive of exposure at work; mean urinary cotinine levels=12.8 ng/ml (7.5 at home and 11 at work)
Thompson et al., 1995[55]	Cross-sectional study, 20 801 US employees from 114 work sites	52.4% reported being exposed to SHS at work
Kurtz et al., 1996[56]	Questionnaire-based cross-sectional survey, 675 Afro-American students enrolled in grades 5–12 in an urban public school district in Detroit, Michigan	Smoking rates higher among students with parents who smoked; 48% reported parental smoking, 46% reported maternal smoking
Brenner et al., 1997[57]	Cross-sectional survey of 974 predominantly blue-collar employees in a south German metal company	>60% non-smoking blue-collar workers were affected by passive smoke at work; 52% non-smoking white-collar workers were exposed if smoking was allowed in work area, 18% if smoking was not allowed
Steyn et al., 1997[46]	Questionnaire-based cross-sectional study, 394 pregnant women attending antenatal services in Johannesburg, Cape Town, Port Elizabeth, and Durban in urban South Africa, 1992	Most women who smoked stopped or reduced tobacco use during their pregnancy; 70% lived with at least one smoker in the house

World Health Organization

Table 5.4. *(continued)*

Reference	Study Design and Population	Results
Lam et al., 1998[47]	Questionnaire-based cross-sectional study, 6304 students, aged 12 to 15 years, from 172 classes of 61 schools in China, Hong Kong SAR	53.1% were living in a household with at least one smoker, 35.2% had one smoker only, 9.5% had two, and 2.5% had three or more smokers in the household; 38% of fathers and 3.5% of mothers smoked
Jones et al., 2001[58]	Cross-sectional study, face-to-face interviews with 435 bar staff, waiters, and bar and eating-place managers and owners in Wellington, New Zealand, during the 1999–2000 summer	59% of the workers interviewed were exposed to SHS
Olivieri et al., 200[59]	Cross-sectional study, 504 randomly selected Caucasian individuals in Verona, Italy; 375 individuals completed the questionnaire (129 smokers, 79 ex-smokers, 167 never-smokers)	57.6% of those surveyed reported exposure to SHS (76.7% of current smokers, 54.4% of ex-smokers, and 44.3% of never-smokers); 10.8% of never-smokers reported SHS exposure at home, 13.2% reported SHS exposure at work, 12.6% reported SHS exposure at home and work, and 7.8% reported SHS in locations outside the home and work
Cameron et al., 2003[60]	Cross-sectional study, 1078 members of the Victorian Branch of the Australian Liquor, Hospitality and Miscellaneous Workers Union in September 2001	54% of the union members worked in locations that did not completely ban smoking, and 34% reported SHS exposure during their work day
Cornelius et al., 2003[61]	Cross-sectional study, 196 low-socioeconomic-status mothers and their children aged 6 years	Based on mother self-reports, 85% of the children had daily SHS exposure, and 71% lived in a household with smokers; urine cotinine measures indicated that 79% of the children were exposed to SHS
Jordan et al., 2005[62]	Cross-sectional study, 574 junior high and high school students from seven schools in an Ohio metropolitan area	54% of the students surveyed reported SHS exposure in the week prior to the survey, and 30% reported 3 or more hours of SHS exposure in the week prior to the survey; the students' homes, inside cars, and someone else's home or apartment were the three most common locations of exposure
Boyaci et al., 2006[63]	Cross-sectional study, 188 primary school students in the Korfez District in Kocaeli, Turkey, May 2004	Based on self-reports, 72.3% of the students lived in households with smokers, and 34.6% had daily SHS exposure; measured urine cotinine levels (>10ng/mL) indicated that 76% of the students were exposed to SHS
Delpisheh et al., 2006[64]	Community-based cross-sectional study, 245 children aged 5 to 11 years attending 10 primary schools in Liverpool	61.4% of the children lived in a smoking household; the average salivary cotinine concentration was 1.6 (+/- SD=+/-0.4); for boys it was 1.9 (+/- 0.4), and for girls it was 1.2 (+/-0.2)
Anuntaseree et al., 2007[65]	Prospective-cohort study of Thai children, follow-up interview of 725 infants aged 1 year in the Songkhla district, Thailand	Based on self-reports, 73.3% of infants lived in households with smoking; prevalence of father and mother smoking in the presence of an infant=63.6%; based on measured urinary cotinine, 40.7% of the infants had SHS exposure (detectable urinary cotinine), and 25 infants had urinary cotinine levels in the range of an adult heavy smoker
Dostal et al., 2007[66]	Pregnancy-outcome study on all pregnant women delivering in the Teplice and Prachatice district, Czech Republic, between 1994 and 1999; postnatal follow up questionnaires of 443 mothers of children aged 3 and 685 mothers of children aged 4.5 years	30.1% of the children surveyed lived in a household with one smoker, and 41.6% lived in a household without smokers; based on measured urine cotinine concentration, 48.2% of the children were exposed to SHS (n=523)
Lee et al., 2008[67]	Cross-sectional study, 1858 participants aged 18 to 24 years in Florida	64% reported visiting a bar or nightclub in the previous month and being exposed to SHS; 46% reported SHS exposure in automobiles; 15% reported SHS exposure in the workplace; 9% reported living with at least one smoker

they offer confirming evidence of the high prevalence of SHS in such countries as the Islamic Republic of Iran,[45] South Africa,[46] and Hong Kong SAR.[47]

Data from a 1988 nationwide survey show that about one half of the children in the United States under the age of 5 are exposed to tobacco smoke.[22] For more than one quarter of them, exposure begins before birth. The survey data indicate that 42% of the children in this age range live in a household with a smoker. The probability of children's exposure to tobacco smoke in groups with the lowest income and maternal education was double that in groups with the highest income and maternal education.

A study of children in North Carolina (United States) found that non-household sources of exposure may become increasingly important as a child ages.[68] The proportion of the children in the study between the ages of 3 weeks and 1 year who were reported to be exposed to SHS increased from 39% to 63%. This increase was accounted for by greater exposure to smoke from both household and non-household smokers, both at home and in other locations. These findings imply that any control strategy devised for limiting children's exposure to SHS must address both the home and other locations.[69] Data on infants in China also point to the importance of the home in exposure to SHS. A study of paternal smoking and birth weight in Shanghai carried out by Zhang et al.[70] in 1986–1987 found that 58% of newborn babies were exposed to SHS, primarily by the father smoking and less frequently by the mother. The study did not consider exposure to SHS from other sources.

Results of studies from several countries showed that 40% to 70% of older children are exposed to SHS. For example, Ware et al.[49] studied schoolchildren in six US communities and reported that 68% of the children 6 to 9 years of age were exposed to SHS in 1984. Using data from the 1988 National Health Interview Survey on Child Health in the United Kingdom, Somerville et al.[20] reported that 42% and 60% of children 5 to 11 years of age in England and Scotland, respectively, were exposed to SHS from parental smoking in 1988. Dijkstra et al.[51] reported that 66% of children 6 to 12 years of age in the Netherlands suffered from SHS exposure in 1990. Sherrill et al.[71] reported that 40% of children 9 to 15 years of age in New Zealand were exposed to SHS in 1992.

The majority of studies measuring the costs of exposure of children and adults to SHS have been conducted in industrialized countries or in urban areas in developing countries. Many of the reports reflect past patterns of exposure in industrialized countries where SHS exposures have recently declined. These studies confirm the prediction of widespread SHS exposure from the prevalence estimates of active smoking. Both the data on active smoking and the surveys of involuntary exposure to SHS document the fact that women and children are the predominant exposed groups.

Health Effects of SHS

Overview

Direct evidence of the health risks of SHS comes from epidemiological studies that have assessed the association of SHS exposure with disease outcomes. Judgements about causality between SHS exposure and health outcomes are based not only on this epidemiological evidence, but also on the extensive evidence derived from epidemiological and toxicological investigations of the health consequences of active smoking. The literature on SHS and health has been reviewed periodically, beginning as early as the 1971 report of the US Surgeon General.[72] Particularly significant early syntheses were the 1986 report of the US Surgeon General on involuntary smoking[10] and a report of the US National Research Council, also published in 1986;[73] the 1992 risk assessment report published by the US Environmental Protection Agency (EPA);[74] the comprehensive review of the California EPA, published in 1997;[75] the report of the Scientific Committee on Tobacco in the United Kingdom, published in 1998;[6] and the WHO report on the international consultation on environmental tobacco smoke and child health, published in 1999.[3] Each of these studies systematically evaluated the evidence to reach overall conclusions with regard to the relationship between SHS and disease. In recent years, the International Agency for Research on Cancer (IARC),[7] the California EPA,[8] the Office of the US Surgeon General,[9] and WHO[76] have published reports and/or guidelines on the health effects of SHS exposure. Principal conclusions are provided in Table 5.5.

Causal conclusions were reached as early as 1986, when involuntary smoking was found by IARC,[77] the US Surgeon General, and the US National Research Council to be a cause of lung cancer in non-smokers. Researchers at each of these agencies interpreted the available epidemiological evidence in the context of the wider understanding of active smoking and lung cancer. In spite of somewhat differing approaches for reaching a conclusion, the findings of the three studies were identical: all found that involuntary smoking is a cause of lung cancer in non-smokers. In 1986, the reports of the US Surgeon General and the National Research Council also addressed the then-mounting evidence on adverse respiratory effects of SHS exposure on children. Subsequent reports, as mentioned above, identified further effects of SHS exposure, and the most recent reports have classified SHS as the cause of a number of adverse effects on exposed children (Table 5.5).

In this section, we provide an overview of the now extensive data on adverse health effects of SHS on women and children, drawing on these synthesis reports and other reviews.[5] We review the evidence separately for women and children. The available studies on SHS exposure and lung cancer among women and children in Asian and Pacific Rim countries are listed in Table 5.6a; studies on SHS exposure and other respiratory effects in these countries are listed in Table 5.6b. The evidence in these tables is only part of the evidence on SHS, and it should not be interpreted in isolation from the totality of the evidence, which includes studies from many other countries.

Table 5.5. Adverse Health Effects of Exposure to Tobacco Smoke

Health Effect	SGR 1984	SGR 1986	EPA 1992	CALIF. EPA 1997	UK 1998/ 2004	WHO 1999	IARC 2004	CALIF. EPA[a] 2005	SGR 2006
Increased prevalence of chronic respiratory symptoms	Yes/a	Yes/a	Yes/c	Yes/c	Yes/c	Yes/c		Yes/c	Yes/c
Decrement in pulmonary function	Yes/a	Yes/a	Yes/a	Yes/a	Yes/a[b]	Yes/c		Yes/a	Yes/c
Increased occurrence of acute respiratory illnesses	Yes/a	Yes/a	Yes/a	Yes/c		Yes/c		Yes/c	Yes/c
Increased occurrence of middle-ear disease		Yes/a	Yes/c	Yes/c	Yes/c	Yes/c		Yes/c	Yes/c
Increased severity of asthma episodes and symptoms			Yes/c	Yes/c		Yes/c		Yes/c	Yes/c
Risk factor for new asthma			Yes/a	Yes/c				Yes/c	Yes/c
Risk factor for sudden infant death syndrome (SIDS)				Yes/c	Yes/a	Yes/c		Yes/c	Yes/c
Risk factor for lung cancer in adults		Yes/c	Yes/c	Yes/c	Yes/c		Yes/c	Yes/c	Yes/c
Risk factor for breast cancer for younger, primarily post-menopausal women								Yes/c	
Risk factor for nasal sinus cancer								Yes/c	
Risk factor for heart disease in adults				Yes/c	Yes/c			Yes/c	Yes/c

Note: Yes/a=association; Yes/c=cause.
Source: Adapted from Ref. 9.
[a]   Only effects causally associated with SHS exposure are included.
[b]   Added in 2004.

Table 5.6a. **Studies Investigating SHS Exposure and Lung Cancer in Asia and the Pacific Rim**

Reference	Study Design and Population	Results
Koo et al., 1985[78]	Case–control study, 78 cases of never-smoked females from 1977 to 1980 and 137 never-smoked female controls in Hong Kong SAR	No significant increase in relative risk (RR), RR squamous-cell=1.75, AR(%)=34.7; RR large-cell=1.44, attributable risk (AR)=23.8; RR small-cell=1.10, AR=6.6; RR adenocarcinoma=7.2, AR=7.2;
Lam et al., 1987[79]	Case–control study, 445 Chinese female lung cancer patients confirmed pathologically and 445 age-matched Chinese female healthy neighborhood controls from 1983 to 1986 in Hong Kong SAR	RR=1.65 (*P*<0.01, 95% CI=1.16, 2.35), RR for adenocarcinoma-only cell type significant=2.12 (*P*=0.01, 95% CI=1.32, 3.39); both RRs had significant trends with daily amount smoked by husband
Koo et al., 1987[78,80]	Case–control study, 88 never-smoked female lung cancer patients from 1981 to 1983 and 137 never-smoked district controls in Hong Kong SAR	No dose-response relationships: odds ratio (OR)=1.83 (95% CI=0.65, 5.11) for 1–10 cigarettes/day smoked by each household member (adjusted for age, number of live births, schooling, years since exposure ceased); OR=2.56 (95% CI=1.06, 6.19) for 11–20 cigarettes/day; OR=1.21 (95% CI=0.51, 2.86) for 21+ cigarettes/day
Wu-Williams et al., 1990[81]	Hospital-based case–control study, 965 female cases and 959 age/frequency-matched controls from 1985 to 1987 in the Shenyang and Harbin districts, China	RR=0.7 (95% CI=0.6, 0.9) for non-smokers who lived with a spouse who smoked in Harbin; no dose-response relationship except for father's smoking in the presence of index case
Liu et al., 1991[82]	Hospital-based case–control study, 110 newly diagnosed lung cancer patients and 426 age, sex, occupation, and resident-matched controls from November 1985 to December 1986, China	Non-smoking females OR=0.77 (95% CI=0.30, 1.96)
Liu et al., 1993[83]	Hospital based case–control study, 224 male and 92 female incident lung cancer cases and individually matched hospital controls from June 1983 to June 1984 in Guangzhou, China	OR=2.9 (95% CI=1.2, 7.3) for >20 cigarettes/day smoked by husband, OR=0.7 (95% CI=0.2, 2.2) for 1–19 cigarettes/day; C^2=4.5, *P*=0.03 for trend test
Du et al., 1996[84]	606 000 cases of lung cancer deaths over the past 9 years in Guangzhou, China; two studies: 1. 120 participants (28 males and 92 females), 2. 75 never-smoking females	SHS exposure not statistically associated
Gao, 1996[85]	Review of epidemiological investigations	No association with SHS exposure
Koo and Ho, 1996[86]	Four epidemiology studies over the past 15 years in Hong Kong SAR: 1. Retrospective study of 200 cases and 200 neighborhood controls 2. Cross-sectional study measuring NO_2 of 362 children and their mothers 3. Site monitoring of 33 homes of airborne carcinogens 4. Telephone survey of 500 women's dietary habits and air-pollutant exposures	SHS exposure moderately high (36% have current smokers at home)
Ko et al., 1997[87]	Hospital-based case–control study, 117 interviewed female patients suffering from lung cancer (including 106 non-smokers) and 117 individually matched hospital controls from 1992 to 1993 in Kaohsiung, Taiwan, China	OR=1.3 (95% CI=0.7, 2.5) for those with spouse who smoked (socioeconomic status, residential area, and education-adjusted), OR=1.0 (95% CI=0.4, 2.3) for cohabitant who smoked
Wang and Zhou, 1996[88]	Hospital-based case–control study, 135 newly diagnosed lung cancer cases and 135 age- and sex-matched controls from April 1992 to May 1994 in Shenyang, China	No association with SHS exposure; OR=2.25 (95% CI=1.01, 5.17) for family history of cancer
Wang et al., 1996[89]	Case–control study, 390 lung cancer cases (291 males, 99 females) and 390 individually matched controls from April 1992 to May 1994 in Guangdong, China	Females predominantly had adenocarcinoma (squamous cell carcinoma/adenocarcinoma=1:2.7) and were diagnosed at an earlier age than males, (*P*<0.0001); exposure to SHS in home and work an independent risk factor
Wang and Zhou, 1997[90]	Meta-analysis of six case–control studies, 767 cases and 1193 controls from Shanghai, Guangzhou, Shenyang, Harbin, Xuanwei, and Hong Kong SAR	Overall OR=0.91 (95% CI=0.75, 1.10), C^2=4.51, *P*>0.25, no significant dose–response relationship

World Health
Organization

Table 5.6a. *(continued)*

Reference	Study Design and Population	Results
Shen et al., 1998[91]	Case–control study, 70 adenocarcinoma lung cancer cases and 70 controls in Nanjing, China	No statistical association with SHS exposure; risk factors include chronic lung disease (OR=3.90) and family history of tumor (OR=4.36)
Jee et al. 1999[92]	Cohort study, 157 436 non-smoking married women aged 40 to 88 years who were health-insurance subscribers in the Republic of Korea, 3.5 years of follow-up	79 incident and prevalent cases of lung cancer among non-smoking wives; risk of developing lung cancer increased with increasing duration and amount of cigarettes smoked: RR=1.30 (95% CI=0.6, 2.7) for the wives of former smokers, RR=1.90 (95% CI 1.0-3.5) for the wives of current smokers (adjusted for age, socioeconomic status, occupation, residency, and vegetable intake)
Rapiti et al., 1999[93]	Hospital based case–control study, 58 non-smoking histologically confirmed cases (17 men, 41 women) and 123 non-smoking non-matched controls (56 men, 67 women) from 1991–1992 in Chandigarh, India	No significant association found between risk and years of spousal smoking; RR=1.1 (95% CI=0.5, 2.6) for women whose husbands smoked (adjusted for gender, age, religion, and residence)
Zhong et al., 1999[94]	Population-based case–control study, 504 non-smoking female lung cancer cases aged 35 to 69 and 601 non-smoking frequency-matched-for-age controls from Shanghai, China	RR=1.2 (95% CI=0.8, 1.7) for women exposed to SHS at home; RR=1.9 (95% CI=0.9, 3.7) for women exposed to SHS in the workplace (adjusted for age, income, vitamin C intake, respondent status, smokiness of kitchen, family history of lung cancer, and high-risk occupation)
Lee et al., 2000[95]	Hospital-based case–control study, 268 non-smoking female lung cancer cases and 445 non-smoking female age- and date-of-admission matched controls from 1992–1998 in Kaohsiung, Taiwan, China	Significant associations between increased risk and a variety of sources of SHS exposure; RR=2.2 (95% CI=1.5, 3.3) for women whose husbands smoke in their presence; RR=2.0 (95% CI=1.2, 3.5) for women with 41 to 60 years of SHS exposure; RR=2.8 (95% CI=1.6, 4.8) for women with > 60 years of SHS exposure
Wang et al., 2000[96]	Case–control study, 233 cases (33 men, 200 women) aged 30 to 75 and 521 controls frequency-matched for age, gender, and residence from 1994–1998 in two rural prefectures of China	Significant increase in risk associated with SHS exposure in childhood, but no significant increase in adulthood; RR=1.52 (95% CI=1.1, 2.2) for individuals exposed to SHS during childhood; RR=0.9 (95% CI=0.6, 1.4) for individuals exposed to SHS in adulthood (adjusted for age, social class, prefecture, and other potential confounders)
Zhou et al., 2000[97]	Population-based case–control study, 72 lifetime non-smoking female lung cancer cases aged 35 to 69 and 72 age-matched healthy females in April–December 1995 living in Shenyang, China	No significant increase in risk associated with husband's smoking status; RR=1.11 (95% CI=0.65, 1.88) for women whose husbands smoke
Nishino et al., 2001[98]	Prospective-cohort study, 9675 Japanese non-smoking women over 40 years of age from three municipalities of Miyagi, Japan; 9 years of follow-up	24 incident cases of lung cancer; no significant increase in risk associated with SHS exposure from other household members; RR=1.8 (95% CI=0.7, 4.6) for women with husbands who smoked (adjusted for age, area, intake of alcohol, vegetables, fruit, meat, and history of lung disease)
Seow et al., 2002[99]	Hospital-based case–control study, 176 lifetime non-smoker female lung cancer cases less than 90 years of age from 1996–1998 and 663 lifetime non-smoker female age-, hospital-, and date-of-admission matched controls in Singapore	Increased risk with any SHS exposure at home; RR=1.3 (95% CI=0.9, 1.8) for women with any SHS exposure (adjusted for age, birthplace, family history of cancer, soy intake, length of menstrual cycle)
Chan-Yeung et al., 2003[100]	Case–control study, 331 lung cancer cases and 331 age- and sex-matched controls in Hong Kong SAR	Among women, exposure to SHS at home and or at work was a risk factor for lung cancer; OR=3.60 (95% CI=1.52, 8.51) for women exposed to SHS at work and/or at home
Kurahashi et al., 2008[101]	Population-based prospective-cohort study, 28 414 lifelong non-smoking Japanese women aged 40 to 69 years; more than 13 years of follow-up	109 incident cases of lung cancer, of whom 82 developed adenocarcinoma; hazard ratio (HR)=1.34 (95% CI=0.81, 2.21) for all lung cancer incidence in women living with a husband who smokes; HR=2.03 (95% CI=1.07, 3.86) for adenocarcinoma incidence for women living with a husband who smokes

Table 5.6b. Studies Investigating SHS Exposure and Other Respiratory Health Effects in Asia and the Pacific Rim

Reference	Study Design and Population	Outcome	Results
Chen et al., 1986[102]	Prospective-cohort study, 1058 newborns in Shanghai, China	Hospitalization for respiratory illness during first 18 months of life	Significant increase in rate of hospitalization by number of cigarette smoked per day by family members
Chen et al., 1988[103]	Retrospective-cohort study, 2227 children born in one district of Shanghai, China, who did not move out of the district during their first 18 months of life, 1983	Hospitalization and diagnosis of respiratory disease during first 18 months of life via questionnaire	Sex, birth weight, feeding type, and father's education-adjusted incidence density ratio (IDR)=1.79 (95% CI=1.15, 2.79) for 1–9 cigarettes/day; IDR=2.60 (95% CI=1.69, 4.00) for 10+ cigarettes/day
Tupasi et al., 1988[104]	Community-based cohort study, children in selected households less than 5 years of age from April 1981 to March 1982 and September 1982 to September 1983 in Metro Manila, Philippines	Acute respiratory infection (ARI)	RR comparing parental smoking to no parental smoking, mother only, OR=1.2 (95% CI=0.6, 2.1); father only, OR=0.7 (95% CI=0.6, 0.9); both parents OR=1.0 (95% CI=0.7, 1.4)
Pandey et al., 1989[105]	Prospective-cohort study, 1085 children less than 5 years of age in hill region, Nepal	ARI based on home visits	ARI rate doubled by parent smoking
Azizi, 1990[106]	Cross-sectional study, children 7 to 12 years of age in Kuala Lumpur	Spirometric and peak expiratory flow measurements	Children sharing rooms with adult smokers had significantly lower levels of forced expiratory volume in 25–75 seconds (FEV25-75)
Tupasi et al., 1990[107]	Prospective-cohort study, 1978 children aged less than 5 years in Manila, Philippines	ARI based on weekly interview	OR=1.2, both parents smoking
Vathanophas et al., 1990[108]	Prospective cohort study, 674 children aged less than 5 years in Bangkok, Thailand	ARI based on field-worker surveillance	No significant increase from either parent smoking; risk of lower respiratory infection doubled if family members smoked
Woodward et al., 1990[109]	Nested case–control study, 13 996 reference population from Adelaide, South Australia, 258 cases with respiratory illness scores in top 20%, 231 controls from bottom 20%	Respiratory illness	OR=2.06 (95% CI=1.25, 3.39) for maternal smoking in the first year of child's life, adjusted for parental history of respiratory illness, other smokers in the home, use of group child care, parent's occupation, and levels of maternal stress and social support; OR=1.75 (95% CI=1.03, 3.0) for maternal smoking in first year of child's life, without smoking during pregnancy
Azizi, 1991[110]	Cross-sectional study, 1501 schoolchildren aged 7 to 12 years from July 1987 to October 1987 in Malaysia	Asthma	Link between parental smoking and chest wheeze or whistling and cough, and between smoking in the home and bronchial asthma in young children
Sherrill et al., 1992[71]	Cohort study, 634 children aged 9 to 15 years in New Zealand	Lung function	Parental smoking had serious, progressive effects on FEV1/VC (forced expiratory volume in 25–75 seconds/vital capacity ratio) in children with reported wheeze or asthma; mean reduction=3.9%
Ford, 1993[111]	Questionnaire-based cross-sectional study, 1916 mothers giving singleton births from January 1992 to May 1992 in Canterbury region, New Zealand	Smoking rates	333 mothers smoked during at least some part of their pregnancy; 90% of those who quit did so during the first trimester
Jin et al., 1993[112]	Prospective cohort study, 1007 live births who could be followed to 18 months of age in Shanghai, China	Bronchitis and pneumonia infections	RR=1.3, 1.7, and 2.0 for 1–9, 10–19, and 20–39 cigarettes smoked/day, respectively; dose-response relationship (*P*=0.0002)
Chen, 1994[113]	Retrospective-cohort study, 3285 infants from the Jing An (1163 babies born between 1 June and 31 December, 1981) and Changning (2315 babies born in the last quarter of 1983) districts, the Epidemiologic Studies of Children's Health in Shanghai, China	Low birth weight and hospitalization for respiratory disease in the first 18 months of life	Birth weight < 2500 g: adjusted OR=2.91 (95% CI=0.96, 2.03) for light smokers, and 4.48 (95% CI=2.07, 9.73) for heavy smokers; birth weight > 2500 g: adjusted OR for light smokers=1.4 (95% CI=0.96, 2.03), and 1.61 (95% CI=1.08, 2.41) for heavy smokers

World Health Organization

Table 5.6b. *(continued)*

Reference	Study Design and Population	Outcome	Results
Haby et al., 1994[114]	Cross-sectional study, 2765 schoolchildren aged 8 to 11 years from two rural regions of New South Wales and from Sydney, Australia	Lung function, asthma, other respiratory effects	Forced expiratory volume in 1 second (FEV1), peak expiratory flow rate (PEFR), and forced mid-expiratory flow rate (FEF) all reduced
Flynn, 1994[115]	Questionnaire-based cross-sectional study, 487 Fijian and Indian fourth-grade children with mean age 9.3 years in the Nausori District (rural) of the Fiji Islands, May 1991	Respiratory symptoms in the past 12 months	Prevalence of wheezing > 1 time in the previous 12 months was similar in Fijians (19.8%) and Indians (19.4%); 35.8% of Fijian children had productive cough on most mornings vs 23.9% Indian children, not significant after controlling for prevalence of smoker(s) in the home
Shaw, 1994[116]	Questionnaire-based cross-sectional study, 708 Kawerau schoolchildren aged 8 to 13 years in 1992, New Zealand	Asthma symptoms and risk factors, parent-completed questionnaires	Overall prevalence of current wheeze=21.3%; OR=1.4 (95% CI=1.0, 2.1) for those exposed to SHS from the primary caregiver; multiple factors associated with asthma symptoms
Azizi, 1995[117]	Hospital-based case–control study, 158 children aged 1 month to 5 years hospitalized for incident asthma and 201 controls of children from the same age group hospitalized for causes other than respiratory illness from February 1989 to May 1990 in Malaysia	Asthma and other respiratory illness	Sharing a bedroom with an adult smoker, OR=1.91 (95% CI=1.13, 3.21)
Ponsonby et al., 1996[118]	Population-based cohort study, 6109 live births from 1 May 1988 to 30 April 1993 and their mothers in Tasmania, Australia	Several birth outcomes	Good smoking hygiene (mother not smoking in the same room as baby): OR=1.74 (95% CI=1.30, 2.33) for first birth, OR=1.69 (95% CI=1.27, 2.23) for low birth weight, OR=1.39 (95% CI=1.02, 1.90) for private health-insurance status
Rahman et al., 1997[119]	Prospective cohort study, 965 children less than 5 years of age from July 1993 to October 1993 in Bangladesh	Acute respiratory infection	ARI-positive children more than twice as likely as ARI-negative children to have a parent who smoked; OR=2.43, $P<0.001$
Behera et al., 1998[120]	Cross-sectional study, 200 schoolchildren from northern India	Lung function	FEF 50% significantly less in passive smokers whose households used mixed fuels; peak expiratory flow rate (PEFR%) and forced expiratory volume in 25 seconds (FEF 25%) significantly less in passive smokers whose households used liquefied petroleum gas for fuel
Deshmukh et al., 1998[121]	Community-based cohort study, 210 pregnant women from an urban community in Nagpur, India	Several maternal factors	Significant risk for low birth weight: OR=3.14
Lam et al., 1998[47]	Cross-sectional study, survey administered to sample of 6304 students aged mostly 12 to 15 years from 172 classes of 61 schools in 1994, Hong Kong SAR	Respiratory illness, including nose and throat problems, cough and phlegm, and recent wheezing	OR=1.19 (95% CI=1.01, 1.47) for any cough or phlegm symptoms in children with one smoking household member (adjusted for age, gender, area of residence, type of housing, and correlation within schools and classes); OR=1.38, (95% CI=1.07, 1.79) for two smokers; and OR=1.85 (95% CI=1.19, 2.85) for three smokers (*P* for trend <0.001)
Lister and Jorm, 1998[32]	Cross-sectional study, 4281 children aged 0 to 4 years from the 1989 to 1990 National Health Survey of Australia	Parent-reported chronic or recent asthma and other respiratory effects	Maternal smoking associated with asthma, OR=1.52 (95% CI 1.19, 1.94); and asthma wheeze, OR=1.51 (95% CI=1.26, 1.80); significant positive dose-response relationships; population attributable risk 13%
Chhabra et al., 1998[122]	Questionnaire-based study, 2609 schoolchildren aged 4 to 17 years from two randomly selected schools in Delhi, India	Wheeze	Significant association between the prevalence of wheezing and the presence of smokers in the family (OR=1.62)
Lewis et al., 1998[123]	Cross-sectional study, survey administered to sample of 2304 primary-school children aged 8 to 11 years from industrial and non-industrial areas in 1993, Australia	Wheeze, chronic cough, chest cold	Significant association between passive smoking and chest colds but not between other symptoms and passive smoking; OR=1.68 (95% CI=1.29, 2.19) for chest cold with adult(s) smoking indoors (adjusted for age, gender, PM$_{10}$, SO$_2$, gas heating, maternal allergy); OR=1.16 (95% CI=0.853, 1.59) for wheeze with adult(s) smoking indoors (adjusted)

Table 5.6b. *(continued)*

Reference	Study Design and Population	Outcome	Results
Peters et al., 1998[124]	Cross-sectional study, survey administered in 1992 to 10 615 primary schoolchildren aged 8 to 13 years from two districts of Hong Kong SAR	Physician consultation for wheeze, cough, phlegm	OR=1.57 (95% CI=1.02, 2.43) for wheeze in children with two or more smokers in household (adjusted for age, gender, housing type, area, father's education); OR=1.33 (95% CI=1.08, 1.64) for cough with two or more smokers in household (adjusted); OR=1.33 (95% CI=0.97, 1.83) for phlegm with two or more smokers in household (adjusted)
Belousova et al., 1999[125]	Pooled data from seven cross-sectional studies between 1991 and 1993, surveys administered to a random sample of 6394 students aged 8 to 11 years from seven regions in New South Wales, Australia	Wheeze	Significantly increased risk of recent wheeze for children exposed to maternal smoking; OR=1.33 (95% CI=1.2, 1.5) for wheeze when mothers smoked (adjusted for confounders such as atopy, parental history of asthma, and bronchitis)
Chhabra et al., 1999[126]	Questionnaire-based study, 18 955 schoolchildren aged 5 to 17 years from nine randomly selected schools in Delhi, India	Asthma, wheeze	Presence of smokers in the family a significant risk factor for the development of asthma; OR=1.60 (95% CI=1.48, 1.76) for asthma when there are smokers in the family; OR=1.68 (95% CI=1.54, 1.84) for wheeze when there are smokers in the family
Lam et al., 1999[127]	Cross-sectional study, questionnaire administered to 3480 children aged 8 to 13 years from 30 schools in Hong Kong SAR October 1995 to May 1996	Wheeze, cough, phlegm	OR=1.54, (95% CI=1.28, 1.84) for cough when either parent smoked (adjusted for gender, age, place of birth and living district); OR=1.43 (95% CI=1.21, 1.70) for phlegm when either parent smoked (adjusted); OR=1.21, (95% CI=0.89, 1.41) for wheeze when either parent smoked (adjusted); odds ratios increased with increasing number of smokers in the home
Wang et al., 1999[128]	Cross-sectional study, video, and written questionnaire administered to 165 173 high-school students aged 11 to 16 years in communities of Kaohsiung and Pintong, Taiwan, China, between October 1995 and June 1996	Asthma	Passive smoking was strongly associated with asthma: OR=1.08 (95% CI=1.05, 1.21) for asthma in children exposed to SHS (adjusted for age, gender, parental education, area, income, exercise, active smoking, and alcohol consumption)
Yau et al., 1999[129]	Cohort study, 71 healthy full-term infants aged <24 months living in Taiwan, China	Parent-reported acute lower respiratory illness with wheeze	OR=1.04, (95% CI=0.35, 3.05) for wheeze when either parent smoked
Zhang et al., 1999[130]	Questionnaire-based study of 4108 adults who resided in four districts of three large cities in China, conducted in winter 1988	Cough, phlegm, wheeze	OR=1.18 (95% CI=0.95, 1.46) for cough for women exposed to SHS by one or more household members (adjusted for district, age, occupation, education, indoor ventilation, home coal use, and smoking status); OR=0.96 (95% CI=0.75, 1.24) for phlegm for women exposed to SHS by one or more household members (adjusted); OR=0.62 (95% CI=0.44, 0.87) for women exposed to SHS by one or more household members (adjusted)
Darlow et al., 2000[131]	National cohort of 299 former very low-birth-weight infants born in 1986, aged 7 to 8 years, New Zealand	Asthma incidence	Maternal smoking during pregnancy was a significant predictor for asthma (*P*<0.05), with asthma diagnosis more likely if the mother smoked during pregnancy (*P*<0.005) or currently smoked (*P*<0.01)
Ponsonby et al., 2000[132]	Cross-sectional study, survey administered in 1995 to all children aged 7 years from Tasmania, Australia (6378); survey data linked to 1988 Tasmanian Infant Health Survey data	Asthma	OR=1.03 (95% CI=0.83, 1.26) for ever having asthma when mother or other adult resident was a smoker (adjusted for gender, family history, breastfeeding, gas heat, mother's education, number of members in household)
Qian et al., 2000[133]	Questionnaire-based cross-sectional study, parents of 2060 students aged 5 to 14 years from three urban districts and one suburban district of three cities in China	Asthma, wheeze, cough, phlegm	Significant association between the prevalence of cough and phlegm and parental smoking; OR=1.30 (95% CI=1.05, 1.61) for cough when parents smoked (adjusted for age, gender, ventilation, family history, mother's education, coal use, and area); OR=1.36 (95% CI=1.08, 1.72) for phlegm with parental smoking (adjusted); OR=1.31 (95% CI=0.96, 1.78) for wheeze with parental smoking (adjusted); OR=2.11 (95% CI=0.79, 5.66) for asthma with parental smoking (adjusted)

Table 5.6b. *(continued)*

Reference	Study Design and Population	Outcome	Results
Young et al., 2000[134]	Prospective-cohort study, 253 infants aged <24 months in Australia	Parent-reported or physician-diagnosed wheeze	OR=2.7 (95% CI=1.3, 5.2) for wheeze with maternal smoking
Gupta et al., 2001[135]	Questionnaire-based cross-sectional study, 9090 students (4367 boys, 4723 girls) aged 9–20 years in Chandigarh, India	Asthma	Observed prevalence of asthma 2.6% for boys and 1.9% for girls; SHS exposure was positively associated with asthma, OR=1.78 (95% CI=1.33, 2.31)
Pokharel et al., 200[136]	Case–control study, 40 children identified as cases of bronchial asthma and 80 age- and sex-matched non-asthmatic controls selected from a population of 2000 schoolchildren surveyed with the International Study of Asthma and Allergy in Children questionnaire from five schools in rural Haryana	Asthma	Passive smoking was found to be a significant risk factor associated with asthma symptoms in rural children, OR=3.33 (95% CI=1.85, 7.65)
Salo et al., 2004[137]	Questionnaire-based cross-sectional study, 5051 seventh-grade students from 22 randomly selected schools in Wuhan, China	Cough, phlegm, wheeze	Strong associations between smoking in the home and cough, as well as smoking in the home and phlegm production; OR=1.74 (95% CI=1.17, 2.60) for cough without cold with two or more smokers in the home; OR=2.25 (95% CI=1.36, 3.72) for phlegm without cold with two or more smokers in the home
David et al., 2005[138]	Cohort study of Singaporeans of Chinese ethnicity aged 45 to 74 at enrollment; 35 000 never-smokers interviewed regarding SHS exposure before and after the age of 18	Chronic cough, phlegm, and asthma diagnosis	Living with a smoker before the age of 18 increased the odds of chronic dry cough and phlegm; OR=2.14 (95% CI=1.29, 4.32) for chronic dry cough when living with one or more smokers before the age of 18; OR=1.25 (95% CI=1.02, 1.53) for phlegm when living with one or more smokers before age 18; OR=1.08 (95% CI=0.94, 1.23) for asthma diagnosis when living with one or more smokers before age 18 (adjusted for age, sex, dialect group, and current and past exposure to smokers at home and at work after the age of 18)
Gupta et al., 2006[139]	Population-based study of asthma prevalence in adults in India; 62 109 non-smokers questioned on childhood and adult exposure to SHS at home	Asthma	Asthma prevalence was higher among individuals exposed to SHS than among those not those not exposed to SHS (2.2% vs 1.9%, *P*<0.05); SHS exposure during childhood and during both childhood and adulthood were significantly associated with asthma prevalence; OR=1.69 (95% CI=1.38, 2.07) for asthma with exposure to SHS during both childhood and adulthood
Dong et al., 2007[140]	Questionnaire-based cross-sectional study, 6053 kindergarten-aged children in 15 districts of northern China	Persistent cough, persistent phlegm, asthma symptoms, current asthma, wheeze, and wheeze without asthma	SHS exposure was significantly associated with respiratory symptoms and diseases in childhood; OR=1.54 (95% CI=1.32, 1.80) for persistent cough in children with parental smoking; OR=1.61 (95% CI=1.28, 2.02) for persistent phlegm in children with parental smoking; OR=1.38 (95% CI=1.16, 1.64) for wheeze in children with parental smoking; OR=1.42 (95% CI=1.18, 1.70) for wheeze without asthma in children with parental smoking (adjusted for age, sex, family history of allergy, family history of asthma, body mass index, breastfeeding, parental education, and study district)
Sharma and Bang, 2007[141]	Questionnaire-based cross-sectional study, 8470 schoolchildren, aged 6 to 7 years and 13 to 14 years from 10 villages on the outskirts of Delhi, India, using a Hindi version of the International Study of Asthma and Allergies in Childhood survey	Wheeze	Maternal and paternal smoking are both independently associated with wheeze occurrence; OR=1.9 (95% CI=1.4, 2.6) for wheeze in children exposed to maternal smoking; OR=1.7 (95% CI=1.4, 2.2) for wheeze in children exposed to paternal smoking; OR=2.0 (95% CI=1.1, 3.5) for wheeze in children exposed to maternal smoking during infancy

Adverse Effects of SHS Exposure on Children

The first epidemiological studies of SHS focused on respiratory effects. In its 1999 consultation, WHO concurred with other reviewing bodies about the effects of SHS on children (Table 5.5). Exposure to SHS was found to be a cause of slightly reduced birth weight, lower respiratory tract illnesses, chronic respiratory symptoms, middle-ear disease, and reduced lung function. Maternal smoking was characterized as a major cause of sudden infant death syndrome (SIDS), but there was inconclusive evidence on the risk from postnatal exposure to SHS. The conclusions of reports from the California EPA and the United Kingdom's Scientific Committee on Tobacco were similar (Table 5.5), and subsequent reports have identified additional adverse effects (Table 5.5). The individual effects are considered briefly below.

> *SHS exposure from either maternal or paternal smoking may lead to postnatal health effects, including increased risk for SIDS, reduced physical development, decrements in cognition and behaviour, and increased risk for childhood cancers.*

Researchers have demonstrated that active smoking by mothers results in a variety of adverse health effects on children, postulated to result predominantly from transplacental exposure of the fetus to tobacco smoke components. Maternal smoking reduces birth weight substantially[142] and increases risk for SIDS, an association considered causal in the 1999 WHO consultation and the 2004 US Surgeon General's report.[143] Exposure to SHS by non-smoking mothers is associated with reduced birth weight as well, although the reduction is far less than that resulting from active maternal smoking during pregnancy. In a 1999 meta-analysis, the reduction of birth weight associated with paternal smoking was estimated to be only 28 g.[144] One study found that 70% of urban pregnant

women in South Africa lived with at least one smoker, and approximately 8% to 9% of them actually thought that SHS and active smoking were either good for their health or had no effect on their health or that of their babies.[46]

Postnatal health effects on children resulting from either fetal SHS exposure or exposure of newborns include SIDS and adverse effects on neuropsychological development and physical growth. A number of components of SHS, including nicotine and carbon monoxide, may produce these effects. The evidence accumulated by the time of the 2006 US Surgeon General's report was found sufficient to reinforce the conclusion that SHS exposure is a cause of SIDS[9] (Table 5.5). The 2005 California EPA report also concluded that a causal relationship exists between SHS exposure and SIDS. The reports noted not only the epidemiological evidence, but findings of animal models that indicate potential mechanisms. The California EPA report estimates that 10% of SIDS deaths are attributable to SHS exposure.

Possible longer-term health effects of fetal SHS exposure include increased risk for childhood cancers of the brain, leukaemia, and lymphomas. A 2000 meta-analysis of the evidence on childhood cancer through the time of the 1999 consultation, subsequently reported elsewhere, did not show a significant association of SHS exposure with overall risk for childhood cancer or leukaemia.[145]

Non-fatal perinatal health effects of maternal smoking include reduced fetal growth, growth retardation, and congenital abnormalities. In most studies of non-fatal perinatal health effects of SHS, paternal smoking has been used as the exposure measure. Low birth weight was first reported in 1957 to be associated with maternal cigarette smoking during pregnancy,[146] and the association is now considered to be causal.[8,9]

Martin and Bracken demonstrated a strong association between maternal smoking and growth retardation in their 1986 study,[147] and several more-recent studies provide support for their findings.[148,149] The few studies conducted to assess the association between paternal smoking and congenital malformations [70,150,151] have demonstrated risks for exposed children ranging from 1.2 to 2.6 times that for non-exposed children. The most consistent associations are with the central nervous system and neural tube defects. However, because active

World Health Organization

smoking may have effects on sperm, we cannot infer a causal association between SHS from paternal smoking and congenital malformations of children.[9]

SHS exposure from either maternal or paternal smoking may also lead to decrements in cognition and behaviour and increased risk for childhood cancers. However, evidence on cognition and behaviour is limited and is not considered in this review.

Maternal smoking during pregnancy has been causally associated with SIDS (the unexpected death of a seemingly healthy infant while asleep), but the studies measured maternal smoking after pregnancy, along with paternal smoking and household smoking generally. Effects of SHS exposure after birth and maternal smoking during pregnancy cannot be readily separated in many of these studies, but SHS exposure from paternal smoking alone may not have the complicating consequences of maternal smoking during pregnancy.

SHS exposure has also been evaluated as a risk factor for the major childhood cancers. The evidence is limited and does not yet support conclusions about the causality of the observed associations. However, in a meta-analysis conducted for the 1999 WHO consultation and subsequently published elsewhere,[145] the pooled estimate of the relative risk for any childhood cancer associated with maternal smoking was 1.11 (95% confidence interval (CI) = 1.00, 1.23), and that for leukaemia was 1.14 (95% CI = 0.97, 1.33).[9] This meta-analysis was updated for a 2004 IARC monograph,[7] and the estimates showed no statistically significant associations for all lymphatic and haematopoietic neoplasms (relative risk (RR) = 1.0, 95% CI = 0.9, 1.2), for non-Hodgkins lymphoma or total lymphomas (RR = 1.1, 95% CI = 0.9, 1.5), or for all leukaemias, acute leukaemia, or acute lymphocytic leukaemia (RR = 1.1, 95% CI = 0.8, 1.3). The 2006 US Surgeon General's report found the evidence on SHS and childhood cancer to be suggestive of a possible causal association.[9]

Lower respiratory tract illnesses, including bronchitis and pneumonia, are extremely common during childhood. Studies of involuntary smoking and lower respiratory illnesses in childhood, including the more severe illnesses bronchitis and pneumonia, provided some of the earliest evidence on the adverse effects of SHS.[152,153] This association presumably represents an increase in frequency or severity of illnesses that are infectious in

etiology and not a direct response of the lung to the toxic components of SHS. Investigations conducted throughout the world have demonstrated an increased risk of lower respiratory tract illness in infants whose parents smoke.[8,9] These studies also indicate a significantly increased frequency of bronchitis and pneumonia during the first year of life in children whose parents smoke. The 2006 US Surgeon General's report[9] includes a quantitative review of this information, combining data from more than 50 studies. Overall, the approximate increase in risk of illness if either parent smokes is 50%; the risk is slightly higher with maternal smoking. More data are needed concerning differences between male and female children.

Although the health outcome measures vary somewhat among the studies, the relative risks associated with involuntary smoking are similar, and dose-response relations with extent of parental smoking are demonstrable. Although most of the studies have shown that maternal smoking underlies most of the increased risk of parental smoking, studies from China show that paternal smoking alone can increase incidence of lower respiratory illness.[154,155] These studies do not readily identify an effect of SHS after the child's first year of life, and during the first year of life the strength of the effect may reflect higher exposures resulting from the time-activity patterns of young infants, which place them in proximity to cigarettes smoked by their mothers.

Effects of exposure to tobacco smoke on the airways in utero may also play a role in the risk of lower respiratory illnesses due to postnatal exposure. Infants of mothers who smoke during pregnancy have shown evidence of damage to their airways during gestation on lung function testing shortly after birth, and this damage may increase the likelihood of developing more-severe respiratory infections.[5]

Respiratory Symptoms and Illness in Children

The evidence on the association of respiratory symptoms and illnesses in children with SHS exposure comes from numerous surveys and also from cohort studies. Data from surveys demonstrate a greater frequency of the most common respiratory symptoms—coughing, phlegm, and wheezing—in the children of smokers[8,9,156] (Table 5.7). The subjects of these studies have generally been schoolchildren, and the less prominent effects of SHS, in comparison with those found in the studies of lower respiratory illness in infants, may reflect lower exposures to SHS by older children, who spend less time with their parents.

By the mid-1980s, results from several large studies provided convincing evidence that involuntary exposure to SHS increases the occurrence of cough and phlegm in the children of smokers, although earlier data from smaller studies had been ambiguous. A 1984 study of 10 000 schoolchildren in six US communities (the Harvard Six Cities Study) found that smoking by parents—primarily smoking by mothers—increased the frequency of persistent cough in their children by about 30%.[49] In a survey of 15 709 English children aged 8 to 19 years, the prevalence of frequent cough among non-smoking children was significantly higher if either the father or the mother smoked.[157] The preponderance of the early evidence also indicated an excess of chronic wheezing associated with involuntary smoking. In a survey of 650 schoolchildren in Boston, one of the first studies on this association, persistent wheezing was the most frequent symptom;[158] the prevalence of persistent wheezing increased significantly as the number of smoking parents increased. In the Six Cities Study, the prevalence of persistent wheezing during the previous year was significantly higher if the mother smoked.[49]

Although involuntary exposure to tobacco smoke has been associated with wheezing, evidence for association with childhood asthma was initially conflicting. Exposure to

SHS might cause asthma as a long-term consequence of the increased occurrence of lower respiratory infection in early childhood or through other pathophysiological mechanisms, including inflammation of the respiratory epithelium.[9,159] The effect of SHS may also reflect, in part, the consequences of in utero exposure. Assessment of airway responsiveness shortly after birth has shown that infants whose mothers smoke during pregnancy have greater airway responsiveness than that of infants whose mothers do not smoke.[9] Maternal smoking during pregnancy also reduces ventilatory function measured shortly after birth.[160] These observations suggest that in utero exposure from maternal smoking may affect lung development, perhaps reducing airway size. Additionally, childhood asthma is considered to have a strong genetic basis, and SHS exposure may increase or hasten incidence in a genetically predisposed subgroup of the population.

While the underlying mechanisms remain to be fully characterized, the epidemiological evidence linking SHS exposure and childhood asthma is substantial.[8,9,161] The 2006 US Surgeon General's report[9] provides a full review of the evidence, including the large number of cross-sectional studies and the smaller number of cohort studies. The cross-sectional studies cannot directly address SHS exposure as a cause of asthma onset, because the existence of prevalent asthma reflects both incidence and maintenance of the asthmatic condition. Nonetheless, the prevalence studies provide firm evidence that prevalent asthma is associated with SHS exposure at home. The report considered 41 cross-sectional studies that included quantitative risk information. Overall, if either parent

Table 5.7. Summary of Pooled Random-Effects Odds Ratios with 95% Confidence Intervals

Effect	Either Parent Smokes			One Parent Smokes			Both Parents Smoke			Only Mother Smokes			Only Father Smokes		
	OR	95% CI	n	OR	95% CI	n	OR	95% CI	n	OR	95% CI	n	OR	95% CI	n
Asthma	1.21	1.10–1.34	21	1.04	0.78–1.38	6	1.50	1.29–1.73	8	1.36	1.20–1.55	11	1.07	0.92–1.24	9
Wheeze	1.24	1.17–1.31	30	1.18	1.08–1.29	21	1.47	1.14–1.90	11	1.28	1.19–1.38	18	1.14	1.06–1.23	10
Cough	1.40	1.27–1.53	30	1.29	1.11–1.51	15	1.67	1.48–1.89	16	1.40	1.20–1.64	14	1.21	1.09–1.34	9
Phlegm	1.35	1.13–1.62	6	1.25	0.97–1.63	5	1.46	1.04–2.05	5						
Breathlessness	1.31	1.08–1.59	6												

Source: Ref. 156.

smoked, the pooled odds ratio was 1.23, compared with the odds if neither smoked. Household exposure to SHS was also associated with wheezing. The evidence was judged to be sufficient to infer a causal relationship between parental smoking and ever having asthma.[9]

The report separately reviewed the seven cohort studies that addressed asthma incidence, as well as 21 case–control studies. Interpretation of the cohort-study findings is complicated by the array of outcome measures and the heterogeneity of effect by age of the children. The quantitative meta-analysis yielded a pooled odds ratio of 1.31, statistically significant, for children during the first 5 to 7 years of life; for children in the school years, the estimate was only 1.13. The case–control studies of prevalent asthma showed a 40% increase in association with smoking by either parent, a 50% increase for maternal smoking, but no increase for paternal smoking. Acknowledging the complexities of interpreting the cohort data, the 2006 report concluded that the evidence was suggestive, but not sufficient to infer a causal relationship between SHS exposure from parental smoking and onset of childhood asthma. The report also noted that SHS exposure can exacerbate childhood asthma.[9]

During childhood, lung function increases more or less in parallel with increase in height. On the basis of the primarily cross-sectional data available at the time, the 1984 report of the US Surgeon General[162] concluded that the children of parents who smoked had somewhat reduced lung function in comparison with children of non-smokers, but the long-term consequences of the reduction were regarded as unknown. On the basis of further longitudinal evidence, the 1986 report[10] concluded that involuntary smoking reduces the rate of lung function growth during childhood. Evidence from cohort studies has continued to accumulate.[8] The WHO consultation noted the difficulty of separating the effects of in utero SHS exposure from those of childhood exposure, because most mothers who smoke while pregnant continue to do so after the children are born.[3]

Meta-analyses of the cross-sectional data provide an indication of the magnitude of the effect of SHS exposure on lung function.[9,163] The 2006 US Surgeon General's report pooled 26 studies and found that the effect of SHS exposure was greatest for flow measures (the mid-expiratory and end-expiratory flow rates), approximately 4% to 5%, and less for the forced expiratory volume in one second (FEV1), approximately 1%. The effect of SHS exposure was greatest

if both parents smoked and was robust to adjustment for potential confounding factors.

In summary, the cohort studies show that lung function during childhood is adversely affected by maternal smoking during pregnancy and further impaired by exposure after birth. Studies of lung function shortly after birth show increased airway resistance and airway responsiveness in children exposed in utero.[9] These in utero effects appear to have implications for later lung growth and development.

The first major epidemiological studies on SHS and lung cancer were reported in 1981. Hirayama reported on a prospective-cohort study of 91 540 non-smoking women in Japan, which found that standardized mortality ratios for lung cancer increased significantly with the amount smoked by their husbands.

Other Effects

Numerous studies have addressed SHS exposure and middle-ear disease in children. Positive associations between SHS and otitis media have been consistently demonstrated in prospective-cohort studies, but not as consistently in case–control studies. This difference in findings may reflect the focus of the cohort studies on the first two years of life, the peak age of risk for middle-ear disease. The case–control studies have been directed at older children, who are at lower risk for otitis media. Exposure to SHS has been most consistently associated with recurrent otitis media, not with incident or single episodes. In their 1997 meta-analysis, Cook and Strachan[156] found a pooled odds ratio of 1.48 (95% CI = 1.08, 2.04) for recurrent otitis media if either parent smoked, 1.38 (95% CI = 1.23, 1.55) for middle-ear effusions, and 1.21 (95% CI = 0.95,

1.53) for outpatient or inpatient care for chronic otitis media, or "glue ear".

The 2006 US Surgeon General's report considered 61 reports based on 59 studies and updated the 1997 meta-analysis, covering multiple outcomes, including acute and recurrent otitis media, middle-ear disease, and adenotonsillectomy. The evidence was sufficient to infer a causal relationship between parental smoking and middle-ear disease in children, including acute and recurrent otitis media and chronic middle-ear effusion. The evidence was inadequate to infer the presence or absence of a causal relationship between parental smoking and an increased risk of adenoidectomy or tonsillectomy.[9]

Health Effects of SHS Exposure on Adults

In 1981, reports from Japan[164] and Greece[165] indicated increased risk of lung cancer in non-smoking women who were married to cigarette smokers. Subsequently, the association of SHS with lung cancer risk in never-smokers has been examined in more than 50 investigations conducted in the United States and other countries, including China. A causal association between involuntary smoking and lung cancer derives biological plausibility from the presence of carcinogens in sidestream smoke and the lack of a documented threshold dose for respiratory carcinogenesis in active smokers.[10,77] Moreover, genotoxic activity—the ability to damage DNA—has been demonstrated for many components of SHS.[166–168] Experimental and real-world exposure of non-smokers to SHS led to their excreting 4-(methylnitrosamino)-1-(3-pyridyl)-1-butanol (NNAL), a tobacco-specific carcinogen, in their urine.[169,170] Non-smokers, including children, exposed to SHS also have increased concentrations of adducts of tobacco-related carcinogens, such as detectable binding of the carcinogens to DNA of white blood cells.[171,172] Mauderly et al., using an animal model, found that whole-body exposure of rats to cigarette smoke increases the risk of neoplastic proliferative lung lesions and induces lung cancer.[173]

The first major epidemiological studies on SHS and lung cancer were reported in 1981. Hirayama[164] reported on a prospective-cohort study of 91 540 non-smoking women in Japan, which found that standardized mortality ratios for lung cancer increased significantly with the amount smoked by the women's husbands. The findings could not be explained by confounding factors and were unchanged when follow-up of the study group was extended.[174] On the basis of the same cohort, Hirayama also reported significantly increased risk for non-smoking men married to women who smoked 1 to 19 cigarettes and 20 or more cigarettes daily.[174] In 1981, Trichopoulos et al.[165] also reported increased lung cancer risk in non-smoking women married to cigarette smokers. These investigators conducted a case–control study in Athens, Greece, which included cases of adenocarcinoma and controls. The positive findings reported in 1981 were unchanged with subsequent expansion of the study population and consideration of diet.[175] By 1986, the evidence had mounted, and the three synthesis reports published in that year concluded that SHS was a cause of lung cancer.[10,73,77]

In 1992, the US EPA[74] published its risk assessment of SHS as a carcinogen. The agency's evaluation drew on the toxicological evidence on SHS and the extensive literature on active smoking. A meta-analysis of the 31 studies published to that time was central to the decision to classify SHS as a Group A carcinogen, i.e. a known human carcinogen. The meta-analysis considered the data from the epidemiological studies by tiers of study quality and location and used an adjustment method for misclassification of smokers as never-smokers. Overall, the analysis found a significantly increased risk of lung cancer in never-smoking women married to smoking men; in the studies conducted in the United States, the estimated relative risk was 1.19 (90% CI = 1.04, 1.35).

The meta-analysis included pooled estimates by geographical region. The data from China and Hong Kong SAR were notable for not showing the increased risk associated with SHS that was found in other regions. The epidemiological characteristics of lung cancer in women in this region of the world have been distinct, with a relatively high proportion of lung cancers in non-smoking women. Explanations for this pattern have centred on exposures to cooking fumes and indoor air pollution from coal-fuelled space heating.

Hackshaw et al. carried out a comprehensive meta-analysis in 1997,[176] which included 37 published studies. They estimated the excess risk of lung cancer for smokers married to non-smokers as 24% (95% CI = 13%, 36%). Adjustment for potential bias and confounding by diet did not alter the estimate. This meta-analysis was part of the basis for the conclusion by the UK Scientific Committee on Tobacco and Health[6] that SHS is a cause of lung cancer. A subsequent IARC meta-analysis[7] that included 46 studies and 6257 cases yielded similar results: 24% (95% CI = 14%, 34%). Incorporating the results from a cohort study with null results overall but only 177 cases[177] did not change the findings.[178]

In 1998, Repace et al.[179] developed a model of workers' risk of lung cancer and heart disease arising from SHS exposure. The pharmacokinetics model incorporated nicotine as an indicator of exposure and cotinine as a measure of dose. It estimated that 400 lung cancer deaths result annually from workplace SHS exposure, with a smoking prevalence rate of 28% among people in the workplace. The California EPA estimates that at least 3423, and perhaps as many as 8866, lung cancer deaths were caused by SHS across the United States in 2003. Of the 3423 deaths, 967 were caused by non-spousal exposures to SHS, and 2456 were caused by spousal exposure.[8] These US estimates imply a substantial burden of lung cancer in never-smoking women around the world from SHS exposure.

Causal associations have long been demonstrated between active smoking and fatal and non-fatal coronary heart disease (CHD).[180] The risk of CHD in active smokers increases with the amount and duration of cigarette smoking and decreases relatively quickly with cessation. Active cigarette smoking is considered to (1) increase the risk of cardiovascular disease by promoting atherosclerosis; (2) increase the tendency to thrombosis; (3) cause spasm of the coronary arteries; (4) increase the likelihood of cardiac arrhythmias; and (5) decrease the oxygen-carrying capacity of the blood.[180] The 2006 US Surgeon General's report[9] summarized the pathophysiological mechanisms by which SHS might increase the risk of heart disease. It is biologically plausible that SHS could also be associated with increased risk for CHD through the same mechanisms considered relevant for active smoking, although the passive smoker's lower exposures to smoke components have raised questions regarding the relevance of those mechanisms.[9]

In 2005, Barnoya and Glantz[181] summarized the pathophysiological mechanisms by which SHS exposure might increase the risk of heart disease. They suggest that SHS, like active smoking, may promote atherogenesis, increase the tendency of platelets to aggregate and thereby

promote thrombosis, impair endothelial cell function, increase arterial stiffness leading to atherosclerosis, reduce the oxygen-carrying capacity of the blood, and alter myocardial metabolism. In a 2004 study, Rubenstein et al. found that sidestream smoke was 50% more potent than mainstream smoke in activating platelets.[182] Glantz and Parmley also proposed that carcinogenic agents such as polycyclic aromatic hydrocarbons found in tobacco smoke promote atherogenesis by effects on cell proliferation.[183] Exposure to SHS may also worsen the outcome of an ischaemic event in the heart; animal data have demonstrated that SHS exposure increases cardiac damage following an experimental myocardial infarction.

The American Heart Association's Council on Cardiopulmonary and Critical Care concluded that exposure to SHS both increases the risk of heart disease and is a major preventable cause of CHD and death.

Experiments on rabbits and cockerels have demonstrated that not only does exposure to SHS at doses similar to those of exposure for humans accelerate the growth of atherosclerotic plaques through the increase of lipid deposits, it also induces atherosclerosis. There is impressive and accumulating evidence that SHS can also quickly affect vascular endothelial cell functioning.[184–186] Otsuka et al. found that 30 minutes of exposure to SHS by healthy young volunteers compromised coronary artery endothelial function in a manner that was indistinguishable from that of habitual smokers, suggesting that endothelial dysfunction may be an important mechanism by which exposure to SHS increases risk of CHD.[185]

Epidemiological data in the 1985 report of Garland et al.,[187] based on a cohort study in Southern California, first raised concern that SHS may increase risk for CHD. More than 20 studies, including 11 cohort studies, 12 case–control studies, and one cross-sectional study, have examined the association between exposure to SHS and CHD.[9] These studies assessed both fatal and non-fatal CHD outcomes, and most used self-administered questionnaires to assess SHS exposure. They covered a wide range of populations, both geographically and racially: many were conducted within the United States, and others were conducted in Europe (Scotland, Italy, and the United Kingdom), Asia (Japan and China), South America (Argentina), and the South Pacific (Australia and New Zealand). The majority of the studies measured the effect of SHS exposure from spousal smoking; however, some also assessed exposures from smoking by other household members or occurring at work or in transit. Several studies included measurement of exposure biomarkers.

The risk estimates for SHS and CHD outcomes vary in these studies, ranging from null to modest and significant increases in risk, with the risk for fatal outcomes generally higher. In a 1997 meta-analysis, Law et al.[188] estimated the excess risk from SHS exposure to be 30% (95% CI = 22%, 38%) at the age of 65. The American Heart Association's Council on Cardiopulmonary and Critical Care concluded that exposure to SHS both increases the risk of heart disease and is a major preventable cause of CHD and death.[189] This conclusion was echoed in 1998 by the UK Scientific Committee on Tobacco and Health.[6] In 2005, the California EPA[8] concluded that there is an overall risk of 30% for CHD due to exposure to SHS, and the 2006 US Surgeon General's report found that pooled relative risks from meta-analyses indicate a 25% to 30% increase.[9]

Only a few cross-sectional investigations provide information on the association between respiratory symptoms in non-smokers and involuntary exposure to tobacco smoke. These studies have primarily considered exposure outside the home. Consistent evidence has been found of an effect of SHS exposure on acute respiratory symptoms in adults. Analysis of National Health Interview Survey data showed that a pack-a-day smoker increases respiratory-restricted days for a non-smoking spouse by about 20%.[190] After results for personal smoking were controlled, a study of determinants of daily respiratory symptoms in student nurses in Los Angeles showed that a smoking room-mate significantly increased the risk of an episode of phlegm.[191] Consistent evidence of an effect of SHS exposure on chronic respiratory symptoms in adults has not been found. Overall, symptoms of chronic cough and dyspnea have been more consistently associated with exposure to SHS than have the symptoms of chronic phlegm and wheezing.[9]

Neither epidemiological nor experimental studies have firmly established the role of SHS in exacerbating asthma in adults.[192] The acute responses of asthmatics to SHS have been assessed by exposing subjects to tobacco smoke in a chamber. This experimental approach cannot be readily controlled, because of the impossibility of blinding subjects to exposure to SHS. However, suggestibility does not appear to underlie physiological responses of asthmatics to SHS.[193]

A 2003 population-based case–control study by Jaakkola et al.[194] investigated the association between SHS exposure and the onset of adult asthma in the Pirkanmaa district of Finland. The researchers recruited all incident cases of asthma in the district and selected population-based controls. After excluding current or previous smokers, they had 239 lifetime non-smoking cases and a comparison group of 487 lifetime non-smoking controls. They found that the risk of asthma among those exposed to SHS in the home and the workplace was twice as high as the risk among those who were not exposed.

The 2006 US Surgeon General's report concluded that the evidence is suggestive but not sufficient to infer a causal relationship between SHS exposure and adult-onset asthma or a worsening of asthma control.[9]

With regard to involuntary smoking and lung function in adults, SHS exposure has been associated in cross-sectional investigations with reduction of several lung function measures. However, the findings have not been consistent, and methodological issues constrain interpretation of them. The 2006 US Surgeon General's report states that the evidence is suggestive but not sufficient to infer a causal association in the effects of SHS exposure on lung function in adults.[9] However, further research is warranted, because of widespread exposure in workplaces and homes.

Interventions to Control SHS Exposure

The scientific evidence on adverse health effects of smoking and SHS exposure provides a strong rationale for the development of tobacco control measures. Since the publication of the first studies linking tobacco use to specific diseases, a number of measures to reduce tobacco use have been promoted, both nationally and internationally.[195,196] In 1970, the World Health Assembly adopted its first resolution related to tobacco, WHA23.32, and the Health Assembly has since adopted 20 resolutions related to tobacco control. In the 1970 resolution text, the Twenty-third World Health Assembly requested that the Director-General of WHO promote the issue of tobacco to all Member States and initiate a number of control measures, including a review of educational methods to prevent smoking initiation among youth, assembling an expert group to recommend actions to discourage smoking, and making the health consequences of smoking the topic of a future World Health Day. Eight years later, the Thirty-first World Health Assembly adopted resolution WHA31.56, the first resolution to include text related to the protection of the rights of non-smokers. In it, the Health Assembly urged Member States to adopt wide-ranging tobacco control measures to "protect the rights of non-smokers to enjoy an atmosphere unpolluted by tobacco smoke".[197]

Further support for measures protecting non-smokers from SHS exposure came in 1986, in the conclusions on disease causation reached by the US Surgeon General in *The Health Consequences of Involuntary Smoking,*[10] the US National Research Council,[73] and the IARC.[77] Accordingly, the Thirty-ninth World Health Assembly adopted the first resolution that provided recommendations related to SHS. In the final text, the Health Assembly proposed a comprehensive tobacco control strategy for Member States, the first element of which pertained to the protection of non-smokers from exposure to tobacco smoke in public places, workplaces, restaurants, transport, and entertainment venues.[197] Finally, in 1996, the Health Assembly adopted resolution WHA49.17, which requested the Director-General of WHO to develop the WHO Framework Convention on Tobacco Control (WHO FCTC). In 2003, the Fifty-sixth World Health Assembly unanimously adopted this global treaty for tobacco control.[198] Article 8 of the WHO FCTC, *Protection from exposure to tobacco smoke,* calls for legislation to protect non-smokers from exposure to tobacco smoke and requires the more than 170 Parties to implement smoking restrictions in public places.[199] The 2006 US Surgeon General's report provided further evidence of the disease causation of SHS exposure. The report concluded that there is no risk-free level of exposure to SHS and that even brief exposure can cause harm.[9] Noting the harms of SHS as demonstrated

in reports like this one, the Parties to the WHO FCTC adopted guidelines for implementing Article 8 in 2007. These guidelines include direction for Parties to provide universal protection from tobacco smoke in all indoor public places, indoor workplaces, and public transportation. The listed recommendations include raising public awareness and support, adopting necessary legislative measures, and monitoring the enforcement and impact of such measures.

> *Women around the world may be disproportionately affected by SHS exposure if they spend most of their time with a smoker in the home. In addition, in many countries, gender differences in power may prevent women from requesting that male smokers refrain from smoking around them.*

The WHO FCTC has prompted many countries to implement smoking bans in public places and workplaces to protect the health of non-smokers. These initiatives are a necessary but only partial step towards fully protecting non-smokers from SHS, as adults and children spend a great deal of time in their homes, an environment beyond the reach of regulation. Women and children cannot be fully protected from inhaling SHS, and separating smokers from non-smokers in the same air space, cleaning the air, and increasing ventilation are inadequate for protecting against SHS exposure.[9]

Target Populations

All non-smokers are vulnerable to the adverse effects of SHS exposure and therefore deserve the right to protection against it. In this chapter, however, we focus on two subgroups, women and children, as they are heavily exposed to SHS in many countries and are particularly susceptible.

Women may be susceptible to the adverse health effects of SHS exposure in part because of substantial exposure at home. Women around the world may be disproportionately affected by SHS exposure if they spend most of their time with a smoker in the home. In addition, in many countries, gender differences in power relations may prevent women from requesting that male smokers refrain from smoking around them.

Children and infants are particularly susceptible to the adverse effects of SHS. Children inhale more of the toxic chemicals in smoke per unit body weight than adults do because they breathe faster and are generally more physically active. They may also be less able to metabolize and excrete certain toxic components of SHS, so these components remain in the body for longer periods of time. In addition, unlike adults, infants and children may not be able to remove themselves from smoky places or to voice complaints about SHS exposure.

Some subgroups may have particular susceptibility because of underlying chronic conditions. Women and children with asthma are especially at risk when exposed to SHS, because SHS is an asthma irritant and a leading trigger for asthma episodes.[200] Worldwide, asthma is the most common chronic disease of childhood. The International Study of Asthma and Allergies in Childhood (ISAAC) estimated that asthma prevalence rates range from 5% to 15% in Asian countries,[201] and the US EPA estimates that each year, between 200 000 and 1 million children with asthma in the United States have their condition worsened by SHS exposure.[202]

Table 5.8. Strategies for Prevention of SHS Exposure of Women and Children

Location	Intervention Strategy	
	Community Level	**Individual Level**
Public places and workplaces	Create laws that require all public places to be 100% smoke-free, completely banning smoking in public environments	• Volunteer to monitor and advise smokers not to smoke in enclosed areas • Teach children and adolescents the adverse effects of smoking to prevent smoking initiation • Help smokers quit
Home	Mass-media campaigns about the dangers of SHS exposure to children, the importance of the home as an environment of exposure, and making homes smoke-free. Place health warnings on tobacco packages describing the dangers of SHS exposure to children and adults using a gender-specific approach Incorporate smoking cessation techniques as part of medical training or continuing education to increase clinical counselling on cessation and SHS exposure	• Teach fathers and pregnant women the risk of SHS exposure to children • Show parents how to ask smokers in the family or visitors not to smoke in the house, especially in the presence of children or pregnant women • Health-care providers should enquire about tobacco use in the home, counsel and educate parents and guardians on the adverse health effects of SHS exposure, and provide guidance on means of smoking cessation • Empower women on how to "win" smoke-free homes
Vehicles	Create legislation to ban smoking of tobacco products in vehicles carrying children	• Teach fathers as well as mothers the risk of SHS exposure to children • Teach parents how to ask smokers in the family or visitors not to smoke in the vehicle, especially in the presence of children or pregnant women
Child-care settings/schools	Create legislation that requires all educational, school, and child-care facilities to be 100% smoke-free, completely banning smoking in these facilities	• Teach fathers as well as mothers the risk of SHS exposure to children • Teach child-care providers and schoolteachers about the risk of SHS exposure to children

World Health Organization

Models and Strategies for Intervention

Interventions to protect women and children from the adverse effects of SHS exposure should be developed that target both the locations where they spend time and the groups they are in contact with. The ultimate goal is to create 100% smoke-free environments in the places where women and children live, work, and play, including public places, workplaces, homes, vehicles, child-care settings, and schools. The home is a key micro-environment for children's exposure to SHS, as are vehicles, public places, and schools. The home is a key exposure environment for women as well, and the workplace, transportation environments, and public places are also locations for SHS exposure for women in the workforce. Parents, smoking family members, and smoking spouses, particularly fathers and husbands in Asian countries, are critical targets for interventions, along with others who are in frequent contact with children, including teachers and child-care providers.

Programmes and interventions aimed at influencing health behaviour are most likely to be successful when they are based on a behaviour-change theory. The research and evidence on effective health education and behaviour-change strategies continues to grow, and models and theories continue to evolve. Recently, increasing emphasis is being placed on developing, implementing, and disseminating evidence-based interventions. Current theories of behaviour change can be classified into three broad groups based on their targets: intrapersonal (individual), interpersonal, and community.[203] This framework is useful for categorizing, developing, and understanding interventions aimed at reducing SHS exposure of women and children.

Intrapersonal or individual-level theories focus on the influence of an individual's knowledge, attitudes, beliefs, prior experience, and personality on his or her behaviour. These theories address thoughts, perception, and motivation. Interpersonal-level theories focus on the influence of relationships with other people, such as family, friends, neighbours, or co-workers, on the individual's behaviour. These theories address social norms and social influence. Intrapersonal- and interpersonal-level theories are sometimes referred to together as individual-level theories. Community-level theories focus on the role of organizational settings (schools, churches, workplaces, health-care settings, community groups, and governmental agencies), social and health policies, societal influences, and communities in influencing behaviour. These theories address community mobilization and organizational change. They can guide organization-wide and community-wide health-promotion and education interventions. They complement individually oriented behaviour-change interventions through policy development, sanctions, and shifting community norms.[203]

This framework of behaviour-change theories can be used to inform interventions to reduce or eliminate SHS exposure. A multilevel-intervention approach aimed at both the individual and community levels is needed to reduce SHS exposure of women and children. Table 5.8 lists intervention strategies aimed at these levels. At the community level, intervention strategies such as smoke-free policies are used to influence community norms regarding the acceptability of smoking in the home, workplace, public places, and vehicles, particularly in the presence of children. At the individual level, intervention strategies are used to modify the knowledge, attitudes, and beliefs of individual smokers and non-smokers concerning the dangers of smoking and SHS.

Community-level programmes can use existing social structures such as policy and mass media to reduce SHS exposure of women and children. For areas within the realm of government regulation—public places, workplaces, child-care settings, and schools—smoke-free environments should be mandated by law. Legislation should include methods for implementation and enforcement and penalties for violations. Governments should partner with civil society to raise awareness of the risks of SHS exposure to create an environment for successful implementation.[76] If governments do not take action, nongovernmental agencies and advocates should push the legislative process. Mass media should be used to increase compliance and change public attitudes, publicize legislation, and disseminate information on the health effects of SHS exposure.[204] Messages should be strong, clear, and consistent.[76] Finally, legislation enforcement and impact should be monitored, evaluated, and documented.[198]

For areas outside the reach of government regulation, governmental and nongovernmental agencies should work together to implement educational strategies aimed at encouraging voluntary smoke-free policies.[76] Educational campaigns should be created to disseminate

Table 5.9. Regulation of Smoke-Free Environments in WHO Member States in the South-East Asia and Western Pacific Regions

Country	Health-care Facilities	Educational Facilities	Universities	Government Facilities	Indoor Offices	Restaurants	Pubs and Bars	Other transportation	All Other Indoor Public Places	Overall Compliance With Regulations on Smoke-Free Environments[a]
South-East Asia Region										
Bangladesh	Yes	Yes	No	No	No	No	No	No	No	4
Bhutan	Yes	Yes	Yes	Yes	Yes	Yes	Yes	Yes	Yes	7
Democratic People's Republic of Korea	No	No	No	No	No	No	No	No	No	—
India	Yes	Yes	Yes	Yes	Yes	No	No	No	Yes	5
Indonesia	Yes	Yes	Yes	No	No	No	No	No	No	0
Maldives	Yes	Yes	Yes	Yes	No	No	...	No	No	3
Myanmar	Yes	Yes	Yes	No	No	No	No	No	No	3
Nepal	No	No	No	No	No	No	No	No	No	—
Sri Lanka	Yes	Yes	Yes	Yes	Yes	No	No	Yes	No	8
Thailand	No	Yes	No	No	No	No	No	Yes	Yes	6
Timor-Leste	No	No	No	No	No	No	No	No	No	—
Western Pacific Region										
Australia	No	No	No	No	No	No	No	No	No	—
Brunei Darussalam	Yes	Yes	Yes	No	Yes	Yes	—	Yes	No	5
Cambodia	No	No	No	No	No	No	No	No	No	—
China	No	No	No	No	No	No	No	No	No	—
Cook Islands	No	No	No	No	No	No	No	Yes	No	5
Fiji	Yes	No	No	No	No	No	No	No	Yes	5
Japan	No	No	No	No	No	No	No	No	No	—
Kiribati	No	No	No	No	No	No	No	No	No	—
Lao People's Democratic Republic	Yes	Yes	Yes	No	No	No	No	No	No	7
Malaysia	No	No	No	No	No	No	No	Yes	No	...
Marshall Islands	Yes	Yes	Yes	Yes	Yes	Yes	Yes	Yes	Yes	3
Micronesia (Federated States of)	No	No	No	No	No	No	No	No	No	—
Mongolia	No	No	No	No	No	No	No	No	No	—
Nauru	No	No	No	No	No	No	No	No	No	—
New Zealand	Yes	Yes	Yes	Yes	Yes	Yes	Yes	Yes	Yes	10
Niue	No	No	No	No	No	No	No	No	No	—
Palau	No	No	No	Yes	No	No	No	No	No	7
Papua New Guinea	No	No	No	No	No	No	No	No	No	—
Philippines	Yes	Yes	Yes	No	No	No	No	No	No	3
Republic of Korea	Yes	Yes	No	No	No	No	Yes	Yes	No	6
Samoa	No	No	No	No	No	No	No	No	No	—
Singapore	Yes	Yes	No	No	No	Yes	No	Yes	No	10
Solomon Islands	No	No	No	No	No	No	No	No	No	—
Tonga	No	No	No	Yes	Yes	No	No	No	Yes	7
Tuvalu	No	No	No	No	No	Yes	Yes	Yes	No	5
Vanuatu	No	No	No	No	No	No	No	No	No	—
Viet Nam	Yes	Yes	Yes	Yes	Yes	No	No	Yes	No	1

Source: Ref. 1.

[a] Based on a score of 0–10, where 0 is low compliance. Refer to Ref. 1 for more information.

... Data not reported/not available.

— Data not required/not applicable.

World Health Organization

the dangers of SHS exposure, to stress the importance of the home and vehicles as environments of exposure, and to encourage individuals to make homes and vehicles smoke-free. Health warnings on tobacco packages describing the dangers of SHS exposure could complement educational campaigns.[76]

Individual-level programmes can use behaviour-change theories, such as counselling, to modify the knowledge, attitudes, and beliefs of the populace. Health-care providers should provide information about the adverse health effects of SHS exposure to patients. Smokers should be aided in cessation and taught methods to modify their smoking patterns around non-smokers. In addition, individuals, particularly women, should be taught techniques to create and maintain tobacco-free environments. Finally, interventions should be developed that target special populations such as pregnant women, parents (particularly fathers), guardians, and individuals who work in day-care centres or schools.

Current Interventions

Public places and workplaces. Many countries have begun to implement policies that prohibit or restrict smoking in public places and workplaces. More than 170 Parties have ratified the WHO FCTC, which requires them to protect all people from exposure to tobacco smoke in most public places and on public transport.[199]

Some laws prohibit smoking in many or most public places but allow for smoking rooms or make exceptions, while others prohibit smoking in all enclosed public places, with no exceptions. Some laws are implemented at the national level, while others are implemented at the local or regional level.

On 29 March 2004, Ireland became the first country to implement legislation to make 100% of enclosed workplaces, including restaurants and bars, smoke-free. Since then, several countries, including the United Kingdom, New Zealand, Uruguay, Bermuda, Bhutan, and the Islamic Republic of Iran, have enacted 100% smoke-free laws.[205] Other jurisdictions around the world have enacted similar legislation at the local or regional levels. The United States, for example, does not have a federal policy requiring smoke-free public places, but policies have been developed at the state and local

levels. In 1998, California became the first US state to legislate 100% smoke-free public places; since then, 17 states and multiple municipalities have implemented such legislation.[205] Territories in Canada and Australia have implemented legislation mandating 100% smoke-free public places at the regional level,[205] and many other countries and jurisdictions are making progress towards enacting similar legislation.

The actions in the countries of the South-East Asia and Western Pacific Regions are listed in Table 5.9. National regulations are rapidly changing, and most of the countries in these regions have passed legislation related to controlling SHS exposure, to different extents. Overall, however, the majority of jurisdictions in these countries are without such legislation, leaving women and children vulnerable to SHS exposure in public places.

Studies have found that smoke-free legislation is associated with increased cessation, improved health benefits, and decreased SHS exposure. A review of 26 studies conducted in the United States, Australia, Canada, and Germany found that smoke-free workplaces were associated with a 3.8% reduction in the prevalence of smoking and lower daily cigarette consumption (3.1 fewer cigarettes per day).[206] A study in Pueblo City, Colorado, found that a citywide smoke-free ordinance was associated with a reduction in rates of acute myocardial infarction.[207] Similarly, a study of bar workers in Scotland before and after the implementation of smoke-free legislation found that the legislation was associated with improvements in respiratory symptoms and pulmonary function.[208] Finally, another study in Scotland measuring salivary cotinine levels in schoolchildren before and after the implementation of smoke-free legislation found that the overall average concentration decreased by 39% (from 0.36 ng/mg to 0.22 ng/mg) after smoke-free legislation was put in place. This decrease, however, was significant only among children living in households with lower SHS exposure. Average cotinine concentrations in children living in households with non-smoking parents dropped significantly, by 51%, but average concentrations in children living in households where both parents smoked or only the mother smoked decreased by only 11%, a decrease that was not statistically significant.[209] Smoke-free laws not only provide protection from SHS exposure and lead to improved health, they also help shift the social norms concerning smoking.

World Health Organization

Homes. Because the home is generally considered outside the realm of government regulation, and in many cultures it may not be acceptable for a woman to ask her partner or another male to refrain from smoking in the home, many public health and tobacco control organizations have begun to implement educational campaigns to reduce SHS exposure in the home. In the United States, two community-level educational campaigns were recently introduced to encourage smoke-free homes and vehicles, the US EPA's national Smoke-Free Homes and Cars Program and the American Legacy Foundation's 2005 "Don't Pass Gas" media campaign.[202,210] Similar interventions are being implemented in countries around the world. WHO launched a community-based intervention that used media campaigns, advocacy, and public events to encourage non-smoking by pregnant women, smoke-free schools, and smoke-free homes.[211] In 2000, Ontario, Canada, launched the community-based education programme Breathing Space: Community Partners for Smoke-Free Homes to provide the public with information on the dangers of SHS and to encourage smoke-free homes.[212] Similarly, the Norwegian Cancer Society has led a public-awareness campaign since 1995 aimed at reducing children's SHS exposure in the home and at day-care facilities.[213] Finally, in July 2007, a local organization in Salford, United Kingdom, implemented a Smoke-Free Homes Promise campaign to raise awareness of the dangers of SHS and to encourage smoke-free homes; by October, 1000 homes had signed the promise.[214] In addition to educational programmes, mass-media campaigns and graphic health warnings on tobacco packaging are used to discourage smoking around children and to encourage smoking cessation.[215]

The child-care setting—both formal child day care and informal arrangements involving family and friends—is a major potential source of SHS exposure for infants and children.

Many individual-level interventions that provide physician office counselling or home-based counselling have been evaluated to examine their effect on SHS exposure. Gehrman and Hovell reviewed 19 community interventions published between 1987 and 2002 aimed at reducing SHS exposure among children.[216] In the physician-based interventions, individual counselling was provided in a clinic setting to inform patients about SHS and to recommend methods to reduce exposure. The home-based interventions provided intensive counselling from a nurse or research assistant during home visits. The researchers found that 11 of the 19 interventions resulted in significant reductions in reported SHS exposure. Most of the studies they reviewed, however, measured self-reported exposure, and of the eight studies that used urinary cotinine concentrations to measure exposure, only one reported significant reductions in cotinine levels. Nevertheless, Gehrman and Hovell suggested that individual-level interventions can be effective in reducing children's exposure to SHS, and they concluded that home-based interventions and those based on a behaviour-change theory appeared to be more effective than physician-based interventions or those not explicitly based on a behaviour-change theory.[216]

Klerman reviewed eight US interventions published between 1990 and 2003, four of which were included in the Gehrman and Hovell review.[217] Klerman grouped the studies into two types of interventions: low-intensity, in which a provider in a clinical setting gave information and educational material with little or no follow-up, and high-intensity, in which individuals trained in smoking cessation provided extended counselling in a clinic or home setting. Most of the studies found that both low-intensity and high-intensity interventions had small but significant effects on maternal smoking and the number of cigarettes smoked in the home.[217] Both of these reviews are limited by the small number of studies on SHS exposure interventions, however, and their conclusions are therefore tentative.[216]

Several studies have evaluated individual-level interventions specifically aimed at reducing SHS exposure among children with asthma. Hovell et al.[218] examined the impact of a series of behavioural counselling sessions designed to decrease SHS exposure of asthmatic children and found a significantly greater reduction in self-reported exposure in the intervention group (79%) than in the control group (34%). In 2001, Wilson et al. examined a behavioural-change-based intervention in which nurses administered counselling and feedback to reduce SHS exposure of children 3 to 12 years of age who had asthma.[219] They found that children in the intervention group were 70% less likely than those in the control group to have more than one asthma-related medical visit in the follow-up year, but found no significant effect on urine cotinine levels. Finally, Hovell et al.[220] found that coaching sessions aimed at reducing SHS exposure of Latino children with asthma resulted in significant reductions in urinary cotinine levels and differences in self-reported exposures between the intervention and control groups.[220] There are few evaluations of intervention from developing countries, and it is unlikely that the practice and experience in industrialized areas can be applied directly to them, because of differences in culture, social norms, and structure. To be successful, interventions should be culture-specific.

Vehicles. Private vehicles have traditionally been considered outside the realm of government smoking bans. Recently, however, jurisdictions have begun to implement community-level policies that ban smoking in vehicles carrying children. Three US states (Arkansas, Louisiana, and California), one US territory (Puerto Rico), and a few US cities have passed such legislation. Similar legislation has also been proposed in a dozen other US states and cities. South Australia and Cyprus have introduced similar legislation, and several other jurisdictions, including Queensland, Australia; New South Wales, Australia; Tasmania, Australia; Nova Scotia, Canada; and South Africa, have considered legislation. The majority of jurisdictions worldwide, however, remain without legislation, leaving children reliant on adults to voluntarily restrict smoking in vehicles. Many community-level education programmes stress the importance of vehicles as locations of SHS exposure, particularly of children, and encourage the adoption of voluntary smoke-free-vehicle rules. Also, many of the individual-level physician- and home-based counselling interventions encourage changes in smoking patterns around non-smokers and smoking cessation, which could increase voluntary cessation of smoking in vehicles.

Child-care settings. The child-care setting— both formal child day care and informal arrangements involving family and friends—is a major potential source of SHS exposure for infants and children. Unlike private homes or vehicles, child-care facilities and schools are within the realm of government regulation; in fact, several countries have already begun to implement policies that prohibit smoking in child-care facilities and

schools. In the United States, both federal and state laws prohibit smoking in educational facilities. The Pro Children Act of 1994 prohibits smoking in schools that receive federal funding from the US Department of Education, including Head Start facilities, kindergartens, and elementary and secondary schools.[9] All but four states in the United States (Kentucky, Mississippi, North Carolina, and Wyoming) have enacted laws that restrict smoking in child-care centres. Some states prohibit smoking in child-care facilities at all times, while others prohibit smoking except in ventilated areas within facilities, and still others restrict smoking to designated areas within facilities. Some state laws explicitly apply to both licensed child-care centres and home-based child-care centres, while others do not.[221]

In Ontario, Canada, the Ontario Tobacco Control Act requires all educational institutions, including licensed child-care facilities, to be smoke-free. This law, however, does not cover child care provided in private homes, leaving children cared for in these settings unprotected against SHS exposure.[212] According to the European Public Health Alliance, several countries in Europe, including Austria, Denmark, the Czech Republic, Estonia, Finland, Hungary, Iceland, Latvia, Portugal, and Slovenia, have legislation that specifically bans smoking in schools and educational facilities. Only Hungary and Iceland, however, have legislation that specifically bans smoking in child-care facilities.[222] As countries begin to implement regulations to make public places and workplaces smoke-free, child-care facilities and schools may fall under the workplace regulations.

The scientific evidence on the health risks associated with exposure to SHS is clear, credible, and indisputable. SHS causes premature death and disease in adults and children who do not smoke.[9] The only way to fully protect women and children from the adverse health effects of SHS exposure is to create 100% smoke-free environments in the places where they live, work, and play. Multilevel interventions based on behaviour-change theories should be developed that target both the specific locations where women and children spend their time and specific groups that are in contact with them. At the community level, intervention strategies such as smoke-free policies, information disseminated by mass media, and education campaigns can be used to shift community norms regarding the social acceptability of smoking in the home, the workplace, public places, and vehicles. At the individual level, intervention strategies such as counselling and education based on behaviour-change theory can be used to modify the knowledge, attitudes, and beliefs of individual smokers and non-smokers regarding the dangers of smoking and SHS. Finally, interventions aimed at reducing SHS exposure should be only one part of national plans for comprehensive tobacco control.

Summary

Many countries have passed legislation banning smoking in public places or workplaces, but for some, the ban applies to very limited locations, and enforcement is variable or ineffective. The Parties to the WHO FCTC have an obligation to implement Article 8, which addresses public places and workplaces but does not address the home. To assure smoke-free homes for women and children, broader efforts are needed. Communicating information about SHS by mass media can be a very effective method, as demonstrated by the US EPA case-study, and this should be promoted in other countries. Community projects to improve individuals' knowledge and skills for conducting interventions on SHS exposure are also useful. Every country needs a comprehensive strategy for intervention against SHS exposure, as well as improvement of individual skills through community outreach and education. Health-care providers should also be involved in efforts to protect children from SHS exposure.

As emphasized in WHO FCTC Article 22, *Cooperation in the scientific, technical, and legal fields and provision of related expertise,* interventions against SHS exposure should be part of national plans for tobacco control. These plans should include legislation, health education, and communication, with the following goals: (1) to prevent children from becoming addicted to tobacco; (2) to implement effective cessation programmes; (3) to progressively eliminate tobacco advertising; (4) to enact financial measures to discourage tobacco consumption; and (5) to reduce exposure to SHS in homes. The success of such interventions has been proven in case-studies of countries with long-standing comprehensive tobacco control policies. Widespread implementation of such policies will result in a substantial reduction in the smoking-caused burden of disease.[223,224]

Recommendations

Public policies to eliminate SHS exposure in public places and workplaces, as recommended by WHO,[76] should be increased and enforced. Among the actions recommended are the following:

1. Remove the source—tobacco smoke—through implementation of 100% smoke-free environments. This is the only effective strategy for reducing exposure to tobacco smoke in indoor environments to safe levels and providing an acceptable level of protection from the dangers of SHS exposure. Ventilation and smoking areas, whether separately ventilated from non-smoking areas or not, do not reduce exposure to a safe level of risk and are not recommended.

2. Enact legislation requiring all indoor workplaces and public places to be 100% smoke-free. Laws should ensure equal protection for all. Voluntary policies are not an acceptable means of providing protection. Under some circumstances, universal, effective protection may require specific quasi-outdoor and outdoor workplaces to be smoke-free.

3. Passing smoke-free legislation is not enough. The proper implementation and adequate enforcement of such legislation require relatively small but critical efforts and means.

4. Implement educational strategies to reduce SHS exposure in the home, recognizing that smoke-free workplace legislation increases the likelihood that both smokers and non-smokers will voluntarily make their homes smoke-free.

In addition, gender-specific measures are needed. These may include:

1. Develop Tobacco-Free Family campaigns at the community level that include the active participation of girls and women as well as boys and men.

2. Include prevention of SHS exposure at a time when prospective parents should be receptive to recognizing the potential for harm to the fetus and to

children such as through Maternal Child Health and family planning projects.

3. Carry out studies to develop and test culturally appropriate interventions for different circumstances that are gender-specific and that recognize the diversity of the population by age, ethnicity, region, and socioeconomic level.

4. Use a gender framework to monitor exposure prevalence levels and trends and the health impacts of SHS exposure to assess the impact of legislation, communication, and interventions.

Control measures for SHS exposure and other tobacco-related policies, including taxation, smoking cessation projects, restrictions on youth access to tobacco, and restrictions on international trade, can work together to prevent a tobacco epidemic among women and reduce tobacco use among men. With this underlying principle in mind, as well as sensitivity to the differing populations receiving messages about the dangers of tobacco exposure, researchers and policy-makers should move forward with implementation of SHS control measures.

References

1. *WHO report on the global tobacco epidemic, 2009: implementing smoke-free environments*. Geneva, World Health Organization, 2009.

2. Shafey O et al. *The tobacco atlas*, 3rd ed. Atlanta, GA, American Cancer Society, 2009.

3. *International Consultation on Environmental Tobacco Smoke (ETS) and Child Health. Consultation report*. Geneva, World Health Organization, 1999.

4. *Women and the tobacco epidemic: challenges for the 21st century*. Geneva, World Health Organization, 2001.

5. Samet JM, Neta GI, Wang SS. Secondhand smoke. In: Lippmann M, ed. *Environmental toxicants: human exposures and their health effects*, 3rd ed. Hoboken, NJ, John Wiley & Sons, Inc., 2009:709–761.

6. UK Department of Health. *Report of the Scientific Committee on Tobacco and Health*. London, The Stationery Office, 1998.

7. *Tobacco smoke and involuntary smoking*. Lyon, International Agency for Research on Cancer, 2004 (IARC Monograph 83).

8. *Proposed identification of environmental tobacco smoke as a toxic air contaminant*. Sacramento, CA, California Environmental Protection Agency, Air Resources Board, 2005.

9. *The health consequences of involuntary exposure to tobacco smoke: a report of the Surgeon General*. Rockville, MD, US Department of Health and Human Services, Centers for Disease Control and Prevention, 2006.

10. US Department of Health and Human Services. *The health consequences of involuntary smoking: a report of the Surgeon General*. Washington, DC, US Government Printing Office, 1986 (DHHS Publication No. (CDC) 87–8398).

11. Jenkins RA, Guerin MR, Tomkins BA. *The chemistry of environmental tobacco smoke: composition and measurement*, 2nd ed. Boca Raton, FL, Lewis Publishers, 2000.

12. Jaakkola MS, Jaakkola JJK. Assessment of exposure to environmental tobacco smoke. *European Respiratory Journal*, 1997, 10:2384–2397.

13. Ott WR. Mathematical models for predicting indoor air quality from smoking activity. *Environmental Health Perspectives*, 1999, 107:375–381.

14. Jenkins RA, Counts RW. Occupational exposure to environmental tobacco smoke: results of two personal exposure studies. *Environmental Health Perspectives*, 1999, 107:341–348.

15. Hammond SK. Exposure of US workers to environmental tobacco smoke. *Environmental Health Perspectives*, 1999, 107:329–340.

16. Benowitz NL. Cotinine as a biomarker of environmental tobacco smoke exposure. *Epidemiologic Reviews*, 1996, 18:188–204.

17. Al Delaimy WK. Hair as a biomarker for exposure to tobacco smoke. *Tobacco Control*, 2002, 11:176–182.

18. *Women and health: today's evidence, tomorrow's agenda*. Geneva, World Health Organization, 2009.

19. Coultas DB at al. Salivary cotinine levels and involuntary tobacco smoke exposure in children and adults in New Mexico. *American Review of Respiratory Disease*, 1987, 136:305–309.

20. Somerville SM, Rona RJ, Chinn S. Passive smoking and respiratory conditions in primary schoolchildren. *Journal of Epidemiology and Community Health*, 1988, 42:105–110.

21. Chilmonczyk BA et al. Environmental tobacco smoke exposure during infancy. *American Journal of Public Health*, 1990, 80:1205–1208.

22. Overpeck MD, Moss AJ. *Children's exposure to environmental cigarette smoke before and after birth*. Hyattsville, MD, US Department of Health and Human Services, 1991.

23. Borland R et al. Protection from environmental tobacco smoke in California: the case for a smoke-free workplace. *Journal of the American Medical Association*, 1992, 268:749–752.

24. Burns D, Pierce JP. *Tobacco use in California 1990–1991*. Sacramento, CA, California Department of Health Services, 1992.

25. Jaakkola N, Ruotsalainen R, Jaakkola JJK. What are the determinants of children's exposure to environmental tobacco smoke at home? *Scandinavian Journal of Social Medicine*, 1994, 22:107–112.

26. Jenkins PL et al. Activity patterns of Californians: use of and proximity to indoor pollutant sources. *Atmospheric Environment*, 1992, 26A:2141–2148.

27. Lum S. *Duration and location of ETS exposure for the California population*. Memorandum to L. Haroun, California Air Resources Board, 1994.

28. Pierce JPEN et al. *Tobacco use in California: an evaluation of the tobacco control program, 1989–1993*. La Jolla, CA, Cancer Prevention and Control, University of California, San Diego, 1994.

29. Pletsch PK. Environmental tobacco smoke exposure among Hispanic women of reproductive age. *Public Health Nursing*, 1994, 11:229–235.

30. Yang G et al. *Smoking and health in China: 1996 national prevalence survey of smoking patterns*. Beijing, China Science and Technology Press, 1996.

31. Pirkle JL et al. Exposure of the US population to environmental tobacco smoke: the Third National Health and Nutrition Examination Survey, 1988 to 1991. *Journal of the American Medical Association*, 1996, 275:1233–1240.

32. Lister SM, Jorm LR. Parental smoking and respiratory illnesses in Australian children aged 0–4 years: ABS 1989–1990 National Health Survey results. *Australian and New Zealand Journal of Public Health*, 1998, 22:781–786.

33. Centers for Disease Control and Prevention (CDC). Secondhand smoke exposure among middle and high school students—Texas, 2001. *Morbidity and Mortality Weekly Report*, 2003, 52:152–154.

34. Gu D et al. Cigarette smoking and exposure to environmental tobacco smoke in China: the international collaborative study of cardiovascular disease in Asia. *American Journal of Public Health*, 2004, 94:1972–1976.

35. Nebot M et al. Exposure to environmental tobacco smoke at work and at home: a population based survey. *Tobacco Control*, 2004, 13:95.

36. Martinez-Donate AP et al. Smoking, exposure to secondhand smoke, and smoking restrictions in Tijuana, Mexico. *Revista Panamericana Salud Pública*, 2005, 18:412–417.

37. Maziak W, Ward KD, Eissenberg T. Measuring exposure to environmental tobacco smoke (ETS): a developing country's perspective. *Preventive Medicina*, 2006, 42:409–414.

38. Pickett MS et al. Smoke-free laws and secondhand smoke exposure in US non-smoking adults, 1999–2002. *Tobacco Control*, 2006, 15:302–307.

39. The GTSS Collaborative Group. A cross country comparison of exposure to secondhand smoke among youth. *Tobacco Control*, 2006, 15 (Suppl. 2):ii4–19.

40. Exposure to secondhand smoke among students aged 13–15 years—worldwide, 2000–2007. *Morbidity and Mortality Weekly Report*, 2007, 56:497–500.

41. Perez-Rios M et al. Exposure to second-hand smoke: a population-based survey in Spain. *European Respiratory Journal*, 2007, 29:818–819.

42. Rudatsikira E et al. Prevalence and correlates of environmental tobacco smoke exposure among adolescents in Mongolia. *Indian Journal of Pediatrics*, 2007, 74:1089–1093.

43. Twose J et al. Correlates of exposure to second-hand smoke in an urban Mediterranean population. *BMC Public Health*, 2007, 7:194.

44. Cummings KM et al. Measurement of current exposure to environmental tobacco smoke. *Archives of Environmental Health*, 1990, 45:74–79.

45. Masjedi MR, Kazemi H, Johnson DC. Effects of passive smoking on the pulmonary function of adults. *Thorax*, 1990, 45:27–31.

46. Steyn K et al. Smoking in urban pregnant women in South Africa. *South African Medical Journal*, 1997, 87:460–463.

47. Lam TH et al. Respiratory symptoms due to active and passive smoking in junior secondary school students in Hong Kong. *International Journal of Epidemiology*, 1998, 27:41–48.

48. Kauffmann F, Tessier JF, Oriol P. Adult passive smoking in the home environment: a risk factor for chronic airflow limitation. *American Journal of Epidemiology*, 1983, 117:269–280.

49. Ware JH, Dockery DW, Spiro A, III. Passive smoking, gas cooking, and respiratory health of children living in six cities. *American Review of Respiratory Disease*, 1984, 129:366–374.

50. Greenberg RA et al. Ecology of passive smoking by young infants. *Journal of Pediatrics*, 1989, 114:774–780.

51. Dijkstra L et al. Respiratory health effects of the indoor environment in a population of Dutch children. *American Review of Respiratory Disease*, 1990, 142:1172–1178.

52. Butz AM, Rosenstein BJ. Passive smoking among children with chronic respiratory disease. *Journal of Asthma*, 1992, 29:265–272.

53. Sherrill DL et al. The effects of airway hyperresponsiveness, wheezing, and atopy on longitudinal pulmonary function in children: a 6-year follow- up study. *Pediatric Pulmonology*, 1992, 13:78–85.

54. Cummings M. *Passive smoking study*. Memorandum to D. Collia, OSHA, from K.M. Cummings, Roswell Park Cancer Institute, New York State Department of Health, 1994.

55. Thompson B et al. ETS exposure in the workplace: perceptions and reactions by employees at 114 work sites. *Journal of Occupational and Environmental Medicine*, 1995, 37:1363.

56. Kurtz ME et al. Exposure to environmental tobacco smoke—perceptions of Afro-American children and adolescents. *Preventive Medicine*, 1996, 25:286–292.

57. Brenner H et al. Smoking behavior and attitude toward smoking regulations and passive smoking in the workplace: a study among 974 employees in the German metal industry. *Preventive Medicine*, 1997, 26:138–143.

58. Jones S, Love C, Thomson G, Green R, Howden-Chapman P. Second-hand smoke at work: the exposure, perceptions and attitudes of bar and restaurant workers to environmental tobacco smoke. *Australian and New Zealand Journal of Public Health*, 2001, 25:90–93.

59. Olivieri M et al. Tobacco smoke exposure and serum cotinine in a random sample of adults living in Verona, Italy. *Archives of Environmental Health*, 2002, 57:355–359.

60. Cameron M et al. Exposure to secondhand smoke at work: a survey of members of the Australian Liquor, Hospitality and Miscellaneous Workers Union. *Australian and New Zealand Journal of Public Health*, 2003, 27:496–501.

61. Cornelius MD, Goldschmidt L, Dempsey DA. Environmental tobacco smoke exposure in low-income 6-year-olds: parent report and urine cotinine measures. *Nicotine & Tobacco Research*, 2003, 5:333–339.

62. Jordan TR et al. Adolescent exposure to and perceptions of environmental tobacco smoke. *Journal of School Health*, 2005, 75:178–186.

63. Boyaci H et al. Environmental tobacco smoke exposure in schoolchildren: parent report and urine cotinine measures. *Pediatrics International*, 2006, 48:382–389.

64. Delpisheh A, Kelly Y, Brabin BJ. Passive cigarette smoke exposure in primary schoolchildren in Liverpool. *Public Health*, 2006, 120:65–69.

65. Anuntaseree W et al. Exposure to environmental tobacco smoke among infants in southern Thailand: a study of urinary cotinine. *Bulletin of Environmental Contamination and Toxicology*, 2008, 80:34–37.

66. Dostal M et al. Environmental tobacco smoke exposure in children in two districts of the Czech Republic. *International Journal of Hygiene and Environmental Health*, 2008, 211: 318--325, published online 28 August 2007.

67. Lee DJ et al. Respiratory effects of secondhand smoke exposure among young adults residing in a "clean" indoor air state. *Journal of Community Health*, 2008, 33:117–125.

68. Greenberg RA et al. Passive smoking during the first year of life. *American Journal of Public Health*, 1991, 81:850–853.

69. Samet JM, Lewitt EM, Warner KE. Involuntary Smoking and Children's Health. *Critical Health Issues for Children and Youth*, 1994, 4:94–114.

70. Zhang J et al. A case-control study of paternal smoking and birth defects. *International Journal of Epidemiology*, 1992, 21:273–278.

71. Sherrill DL et al. Longitudinal effects of passive smoking on pulmonary function in New Zealand children. *American Review of Respiratory Disease*, 1992, 145:1136–1141.

72. US Department of Health and Human Services. *The health consequences of smoking. a report of the Surgeon General.* Washington, DC, US Government Printing Office, 1971.

73. National Research Council (NRC), Committee on Passive Smoking. *Environmental tobacco smoke: measuring exposures and assessing health effects.* Washington, DC, National Academy Press, 1986.

74. US Environmental Protection Agency. *Respiratory health effects of passive smoking: lung cancer and other disorders.* Washington, DC, US Government Printing Office, 1992 (EPA/600/006F).

75. *Health effects of exposure to environmental tobacco smoke.* Sacramento, CA, California Environmental Protection Agency, Office of Environmental Health Hazard Assessment, 1997.

76. *Protection from exposure to second-hand tobacco smoke. Policy recommendations.* Geneva, World Health Organization, 2007.

77. *IARC monographs on the evaluation of the carcinogenic risk of chemicals to humans: tobacco smoking.* Lyon, International Agency for Research on Cancer, 1986 (IARC Monograph 38).

78. Koo LC, Ho JH, Lee N. An analysis of some risk factors for lung cancer in Hong Kong. *International Journal of Cancer*, 1985, 35:149–155.

79. Lam TH et al. Smoking, passive smoking and histological types in lung cancer in Hong Kong Chinese women. *British Journal of Cancer*, 1987, 56:673–678.

80. Koo LC. Dietary habits and lung cancer risk among Chinese females in Hong Kong who never smoked. *Nutrition and Cancer*, 1988, 11:155–172.

81. Wu-Williams AH et al. Lung cancer among women in northeast China. *British Journal of Cancer*, 1990, 62:982–987.

82. Liu ZY, He XZ, Chapman RS. Smoking and other risk factors for lung cancer in Xuanwei, China. *International Journal of Epidemiology*, 1991, 20:26–31.

83. Liu Q, Sasco AJ, Riboli E, Hu MX. Indoor air pollution and lung cancer in Guangzhou, People's Republic of China. *American Journal of Epidemiology*, 1993, 137:145–154.

84. Du YX et al. An epidemiological study of risk factors for lung cancer in Guangzhou, China. *Lung Cancer*, 1996, 14 (Suppl. 1):S9–S37.

85. Gao YT. Risk factors for lung cancer among nonsmokers with emphasis on lifestyle factors. *Lung Cancer*, 1996, 14 (Suppl. 1):S39–45.

86. Koo LC, Ho JH. Diet as a confounder of the association between air pollution and female lung cancer: Hong Kong studies on exposures to environmental tobacco smoke, incense, and cooking fumes as examples. *Lung Cancer*, 1996, 14 (Suppl. 1):S47–S61.

87. Ko YC et al. Risk factors for primary lung cancer among non-smoking women in Taiwan. *International Journal of Epidemiology*, 1997, 26:24–31.

88. Wang T-J, Zhou B-S, Shi J. Lung cancer in nonsmoking Chinese women: a case-control study. *Lung Cancer*, 1996, 14 (Suppl. 1):S93–S98.

89. Wang SY et al. A comparative study of the risk factors for lung cancer in Guangdong, China. *Lung Cancer*, 1996, 14 (Suppl. 1):S99–105.

90. Wang TJ, Zhou BS. Meta-analysis of the potential relationship between exposure to environmental tobacco smoke and lung cancer in nonsmoking Chinese women. *Lung Cancer*, 1997, 16:145–150.

World Health Organization

91. Shen XB, Wang GX, Zhou BS. Relation of exposure to environmental tobacco smoke and pulmonary adenocarcinoma in non-smoking women: a case control study in Nanjing. *Oncology Reports*, 1998, 5:1221–1223.

92. Jee SH, Ohrr H, Kim IS. Effects of husbands' smoking on the incidence of lung cancer in Korean women. *International Journal of Epidemiology*, 1999, 28:824–828.

93. Rapiti E et al. Passive smoking and lung cancer in Chandigarh, India. *Lung Cancer*, 1999, 23:183–189.

94. Zhong L et al. A case-control study of lung cancer and environmental tobacco smoke among nonsmoking women living in Shanghai, China. *Cancer Causes & Control*, 1999, 10:607–616.

95. Lee CH et al. Lifetime environmental exposure to tobacco smoke and primary lung cancer of non-smoking Taiwanese women. *International Journal of Epidemiology*, 2000, 29:224–231.

96. Wang L et al. Lung cancer and environmental tobacco smoke in a non-industrial area of China. *International Journal of Cancer*, 2000, 88:139–145.

97. Zhou BS et al. Indoor air pollution and pulmonary adenocarcinoma among females: a case-control study in Shenyang, China. *Oncology Reports*, 2000, 7:1253–1259.

98. Nishino Y et al. Passive smoking at home and cancer risk: a population-based prospective study in Japanese nonsmoking women. *Cancer Causes & Control*, 2001, 12:797–802.

99. Seow A et al. Diet, reproductive factors and lung cancer risk among Chinese women in Singapore: evidence for a protective effect of soy in nonsmokers. *International Journal of Cancer*, 2002, 97:365–371.

100. Chan-Yeung M et al. Risk factors associated with lung cancer in Hong Kong. *Lung Cancer*, 2003, 40:131–140.

101. Kurahashi N, Inoue M, Liu Y et al. Passive smoking and lung cancer in Japanese non-smoking women: a prospective study. *International Journal of Cancer*, 2008, 122:653–657.

102. Chen Y, Li W, Yu S. Influence of passive smoking on admissions for respiratory illness in early childhood. *British Medical Journal (Clinical Research Edition)*, 1986, 293:303–306.

103. Chen Y et al. Chang-Ning epidemiological study of children's health: I: passive smoking and children's respiratory diseases. *International Journal of Epidemiology*, 1988, 17:348–355.

104. Tupasi TE et al. Determinants of morbidity and mortality due to acute respiratory infections: implications for intervention. *Journal of Infectious Diseases*, 1988, 157:615–623.

105. Pandey MR et al. Impact of a pilot acute respiratory infection (ARI) control programme in a rural community of the hill region of Nepal. *Annals of Tropical Paediatrics*, 1989, 9:212–220.

106. Azizi BH, Henry RL. Effects of indoor air pollution on lung function of primary schoolchildren in Kuala Lumpur. *Pediatric Pulmonology*, 1990, 9:24–29.

107. Tupasi TE et al. Community-based studies of acute respiratory tract infections in young children. *Review of Infectious Diseases*, 1990, 12:S940–949.

108. Vathanophas K et al. A community-based study of acute respiratory tract infection in Thai children. *Review of Infectious Diseases*, 1990, 12:S957–965.

109. Woodward A et al. Acute respiratory illness in Adelaide children: breast feeding modifies the effect of passive smoking. *Journal of Epidemiology and Community Health*, 1990, 44:224–230.

110. Azizi BH, Henry RL. The effects of indoor environmental factors on respiratory illness in primary schoolchildren in Kuala Lumpur. *International Journal of Epidemiology*, 1991, 20:144–150.

111. Ford RP et al. Patterns of smoking during pregnancy in Canterbury. *New Zealand Medical Journal*, 1993, 106:426–429.

112. Jin C, Rossignol AM. Effects of passive smoking on respiratory illness from birth to age eighteen months, in Shanghai, People's Republic of China. *Journal of Pediatrics*, 1993, 123:553–558.

113. Chen Y. Environmental tobacco smoke, low birth weight, and hospitalization for respiratory disease. *American Journal of Respiratory Critical Care Medicine*, 1994, 150:54–58.

114. Haby MM, Peat JK, Woolcock AJ. Effect of passive smoking, asthma, and respiratory infection on lung function in Australian children. *Pediatric Pulmonology*, 1994, 18:323–329.

115. Flynn MG. Respiratory symptoms of rural Fijian and Indian children in Fiji. *Thorax*, 1994, 49:1201–1204.

116. Shaw R et al. Risk factors for asthma symptoms in Kawerau children. *New Zealand Medical Journal*, 1994, 107:387–391.

117. Azizi BH, Zulkifli HI, Kasim MS. Protective and risk factors for acute respiratory infections in hospitalized urban Malaysian children: a case control study. *Southeast Asian Journal of Tropical Medicine and Public Health*, 1995, 26:280–285.

118. Ponsonby AL, Couper D, Dwyer T. Features of infant exposure to tobacco smoke in a cohort study in Tasmania. *Journal of Epidemiology and Community Health*, 1996, 50:40–46.

119. Rahman MM, Rahman AM. Prevalence of acute respiratory tract infection and its risk factors in under five children. *Bangladesh Medical Research Council Bulletin*, 1997, 23:47–50.

120. Behera D, Sood P, Singh S. Passive smoking, domestic fuels and lung function in north Indian children. *Indian Journal of Chest Diseases & Allied Sciences*, 1998, 40:89–98.

121. Deshmukh JS et al. Low birth weight and associated maternal factors in an urban area. *Indian Pediatrics*, 1998, 35:33–36.

122. Chhabra SK et al. Prevalence of bronchial asthma in schoolchildren in Delhi. *Journal of Asthma*, 1998, 35:291–296.

123. Lewis P et al. Outdoor air pollution and children's respiratory symptoms in the steel cities of New South Wales. *Medical Journal of Australia*, 1998, 169:459–463.

124. Peters J et al. Economic burden of environmental tobacco smoke on Hong Kong families: scale and impact. *Journal of Epidemiology and Community Health*, 1998, 52:53–58.

125. Belousova EG et al. The effect of parental smoking on presence of wheeze or airway hyper-responsiveness in New South Wales schoolchildren. *Australian New Zealand Journal of Medicine*, 1999, 29:794–800.

126. Chhabra SK et al. Risk factors for development of bronchial asthma in children in Delhi. *Annals of Allergy, Asthma & Immunology*, 1999, 83:385–390.

127. Lam TH et al, Child Health and Activity Research Group (CHARG). Passive smoking and respiratory symptoms in primary schoolchildren in Hong Kong. *Human & Experimental Toxicology*, 1999, 18:218–223.

128. Wang TN et al. Association between indoor and outdoor air pollution and adolescent asthma from 1995 to 1996 in Taiwan. *Environmental Research*, 1999, 81:239–247.

129. Yau KI, Fang LJ, Shieh KH. Factors predisposing infants to lower respiratory infection with wheezing in the first two years of life. *Annals of Allergy, Asthma & Immunology*, 1999, 82:165–170.

130. Zhang J et al. Effects of air pollution on respiratory health of adults in three Chinese cities. *Archives of Environmental Health*, 1999, 54:373–381.

131. Darlow BA, Horwood LJ, Mogridge N. Very low birthweight and asthma by age seven years in a national cohort. *Pediatric Pulmonology*, 2000, 30:291–296.

132. Ponsonby AL et al. The relation between infant indoor environment and subsequent asthma. *Epidemiology*, 2000, 11:128–135.

133. Qian Z et al. Effects of air pollution on children's respiratory health in three Chinese cities. *Archives of Environmental Health*, 2000, 55:126–133.

134. Young S et al. The association between early life lung function and wheezing during the first 2 yrs of life. *European Respiratory Journal*, 2000, 15:151–157.

135. Gupta D et al. Prevalence of bronchial asthma and association with environmental tobacco smoke exposure in adolescent schoolchildren in Chandigarh, north India. *Journal of Asthma*, 2001, 38:501–507.

136. Pokharel PK et al. Risk factors associated with bronchial asthma in school going children of rural Haryana. *Indian Journal of Pediatrics*, 2001, 68:103–106.

137. Salo PM et al. Respiratory symptoms in relation to residential coal burning and environmental tobacco smoke among early adolescents in Wuhan, China: a cross-sectional study. *Environmental Health*, 2004, 3:14.

138. David GL et al. Childhood exposure to environmental tobacco smoke and chronic respiratory symptoms in non-smoking adults: the Singapore Chinese Health Study. *Thorax*, 2005, 60:1052–1058.

139. Gupta D et al. Household environmental tobacco smoke exposure, respiratory symptoms and asthma in non-smoker adults: a multicentric population study from India. *Indian Journal of Chest Disease & Allied Sciences*, 2006, 48:31–36.

140. Dong GH et al. Effects of environmental tobacco smoke on respiratory health of boys and girls from kindergarten: results from 15 districts of northern China. *Indoor Air*, 2007, 17:475–483.

141. Sharma SK, Banga A. Prevalence and risk factors for wheezing in children from rural areas of north India. *Allergy and Asthma Proceedings*, 2007, 28:647–653.

142. *Women and smoking: a report of the Surgeon General*. Rockville, MD, US Department of Health and Human Services, 2001.

143. US Department of Health and Human Services. *The health effects of active smoking: a report of the Surgeon General*. Washington, DC, US Government Printing Office, 2004.

144. Windham GC, Eaton A, Hopkins B. Evidence for an association between environmental tobacco smoke exposure and birthweight: a meta-analysis and new data. *Paediatric and Perinatal Epidemiology*, 1999, 13:35–37.

145. Boffetta P, Tredaniel J, Greco A. Risk of childhood cancer and adult lung cancer after childhood exposure to passive smoke: A meta-analysis. *Environmental Health Perspectives*, 2000, 108:73–82.

146. Study Group on Smoking and Health. Smoking and health: a joint report of the study group on smoking and health. *Science*, 1957, 125:1129–1133.

147. Martin TR, Bracken MB. Association of low birth weight with passive smoke exposure in pregnancy. *American Journal of Epidemiology*, 1986, 124:633–642.

148. Roquer JM et al. Influence on fetal growth of exposure to tobacco smoke during pregnancy. *Acta Paediatrica*, 1995, 84:118–121.

149. Mainous AG, Hueston WJ. Passive smoke and low birth weight. Evidence of a threshold effect. *Archives of Family Medicine*, 1994, 3:875–878.

150. Savitz DA, Schwingl PJ, Keels MA. Influence of paternal age, smoking, and alcohol consumption on congenital anomalies. *Teratology*, 1991, 44:429–440.

151. Seidman DS, Ever-Hadani P, Gale R. Effect of maternal smoking and age on congenital anomalies. *Obstetrics & Gynecology*, 1990, 76:1046–1050.

152. Harlap S, Davies AM. Infant admissions to hospital and maternal smoking. *The Lancet*, 1974, 1:529–532.

153. Colley JR, Holland WW, Corkhill RT. Influence of passive smoking and parental phlegm on pneumonia and bronchitis in early childhood. *The Lancet*, 1974, 2:1031–1034.

154. Strachan DP, Cook DG. Health effects of passive smoking. 1. Parental smoking and lower respiratory illness in infancy and early childhood. *Thorax*, 1997, 52:905–914.

155. Yue Chen BM, Wan-Xian LI, Shunzhang Y. Influence of passive smoking on admissions for respiratory illness in early childhood. *British Medical Journal*, 1986, 293:303–306.

156. Cook DG, Strachan DP. Health effects of passive smoking. 3. Parental smoking and prevalence of respiratory symptoms and asthma in school age children. *Thorax*, 1997, 52:1081–1094.

157. Charlton A. Children's coughs related to parental smoking. *British Medical Journal (Clinical Research Edition)*, 1984, 288:1647–1649.

158. Weiss ST et al. Persistent wheeze: its relation to respiratory illness, cigarette smoking, and level of pulmonary function in a population sample of children. *American Review of Respiratory Disease*, 1980, 122:697–707.

159. Tager IB et al. The natural history of forced expiratory volumes. Effect of cigarette smoking and respiratory symptoms. *American Review of Respiratory Disease*, 1988, 138:837–849.

160. Hanrahan JP et al. The effect of maternal smoking during pregnancy on early infant lung function. *American Review of Respiratory Disease*, 1992, 145:1129–1135.

161. Cook DG, Strachan DP. Parental smoking and prevalence of respiratory symptoms and asthma in school age children. *Thorax*, 1997, 52:1081–1094.

162. *The health consequences of smoking: chronic obstructive lung disease. A report of the Surgeon General*. Rockville, MD, Office on Smoking and Health, US Public Health Service, 1984.

163. Cook DG, Strachan DP, Carey IM. Health effects of passive smoking. 9. Parental smoking and spirometric indices in children. *Thorax*, 1998, 53:884–893.

164. Hirayama T. Non-smoking wives of heavy smokers have a higher risk of lung cancer: a study from Japan. *British Medical Journal (Clinical Research Edition)*, 1981, 282:183–185.

165. Trichopoulos D et al. Lung cancer and passive smoking. *International Journal of Cancer*, 1981, 27:1–4.

166. Lofroth G. Environmental tobacco smoke: overview of chemical composition and genotoxic components. *Mutation Research*, 1989, 222:73–80.

167. Claxton LD et al. A genotoxic assessment of environmental tobacco smoke using bacterial bioassays. *Mutation Research*, 1989, 222:81–99.

168. Weiss B. Behavior as an endpoint for inhaled toxicants. In: McClellan RO, Henderson RF, eds. *Concepts in inhalation toxicology*. New York, NY, Hemisphere Publishing, 1989:475–493.

169. Hecht SS et al. A tobacco-specific lung carcinogen in the urine of men exposed to cigarette smoke. *New England Journal of Medicine*, 1993, 329:1543–1546.

170. Carmella SG et al. Analysis of total 4-(methylnitrosamino)-1-(3-pyridyl)-1-butanol (NNAL) in human urine. *Cancer Epidemiology, Biomarkers & Prevention*, 2003, 12:1257–1261.

171. Maclure M et al. Elevated blood levels of carcinogens in passive smokers. *American Journal of Public Health*, 1989, 89:1381–1384.

172. Crawford FG et al. Biomarkers of environmental tobacco smoke in preschool children and their mothers. *Journal of the National Cancer Institute*, 1994, 86:1398–1402.

173. Mauderly JL et al. Chronic inhalation exposure to mainstream cigarette smoke increases lung and nasal tumor incidence in rats. *Toxicological Sciences*, 2004, 81:280–292.

174. Hirayama T. Cancer mortality in nonsmoking women with smoking husbands based on a large-scale cohort study in Japan. *Preventive Medicine*, 1984, 13:680–690.

175. Trichopoulos D, Kalandidi A, Sparros L. Lung cancer and passive smoking: conclusion of Greek study. *The Lancet*, 1983, 2:677–678.

176. Hackshaw AK, Law MR, Wald NJ. The accumulated evidence on lung cancer and environmental tobacco smoke. *British Medical Journal*, 1997, 315:980–988.

177. Enstrom JE, Kabat GC. Environmental tobacco smoke and tobacco related mortality in a prospective study of Californians, 1960–98. *British Medical Journal*, 2003, 326:1057.

178. Hackshaw A. Passive smoking: paper does not diminish conclusion of previous reports. *British Medical Journal*, 2003, 327:501–502.

179. Repace JL et al. Air nicotine and saliva cotinine as indicators of workplace passive smoking exposure and risk. *Risk Analysis*, 1998, 18:71–83.

180. US Department of Health Education and Welfare. *The health consequences of smoking: a public health service review*. Washington, DC, US Government Printing Office, 1967.

181. Barnoya J, Glantz SA. Cardiovascular effects of secondhand smoke: nearly as large as smoking. *Circulation*, 2005, 111:2684–2698.

182. Rubenstein D, Jesty J, Bluestein D. Differences between mainstream and sidestream cigarette smoke extracts and nicotine in the activation of platelets under static and flow conditions. *Circulation*, 2004, 109:78–83.

183. Glantz SA, Parmley WW. Passive smoking and heart disease: mechanisms and risk. *Journal of the American Medical Association*, 1995, 273:1047–1053.

184. Celermajer DS et al. Passive smoking and impaired endothelium-dependent arterial dilatation in healthy young adults. *New England Journal of Medicine*, 1996, 334:150–154.

185. Otsuka R et al. Acute effects of passive smoking on the coronary circulation in healthy young adults. *Journal of the American Medical Association*, 2001, 286:436–441.

186. Sumida H et al. Does passive smoking impair endothelium-dependent coronary artery dilation in women? *Journal of the American College of Cardiology*, 1998, 31:811–815.

187. Garland C et al. Effects of passive smoking on ischemic heart disease mortality of nonsmokers: a prospective study. *American Journal of Epidemiology*, 1985, 121:645–650.

188. Law MR, Morris JK, Wald NJ. Environmental tobacco smoke exposure and ischaemic heart disease: an evaluation of the evidence. *British Medical Journal*, 1997, 315:973–980.

189. Taylor AE, Johnson DC, Kazemi H. Environmental tobacco smoke and cardiovascular disease. A position paper from the council on cardiopulmonary and critical care, American Heart Association. *Circulation*, 1992, 86:1–4.

190. Ostro BD. Estimating the risks of smoking, air pollution, and passive smoke on acute respiratory conditions. *Risk Analysis*, 1989, 9:189–196.

191. Schwartz J, Zeger S. Passive smoking, air pollution, and acute respiratory symptoms in a diary study of student nurses. *American Review of Respiratory Disease*, 1990, 141:62–67.

192. Weiss ST, Utell MJ, Samet JM. Environmental tobacco smoke exposure and asthma in adults. *Environmental Health Perspectives*, 1999, 107 (Suppl 6):891–895.

193. Shephard RJ, Collins R, Silverman F. "Passive" exposure of asthmatic subjects to cigarette smoke. *Environmental Research*, 1979, 20:392–402.

194. Jaakkola MS et al. Environmental tobacco smoke and adult-onset asthma: a population-based incident case-control study. *American Journal of Public Health*, 2003, 93:2055–2060.

195. *The health consequences of smoking: cancer. A report of the Surgeon General*. Rockville, MD, US, Public Health Service, Office on Smoking and Health, 1982 (DHHS Publication (PHS) 82–50179).

196. US Department of Health and Human Services. *Strategies to control tobacco use in the United States: a blueprint for public health action in the 1990's*. Washington, DC: US Government Printing Office, 1991.

197. World Health Organization. *Tobacco Free Initiative: WHO resolutions*. Geneva, World Health Organization, 2003.

198. *WHO Framework Convention on Tobacco Control (FCTC)*. Geneva, World Health Organization, 2003.

199. *Conference of the Parties to the WHO Framework Convention on Tobacco Control, second session*. Geneva, World Health Organization, 2007.

200. National Heart Lung and Blood Institute, National Asthma Education and Prevention Program. *Guidelines for the diagnosis and management of asthma. Expert Panel Report 3 (EPR-3)* Bethesda, MD, US Department of Health and Human Services, National Institutes of Health, 2007 (NIH Publication 08-5846. 2007).

201. Beasley R et al. ISAAC Steering Committee. Worldwide variation in prevalence of symptoms of asthma, allergic rhinoconjunctivitis, and atopic eczema: ISAAC. *The Lancet*, 1998, 351:1225–1232.

202. US Environmental Protection Agency (EPA). *Smoke-free homes and cars program*. US Environmental Protection Agency, 2007 (http://epa.gov/smokefree/).

203. Glantz SA, Rimer BK, Lewis FM. *Health behavior and health education. theory, research and practice*, 3rd ed. San Francisco, CA, Wiley & Sons, 2002.

204. Levy DT, Chaloupka F, Gitchell J. The effects of tobacco control policies on smoking rates: a tobacco control scorecard. *Journal of Public Health Management and Practices*, 2004, 10:338–353.

205. Koh HK, Joossens LX, Connolly GN. Making smoking history worldwide. *New England Journal of Medicine*, 2007, 356:1496–1498.

206. Fichtenberg CM, Glantz SA. Effect of smoke-free workplaces on smoking behaviour: systematic review. *British Medical Journal*, 2002, 325:188–194.

207. Bartecchi C et al. A reduction in the incidence of acute myocardial infarction associated with a citywide smoking ordinance. *Circulation*, 2006, 114:1490–1496.

208. Menzies D et al. Respiratory symptoms, pulmonary function, and markers of inflammation among bar workers before and after a legislative ban on smoking in public places. *Journal of the American Medical Association*, 2006, 296:1742–1748.

209. Akhtar PC et al. Changes in child exposure to environmental tobacco smoke (CHETS) study after implementation of smoke-free legislation in Scotland: national cross sectional survey. *British Medical Journal*, 2007, 335:545.

210. *Don't pass gas*. American Legacy Foundation, 2005 (www.dontpassgas.com/downloads/dpg_brochure.pdf).

211. Przewozniak K, Zatonski W. *Clearing the air from tobacco smoke pollution: creating healthy and safe environments for children: Poland*. Budapest, World Health Organization Regional Office for Europe, 2004.

212. Gosevitz R, Boadway T. *The duty to protect: eliminating second-hand smoke from public places and workplaces in Ontario*. Toronto, Ontario Medical Association, 2003.

213. Lund KE, Helgason AR. Environmental tobacco smoke in Norwegian homes, 1995 and 2001: changes in children's exposure and parents attitudes and health risk awareness. *European Journal of Public Health*, 2005, 15:123–127.

214. *1000 homes in Salford sign up to Smoke Free Homes campaign*. Salford (UK) City Council, 2007 (http://www.councillor.info/salford/dlancaster/0/default.aspx?pane=cp&md=contentview&mtype=news&itemid=20279&mid=27099).

215. Cunningham R. *Package warnings: overview of international developments*. Toronto, Canadian Cancer Society, 2007.

216. Gehrman CA, Hovell MF. Protecting children from environmental tobacco smoke (ETS) exposure: a critical review. *Nicotine and Tobacco Research*, 2003, 5:289–301.

217. Klerman L. Protecting children: reducing their environmental tobacco smoke exposure. *Nicotine and Tobacco Research*, 2004, 6 (Suppl. 2):S239–S253.

218. Hovell MF et al. Reduction of environmental tobacco smoke exposure among asthmatic children: a controlled trial. *Chest*, 1994, 106:440–446.

219. Wilson SR et al. A controlled trial of an environmental tobacco smoke reduction intervention in low-income children with asthma. *Chest*, 2001, 120:1709–1722.

220. Hovell MF et al. Asthma management and environmental tobacco smoke exposure reduction in Latino children: a controlled trial. *Pediatrics*, 2002, 110:946–956.

221. *State legislated actions on tobacco issues: 2006*. Washington, DC, American Lung Association, 2006.

222. European Public Health Alliance. European smoking bans—evolution of the legislation. *European Public Health Alliance* (http://www.epha.org/a/1941), 2007.

223. Frieden TR, Bloomberg MR. How to prevent 100 million deaths from tobacco. *The Lancet*, 2007, 369:1758–1761.

224. Asaria P et al. Chronic disease prevention: health effects and financial costs of strategies to reduce salt intake and control tobacco use. *The Lancet*, 2007, 370:2044–2053.

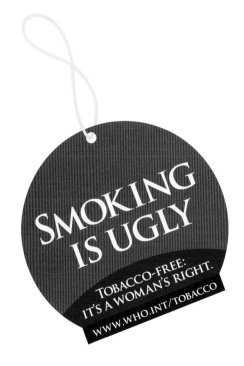

31**MAY:**WORLD**NO**TOBACCO**DAY**

World Health Organization

© WORLD HEALTH ORGANIZATION 2010. THE IMAGES OF WOUNDS, LESIONS OR ULCERATIONS ARE REAL AND SUPERIMPOSED ON THE IMAGE OF THE MODEL DESIGNED BY NOVA S/B.

Chic?
No, throat
cancer.

**Protect women from
tobacco marketing and smoke.**

**SMOKING
IS UGLY**

Why Women and Girls Use Tobacco

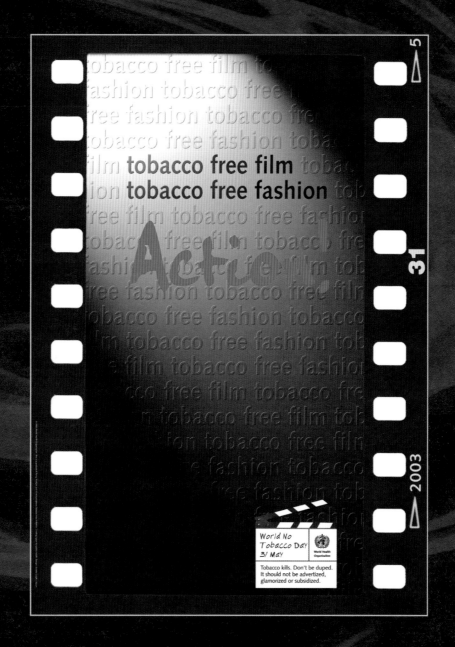

tobacco free film
tobacco free fashion

Action!

World No
Tobacco Day
31 May

World Health
Organization

Tobacco kills. Don't be duped.
It should not be advertized,
glamorized or subsidized.

5

31

2003

6. The Marketing of Tobacco to Women: Global Perspectives

Introduction

Women smokers are likely to increase as a percentage of the total. Women are adopting more dominant roles in society: they have increased spending power, they live longer than men. And as a recent official report showed, they seem to be less influenced by the anti-smoking campaigns than their male counterparts. All in all, that makes women a prime target. So, despite previous hesitancy, might we now expect to see a more defined attack on the important market segment represented by female smokers?[1] Selling tobacco products to women is currently the largest product-marketing opportunity in the world. While marketing tobacco to women in the developing world is a relatively recent phenomenon, the industry benefits from 80 years of experience in enticing women in industrialized countries to smoke. Themes of body image, fashion, and independence resound in marketing strategies and popular media. The tactics used in marketing tobacco in the United States and other industrialized nations now threaten women in the developing world.

This chapter reviews the history of the marketing of tobacco to women in the United States, describes current US and Asian marketing strategies, outlines the changing roles of women in the Asia region as reflected in marketing, reviews research on how marketing affects tobacco use, and presents recommendations for action. The evidence presented highlights the importance of the WHO Framework Convention on Tobacco Control (WHO FCTC) as the leading normative instrument in the effort to reduce the harm from tobacco use among women. In Article 13, *Tobacco advertising, promotion and sponsorship*, the WHO FCTC mandates Parties to undertake a comprehensive ban or, in cases of constitutional limitations, a restriction of all tobacco advertising, promotion and sponsorship. Article 5.3, *General obligations,* directs Parties to protect tobacco control policies from the commercial and vested interests of the tobacco industry.

Marketing Tobacco to Women in the United States

The rich history of the tobacco industry's targeted marketing to women in the United States provides insight into current and future industry marketing tactics in other parts of the world. At the beginning of the present century, the industry faced formidable odds, as few women smoked. Those who did were labelled "defiant" or "emancipated". The Lorillard Company first used images of women smoking in its 1919 advertisements to promote the Murad and Helman brands, but public outcry ensued. In 1926, however, Chesterfield entered the women's market with billboards showing a woman asking a male smoker to "Blow Some My Way" and achieved a 40% increase in sales over two years.[2]

Links to fashion and slimness soon followed. In 1927, Marlboro premiered its "Mild as May" campaign in the sophisticated fashion magazine *Le Bon Ton*, and in 1928, Lucky Strike launched a campaign to get women to "Reach for a Lucky instead of a sweet".[3] These ads featured copy that directly associated smoking with being thin: "Light a Lucky and you'll never miss sweets that make you fat" and "AVOID that future shadow, when tempted. Reach for a Lucky", accompanied by a silhouette of a woman with a grossly exaggerated double chin. Another ad showing a slim woman's body and then an obese woman's shadow said, "Is this you five years from now? When tempted to over-indulge, reach for a Lucky instead. It's toasted".

Marketing Lucky Strikes as a weight-reduction product increased sales by over 300% in the first year and eventually moved the brand's rank from third to first.[4] Actresses and opera stars were hired to promote Lucky Strikes, and American Tobacco paid debutantes and models to smoke in public.[3] American Tobacco's public relations specialist, Edward Bernays, worked with fashion magazines to feature photographs of ultra-slim Paris models wearing the latest fashions. He also convinced the fashion industry to choose green, the colour of the Lucky Strike package, as fashion colour of the year.[5] An American Tobacco executive likened the women's market to "opening a gold mine right in our front yard".[5]

By the end of the 1920s, cigarette ads regularly featured women with their new "symbols of freedom". Cigarette ads appeared in women's fashion magazines, including

 World Health Organization

Vogue, Vanity Fair, and *Harper's Bazaar*.[6] The new era of targeted marketing of tobacco to women was under way.

The late 1960s and early 1970s brought further development of women's brands. Philip Morris launched Virginia Slims with the biggest marketing campaign in company history, "You've come a long way, baby".[7] Its advertising stressed themes of glamour, thinness, and independence. In 1970, Brown & Williamson premiered the fashion cigarette Flair, and Liggett & Myers introduced Eve.

Since that time, other niche brands have appeared, yet women's brands account for only 5% to 10% of the cigarette market.[8] The majority of women smokers (women represent 50% of the market share) smoke gender-neutral brands such as Marlboro and Camel. To understand how the tobacco industry markets its products to women, it is necessary to look at the components of modern-day marketing and their individual and synchronistic functions.

Components of Modern Marketing

Tobacco companies market their products to women as a segment of an overall marketing strategy. The women's market is further segmented by specific subgroup characteristics, as this quote from an American Tobacco Company document reveals:

> There is significant opportunity to segment the female market on the basis of current values, age, lifestyles and preferred length and circumference of products. This assignment should consider a more contemporary and relevant lifestyle approach targeted toward young adult female smokers.[9]

Modern marketing strives to attach symbolic meaning to specific tobacco brands by carefully manipulating the brand name, packaging, advertising, promotion, sponsorship, and placement in popular culture. The purpose of tobacco marketing is to associate its product with psychological and social needs that the consumer wants to fulfil, some of which emanate from the restructuring of social reality that advertising itself provides. Marketing is more successful when its components work in a synchronized fashion, surrounding the target consumers with stimuli from multiple sources.

Brand Name and Packaging

Cigarette brands project distinctive identities.[10] The attraction of a particular brand of cigarettes is affected by its name, logo, and package colours, because they signal an overall image that cues the attitude of potential customers towards the product.[11–13] Brands may use the image to attract women to particular features (e.g. "Slims" to weight control) or to negate negative feelings such as smoking being inappropriate for women (e.g. "Eve").[14] Brand identity may be particularly important, because women make 80% of the purchasing decisions in the general marketplace.[15]

Tobacco has been called the ultimate "badge product", because it is like a name badge that sends a message every time it is seen.[16] It is used many times a day, frequently in social settings. Its package design and brand are visible every time it is used, conveying a particular image. This visual image is enough to stimulate purchase of a brand without recalling its name.[17] Packaging affects consumer attitude to a product and influences brand choice.[18,19] The colour and graphics of the package transfer attributes they symbolize to the product. Blue and white are often used for health products because they send a signal of cleanness and purity.[18] Red is a popular colour for tobacco packaging because it connotes excitement, passion, strength, wealth, and power.[19,20] Red also aids recall of a product.[12,13]

Other colours frequently used in tobacco packaging send different signals,[19, 20] as shown below:

Colour	Shade	Signals
Blue	Light:	calm, coolness, insecurity
	Intense:	loyalty, honesty, royalty, restlessness
	Dark:	tranquillity
Green		coolness, restlessness, nature, cleanliness, youth
Purple	Light:	femininity, freshness, springtime
	Dark:	wealth, elegance, serenity
Pink		femininity, innocence, relaxation
Orange		warmth, fame, friendliness, security, appetite stimulation
Yellow	Light:	freshness, intelligence
	Bright:	optimism, sunshine
	Gold:	wealth, esteem, status

Packaging works most effectively when its symbolic signals (attributes) match the brand's positioning (the image created for the target audience) and are carried through in advertising and promotions.[18,19] When the copy and colour attributes appear in advertisements, they act as stimuli to enhance recall and retention of the brand.[12]

Advertising

Tobacco advertisements are commercial messages that appear in print, on radio or television, and on outdoor signs (in countries that do not restrict them). In 1996, the tobacco industry spent US$ 578 million in the United States to advertise cigarettes, 11% of total advertising and promotion expenditures in the country.[20] Advertising serves several purposes. It builds a brand's image and raises awareness of it.[17] Advertising preconditions the consumer to buy, formulating the attitudes needed for considering a purchase. An attitude about a brand has two parts: a cognitive or logical component that holds beliefs about the benefit of the product, and an affective component in which emotions energize behaviour.

Products project a psychological and social meaning to the consumer who buys them.[21] Smokers and potential smokers who identify with the projected images may purchase the brand as a means of "adopting" the behaviours or attributes portrayed in the ads.[22] Themes such as glamour, romance, and independence appeal to buyers' self-image and may affect their structuring of social reality. When a role, such as smoking, is new to consumers, they may rely on the social meaning of the product portrayed in advertising to guide how it is used. Brand images may appeal to the socially insecure by appearing to pose solutions to identity problems.[10,23] Viewing ads that feature attractive models and elegant surroundings may generate pressure to conform to the lifestyle portrayed.[24]

In addition to attracting new purchasers, advertising is used to reduce fears about smoking and to encourage brand loyalty. It attempts to reduce health fears by presenting figures on lower nicotine and tar content of particular brands, with the implication that these brands are better for health. In fact, the industry has aimed low-tar brands at women, because its research shows that women are generally more concerned with health issues than men are.[25] Positive imagery (e.g. dazzling blue skies and white-capped mountains, models engaged in sporting

pursuits) is commonly used in advertised messages. Such advertising also attracts repeat purchasers, reinforcing preferences so that brand switching is less likely.[26,27]

Examples of Cigarette Advertising

Cigarette brands targeted to women project themes of thinness, style, glamour, sophistication, sexual attractiveness, social inclusion, athleticism, liberation, freedom, and independence. Advertisements for Capri cigarettes (Brown & Williamson) use the slogan, "She's gone to Capri and she's not coming back". The ads, set in a romantic island scene, feature thin models in glamorous or romantic poses, usually holding the ultra-slim cigarette.

Modern marketing strives to attach symbolic meaning to specific tobacco brands by carefully manipulating the brand name, packaging, advertising, promotion, sponsorship, and placement in popular culture.

Virginia Slims (Philip Morris) has used various themes. "You've come a long way, baby" often portrays scenes from women's advances in society or shows a woman taking a dominant role with a man. Glamour and business appeal are used to advertise Virginia Slims clothing and calendar promotions. Misty (American Tobacco Company), advertised heavily in women's magazines, uses "slim 'n sassy's slim price too" copy. Attractive women hold the slim cigarette. Gender-neutral brands such as Merit (Philip Morris) have featured couples. Marlboro (Philip Morris) has its quintessential Marlboro Man cowboy, who exudes independence, freedom, and strength. It also uses peaceful outdoor scenes shot in open surroundings. Strong colours such as red and deep blue are used in the ads that encourage one to "Come to Marlboro country".

Some brands have focused on the product itself, such as Winston's (R. J. Reynolds) ads that proclaim "No additives, no bull". Carlton (Brown & Williamson) makes the claim that "Carlton is lowest" in tar and nicotine, using blue and white colour schemes. Menthol brands such as Kool (Brown & Williamson) and Newport (Lorillard) use blues and greens to signify coolness and healthfulness, often showing activities near water. Discount brands such as Basic (Philip Morris), Doral (R. J. Reynolds), and GPC (Brown & Williamson) frequently appear in women's magazines, touting their reasonable cost and simple features. Ads for Basic have also shown how their product fits in: "Your basic 3-piece suit". Camel (R. J. Reynolds) was known for the funky cartoon character, Joe Camel, who was shown as the life of the party in bars— "Joe's Place"—or the man-about-town. For a brief period in 1994, R. J. Reynolds introduced Josephine Camel and her female friends, noting that "There's something for everyone at Joe's Place". Joe Camel was withdrawn from Camel ads by Reynolds in 1997 because of a pending lawsuit after years of protest from medical, legislative, and public-interest groups about using a cartoon character to market cigarettes.

In addition to attracting new purchasers, advertising is used to reduce fears about smoking and to encourage brand loyalty. It attempts to reduce health fears by presenting figures on lower nicotine and tar content of particular brands, with the implication that these brands are better for health.

Advertising, then, uses factual material or suggestive imagery to influence attitudes and beliefs.[28] These attitudes and beliefs form the basis of consumer action, which takes place when a behavioural prompt, such as a product promotion, stimulates the consumer.[29] Advertising builds awareness, attitudes, and perceptions over the long term.

Promotions

Promotions aim for more-immediate action on the part of the consumer.[30] They can be quite varied and include coupons, multiple-pack discounts ("Buy two, get one free"), promotional allowances paid to retailers, point-of-sale displays, free samples, value-added promotions offering free merchandise such as lighters or clothing, endorsements, and placement in movies and television. In 2005, the tobacco industry in the United States spent US$ 13.11 billion on advertising and promotions.[27]

More than 40% of the total expenditures on advertising and promotions went to retailer promotional allowances, which pay retailers for stocking brands and devoting specific shelf space to them. Allowances also pay for cooperative advertising and cover the costs of retail/wholesale sales incentives. Point-of-sale promotions place cigarettes in convenient retail locations, such as at the ends of aisles or in displays at the checkout counter.

Promotions are used to convince consumers to try a product, build purchase volume, encourage brand switching, win customer loyalty, and enhance corporate image.[3,26,28,31] Value-added promotions, which offer extra specialty items, stimulate short-term sales.[28] They also offer a promotion boost, however, since consumers wear or use the branded clothing or accessories, serving as free "walking billboards" for the companies. These items do not carry the health warnings required in advertisements.

Discount coupons may be especially effective for reaching women and young children, who may be sensitive to lower prices than men are.[32] Jurisdictions that increase taxes on tobacco should expect to see the price increase offset somewhat by increases in discounts, as was reported in California and Arizona after their tax increases. The tobacco companies create databases when coupons or other promotions are redeemed by mail. These databases provide demographics used in further marketing. They are also used to alert tobacco users to take action when tobacco control policies are being voted upon. A newer promotional strategy, used by Philip Morris, is to offer discounts on non-tobacco items, such as food or drinks, with a tobacco purchase.[33] As policies restrict direct tobacco promotions further, there may be a proliferation of this alternative discount strategy.

Philip Morris, the manufacturer of Virginia Slims, the most successful women's brand, offers many promotions. For years, Philip Morris has offered a Virginia Slims annual engagement calendar, the Book of Days. Its V-wear catalogues offer clothing items such as blouses, coats, scarves, and accessories in exchange for proofs of purchase from packs of Virginia Slims cigarettes. Each of the catalogues has a theme (e.g. glamour) that is reflected in the catalogue copy, photographs, and print advertising. To obtain the items, one must amass large numbers of proofs of purchase. For example, a black coat lined in raspberry pink requires the purchase of 325 packs,[34] at a cost of US$ 621, based on an average per-branded-pack cost of US$ 1.91.[35] The theme is carried through in stores, where small plastic shopping baskets feature the ad for Virginia Slims, and plastic bags with the VS logo hold purchases. The fall 1998 catalogue carried a "Light up the night" theme for its clothing.

Misty Slims, an American Tobacco Company product, has offered clothing, lighters, and even a Rand McNally outlet-mall shopping guide. R. J. Reynolds' Camel Cash catalogues offer clothing, jewellery, lipstick holders, lighters, and other accessories. Philip Morris's Marlboro brand has a Marlboro Country Store catalogue and unique promotions, such as a seat on the "Marlboro Train" trip or a vacation at the "Marlboro Ranch". Philip Morris spent US$ 200 million on its Marlboro Adventure Team catalogue.[31] In addition to fashion, glamour, and adventure, tobacco company promotions feature themes of independence and liberty. Philip Morris once gave away playing cards featuring the Statue of Liberty, and Brown & Williamson sent its loyal customers crystal Christmas tree ornaments engraved with the Liberty Bell and the Brown & Williamson logo.

Tobacco companies use promotions to target women by carrying through the themes, colours, and packaging from the ads to the promotional items, reinforcing the image of the brand. While the tobacco industry also targets men with these strategies, women represent a special-interest group. The industry advertises and promotes its products to create primary demand for new users to try them; to reinforce purported tobacco benefits and maintain customers, to make the use of tobacco seem normal, to position products in prominent locations, to minimize the risks of use, and to achieve social legitimacy, and create goodwill.[36–39]

Sponsorships

Brand or corporate sponsorship of entertainment, sporting events, and organizations is the fastest-growing form of tobacco marketing. In 1995, tobacco companies spent about US$ 139 million on sports and entertainment sponsorships in the United States.[40] Sponsorship allows a company to reach a niche market economically and embeds advertising within the event or organization by linking product attributes or images to it. For the cost of a 30-second Super Bowl commercial, a company that sponsors a NASCAR Winston Cup team receives more than 30 hours of television exposure.[41]

For years, Philip Morris has offered a Virginia Slims annual engagement calendar, the Book of Days. Its V-wear catalogues offer clothing items such as blouses, coats, scarves, and accessories in exchange for proofs of purchase from packs of Virginia Slims cigarettes.

Sponsorship creates prestige and credibility for tobacco brands through association with important events (e.g. fine arts performances or art exhibitions). Tobacco sponsorship may blunt criticism of the industry, socially legitimize smoking, create gratitude from recipient organizations, and produce allies or neutral feelings about tobacco industry practices.[3,14,42,43] Tobacco companies use sponsorships as a platform for directing other marketing strategies, such as advertising and promotion.[41] They have long been used to reach women.

Sponsorship of women's tennis is the classic example of such targeting. Women's tennis represents the independence, assertiveness, and success attributes sought by brands such as Virginia Slims or its British counterpart, Kim.[14] From 1973 to 1994, Philip Morris sponsored the Virginia Slims professional tennis tour.[40] Television coverage and other media reports of the tournaments helped promote the brand and its logo, and cigarette samples were given away at the entrances to matches.[3] At a Wimbledon match, Martina Navratilova wore a tennis outfit that was made in the colours of Kim packaging and included the Kim logo.[44]

Philip Morris ended its US$ 5 million per year sponsorship of the tour in 1995. The company replaced it with a US$ 3 million per year Virginia Slims Legends Tour, intended to reach older women. The tour included a six-site tournament of former tennis greats, including Billie Jean King, Chris Evert, and Martina Navratilova. It also presented a concert featuring female singers, including Barbara Mandrell and Gladys Knight.[40,45]

While many assume that car racing is of primary interest to men, a recent study estimated that children 12 to 17 years of age make up 14% of the audience at these events, and more than 25% of children 12 to 17 years of age watched auto racing on television in 1996.

Links to the fashion industry appear in sponsorships as well. More cigarettes, a product of R. J. Reynolds, sponsored fashion shows in shopping malls that were tied to advertising in fashion magazines.[3] They also sponsored the More Fashion Awards for designers in the fashion industry.[46] The tobacco industry sponsors family-oriented festivals and fairs for community cultural groups, events that can lead to dependency on tobacco.[38] For example, it supports the Hispanic Cinco de Mayo street fairs in many communities that have Hispanic organizations. Philip Morris's Marlboro brand sponsored 18 major fairs, including large state fairs, in 1995, spending US$ 850 000 to reach 20 million family members.[40] The Newport brand (Lorillard) spent US$ 155 000 to reach more than 15 million attendees at 31 New York City family and children's events in 1996. Events including family festivals, a Fourth of July (Independence Day) celebration, and even the Sierra Club's Earth Awareness Day accepted these sponsorships.[40]

Tobacco companies also support the arts and athletics.[38,40–46] In 1995 alone, Philip Morris spent US$ 1.2 million to sponsor 15 dance companies (e.g. American Ballet Theatre, Dance Theatre of Harlem, and Joffrey Ballet) and two dance events.[40] Tobacco companies have also sponsored performances of the Alvin Ailey Dance Theatre; a photographic exhibit featuring images of the late civil rights leader Dr Martin Luther King; the Vatican Art Exhibit at New York City's Metropolitan Museum of Art; and the Arts Festival of Atlanta (attended by more than 10 million people). Many of these events target communities with significant numbers of Hispanic and Afro-American members.

Sponsorship of music concerts and festivals also offers opportunities to promote tobacco brands. The Kool Jazz Festival is a traditional sponsorship event. Rock concerts have benefited from tobacco support; for example, as part of its Rockin' Ticketmaster Campaign, Camel (R. J. Reynolds) offered discounted tickets to major rock events, advertising the tickets in a two-page pop-out magazine ad that featured Joe Camel handing the reader a pair of tickets. Getting the discounted tickets required sending in 100 proofs of purchase from Camel packs.[47] The industry has also offered support to female rock artists, with the Virginia Slims Woman Thing Music tour, prompting one young musician, Leslie Nuchow, to publicly turn down Philip Morris's support.[48]

Civic-improvement awards targeted to inner-city leaders are sponsored by Brown & Williamson's Kool brand, a menthol cigarette favoured by Afro-Americans. Kool Achiever Awards honour five such leaders annually, presenting a US$ 50 000 donation to a nonprofit, inner-city organization chosen by each person honoured.[42] Major Afro-American organizations, including the National Urban League, the National Association for the Advancement of Colored People, and the National Newspaper Publishers Association, participate in the selection process.[38]

Tobacco companies also sponsor motorsport racing events, such as the NASCAR Winston Cup stock car and drag races, the Indy Car World Series, and the Marlboro Grand Prix. Additionally, individual cars and drivers receive sponsorships. While many assume that car racing is of primary interest to men, a recent study estimated that children 12 to 17 years of age make up 14% of the audience at these events, and more than 25% of children 12 to 17 years of age watched auto racing on television in 1996.[49] These events also reach many women via television broadcasts. In 1992, more than 350 motorsports broadcasts reached audiences—which included women—of more than 915 million people.[50] Tobacco brands received more than 54 hours of television exposure during these broadcasts, and more than 10 000 mentions, having an exposure value of US$ 57 million (Winston, US$ 41 million; Marlboro, US$ 12 million; Camel, US$ 4 million).

NASCAR's own demographic studies (Harris Poll data) estimate that women constitute 39% of its audience.[51] Several NASCAR officials have described this trend:

> We want to continue in our direction of becoming a white-collar sport, where it's mom, dad, and the kids sitting around the TV and rooting for their favourite driver on Sunday.

> Now, racetracks are places you can bring your kids. I wouldn't say that 20 years ago. It's safe, full of families, the drinking has been greatly curtailed and of course it's all over TV.[52]

The sponsorship of motorsport racing events communicates an image of courage, independence, adventure, and aggression.[37] A vice president of marketing for Philip Morris stated, "We perceive Formula One and Indy car racing as adding, if you will, a modern-day dimension to the Marlboro Man".[37] Tobacco companies also support newer forms of racing, such as motorcycle and hydroplane boat races.

Sponsorship of Women's Organizations

Perhaps the most insidious form of tobacco company support is sponsorship of women's organizations. As part of a long-standing strategy to support groups representing racial/ethnic minorities and women—who strive for acceptance and expanded roles in American society—tobacco companies have supported women's organizations for many years. In 1987, Philip Morris gave more than US$ 2.4 million to more than 180 Afro-American, Hispanic, and women's groups, while R. J. Reynolds gave US$ 1.9 million.[42]

Women's groups that promote women's leadership in business and politics have been a special target.

These groups include the National Women's Political Caucus, the Women's Campaign Fund, the Women's Research and Education Institute, the League of Women Voters Education Fund, Women Executives in State Government, the Center for Women Policy Studies, the Center for the American Woman and Politics, the American Association of University Women, and the American Federation of Business and Professional Women's Clubs.[42,43]

In recent years, organizations such as the National Organization for Women, Women's Policy, Inc. (the nongovernment organizational affiliate of the Congressional Caucus for Women's Issues), and the American Medical Women's Association have actively refused tobacco funds and have worked in the area of women's health and tobacco control.

The National Organization for Women accepted funding from Philip Morris in the past to print its meeting programme.[3] A conference drawing half of the nation's female state legislators was held by the Center for American Women and Politics at Rutgers University (New Jersey), using funding from Philip Morris and R. J. Reynolds.[43] In 1987, those companies also provided 10% to 15% (US$ 130 000) of the budget of the National Women's Political Caucus.[42] A former congresswoman, Patricia Schroeder, a member of the caucus's advisory board and a prominent spokesperson for women's rights, employed fellows funded by the Women's Research and Education Institute and presented the caucus's "Good Guy Award" to a vice president of Philip Morris in 1989.[43] Philip Morris also sponsored internships for the Center for Women Policy Studies and provided funding for a national directory of female elected officials.[42]

World Health Organization

Tobacco industry support of minority women's groups is typical of its support for organizations representing racial/ethnic minorities. The industry has funded the National Coalition of 100 Black Women, the Mexican-American National Women's Association, the US Hispanic Women's Chamber of Commerce, and the National Association of Negro Business and Professional Women's Clubs.[43] Philip Morris has funded leadership training programmes for Hispanic women in New York and gave US$ 150 000 in 1987 to the US Hispanic Chambers of Commerce.[42]

A two-year study commissioned by the US Department of Health and Human Services and the Office of National Drug Control Policy found that 89% of the top 200 movie rentals in 1996–1997 contained scenes of tobacco use.

Other minority organizations that have benefited from tobacco company support include the National Council of La Raza, the League of United American Citizens, the National Hispanic Scholarship Foundation, the National Association of Hispanic Journalists, the United Negro College Fund, the National Urban League, the National Newspaper Publishers Association, and the Black Journalists Hall of Fame, and tobacco companies have provided funding for directories of national Afro-American and Hispanic organizations.[42,43,46]

Many of the organizations that have received tobacco industry support claim that the industry supported them, along with individuals, through hiring and promotion processes when no one else would. The Women's Campaign Fund Executive Director noted, "They were there for us when nobody else was. They legitimized corporate giving for women's groups, from my perspective".[43] But this support has not come without receiving something in return. As the leading sponsorship-tracking organization in the United States reported, "Cause marketing is

expected to show a return on investment".[41] Sponsorships buy visibility and credibility that may lead to neutral or supportive stances on tobacco industry positions.[42,43,46] The director of the fellowship programme for the Women's Research and Education Institute stated it this way:

> *I simply think it's part of their way to make themselves look better. They know they're perceived negatively by representatives who are concerned with health issues. To tell you the truth, I'm not that interested. I'm just glad they found us.[42]*

An August 1986 Tobacco Institute memo reflected the buy-in of women's organizations:

> *We began intensive discussions with representatives of key women's organizations. Most have assured us that, for the time being, smoking is not a priority issue for them.[42]*

Women's groups that take tobacco money have rarely supported anti-smoking campaigns.[43] For example, in 1991, the Congressional Caucus on Women's Issues introduced the Women's Health Equity Act. Although the package included 22 bills, six of them on prevention, none of the proposals addressed smoking.[43]

Mainstream minority organizations have also not been in the forefront of activism against tobacco industry practices that target their members. The National Black Monitor, inserted monthly into 80 Afro-American newspapers, ran a three-part series on the industry. The first article in the series called upon Afro-Americans to "oppose any proposed legislation that often serves as a vehicle for intensified discrimination against this industry which has befriended us, often far more than any other, in our hour of greatest need".[42] Another instalment, ghost-written by R. J. Reynolds, argued that "relentless discrimination still rages unabashedly on a cross-country scope against another group of targets—the tobacco industry and 50 million private citizens who smoke".[42]

Sponsorships thus serve many purposes and are a potent addition to advertising and promotion strategies. The marketing of tobacco products has been overwhelmingly successful in the United States. Even while prevalence rates among male smokers were declining by half, women's rates of smoking rose before they declined.[53] In recent years, organizations such as the National Organization for Women, Women's Policy, Inc. (the nongovernment organizational affiliate of the Congressional Caucus for Women's Issues), and the American Medical Women's Association have actively refused tobacco funds and have worked in the area of women's health and tobacco control. These actions and activities by women's organizations are noteworthy and important to document.

Placement of Tobacco in Popular Culture

Tobacco finds it way into popular culture through exposure in films, television, and music. While the tobacco industry states that it no longer pays to have brands placed in popular movies (no expenditures were reported to the Federal Trade Commission in recent years), during the 1980s, Brown & Williamson paid Sylvester Stallone US$ 500 000 to smoke its cigarettes in six films.[54]

Several studies note the pervasiveness of tobacco in popular films. One study that looked at smoking in movies for four decades (1960–1996) found that tobacco depictions in movies increased in the 1990s to levels found in the 1960s.[54] To analyse this trend, the researchers divided the total length of time of each film into 5-minute segments. In the 1990s, one third of the 5-minute time intervals in the films contained a tobacco reference, and 57% of the major characters smoked. Between 1991 and 1996, 80% of the male and 27% of the female leads smoked. The studies also noted the increasing appearance of cigars—all of the five films in their 1996 sample depicted cigar use.

Another study examined the top 10 moneymaking films in each year from 1985 to 1995 and found that 98% of them had references that supported tobacco use, such as showing smoking or smoking paraphernalia.[55] Again, one third of the 5-minute segments portrayed pro-tobacco events, and in 46% of the films, at least one lead character used tobacco. In 1996, a newspaper reported that the 10 top-grossing films of that year all contained tobacco use, as did 17 of the 18 films in distribution.[56] A two-year study commissioned by the US Department of Health and Human Services and the Office of National Drug Control Policy found that 89% of the top 200 movie rentals in 1996–1997 contained scenes of tobacco use.[57] Children's animated feature films also portray tobacco use. Of 50 such films produced between 1937 and 1997, 68%—including all seven such

films released in 1996 and 1997—displayed at least one episode of tobacco use.[58]

Film stars are important marketing vehicles for the tobacco industry and portray tobacco use more frequently than the actual prevalence among users. Also, a known risk factor for youth smoking is overestimating the number of peers who smoke.[54] John Travolta, Gwyneth Paltrow, Winona Ryder, Brad Pitt, Julia Roberts, Whoopi Goldberg, Bill Cosby, and other popular stars who smoke on film have broad appeal beyond the United States, helping to spread the smoking image to countries where tobacco advertising is restricted. Perhaps the ultimate portrayal of tobacco in film is the 1999 release *200 Cigarettes,* which shows young people with little to do other than hang out in bars and clubs smoking.

Television also offers opportunities to show characters smoking. One study of prime-time television in 1984 found smoking taking place at a rate equal to once per hour.[59] A similar study in 1992 found the same rate-per-hour occurrence, with 24% of prime-time programmes on the three major networks depicting tobacco use.[60] Popular music is another venue for portraying tobacco use. Music videos shown on television make a visual connection between tobacco and music. One study found tobacco use portrayed in 19% of the music videos shown on four music video networks.[61] Posters advertising new music releases and the CD covers themselves also show the musicians using tobacco products.

Philip Morris uses music to attract women to smoking. The company has sponsored a live music series, Club Benson & Hedges, at clubs in cities such as Los Angeles and New Orleans. In 1997, Philip Morris launched its own record label, Woman Thing Music, which matched its print ad slogan "It's a woman thing". The CDs, which feature new women performers, are marketed with packs of Virginia Slims. A music tour included auditions in the cities where performances were held. Admission to some of the performances was free, and attendees received Virginia Slims gear.

Women's magazines, too, provide visual smoking messages (discussed later in this chapter). In addition to formal cigarette advertising, advertising for other products, such as clothing and accessories, may feature popular models who are smoking. Stories about popular screen stars or models often include photographs of

World Health Organization

them smoking. It appears that even though the terms of the Master Settlement Agreement in the United States preclude tobacco companies from specifically targeting teens in their advertising, the companies are not only continuing to target youth but are actually reaching more of them. As noted in recent press releases from the American Legacy Foundation, cigarette makers have increased their advertising in magazines that have large teen readerships.

The Internet offers the most modern opportunity to market tobacco products to women. Numerous sites on the Internet offer tobacco products, clothing, and fantasies. *Smoke* magazine (http://www.smokemag.com) offers smoking-related clothing and accessories, and many sites offer tobacco products by mail, some at discount prices and with few or no protections to prohibit sale to minors.

> *The Internet offers the most modern opportunity to market tobacco products to women. Numerous sites on the Internet offer tobacco products, clothing, and fantasies.*

The major tobacco companies operate their own web sites, on which company and product information mingles with promotional material. For example, the Brown & Williamson site includes sections on its sponsorship of community organizations and its programmes to reduce youth use (http://www.bw.com). Its sponsorship of Fishbone Fred, a Grammy-nominated children's performer, is noted on the site. Fred's performance tours include his song "Be Smart, Don't Start", and his *Safety Songs for Kids* cassette is marketed at the Brown & Williamson site.

Thus, messages about tobacco use pervade women's popular culture. These messages boost the advertising and promotion campaigns that tobacco companies use to target women. Popular culture reinforces the themes of marketing campaigns and sends exaggerated messages about the pervasiveness of women's smoking.

Marketing Strategies in the United States

Contemporary tobacco advertisements and promotions reveal marketing patterns carried forward from the beginning of the 1990s. The women's brands continue to market romance, glamour, independence, and the "in-charge" woman. Virginia Slims (Philip Morris) uses the "It's a woman thing" slogan, with ads that portray feisty, but sexy, women making comments about men. One ad shows a woman looking at a trophy and a stuffed moose head, saying to her partner, "The real reason we have garage sales? Your stuff".[62] In this ad, the woman is demonstrating her control over the domestic sphere and mocking her partner's inability to control his spending. *In Style* carries a Virginia Slims ad showing a man and a woman each driving a blue convertible, along with a shot of the woman's foot in a high wedge sandal decorated with fake fruit. The copy reads, "So maybe we define practical a little different than you".[63] Another ad features a woman in a blue dress pushing a guy in a black suit into a pool. It says, "When we ask what you love most about us, answer carefully, and quickly".[64] Again, these ads assert women's difference from men and reinforce their "in-charge" abilities.

Capri (Brown & Williamson) still uses the slogan "She's gone to Capri and she's not coming back" with a photo of a Mediterranean boudoir overlooking the city below.[65] Basic (Philip Morris) uses a "Keep it Basic" theme that shows the pack,[66] while another discount brand, GPC (Brown & Williamson), shows a woman at the edge of a lake at sunset and the words "Best smoke of the day",[67] and Doral (R. J. Reynolds) features a cat staring at an oversized goldfish in a bowl and the words "Imagine getting more than you hoped for. Get your paws on big taste, guaranteed".[68] Themes of relaxation and pleasure from smoking are increasingly appearing in magazine advertisements.

Merit (Philip Morris) touts its ultra-lights with a series of spoof ads—"Discover the rewards of thinking light"—that depict a sumo wrestler in pointe ballet shoes taking a leap[69] and an Eskimo musher and his loaded sled being pulled by a dachshund.[70] Carlton (Brown & Williamson) uses its familiar blue-and-white format to feature its 1 mg of tar: "Isn't it time you started thinking about number one? Think Carlton. With 1 mg. tar, it's the Ultra ultra light".[71] Camel, after withdrawing Joe Camel, turned to parody ads, many of which spoof the

Surgeon General's warnings by including a large "Viewer Discretion Advised" box, noting what out-of-the-norm symbols you can find in the ad. For example, one ad shows a young man behind jail bars and an overweight policeman. The second page reveals, from a back view, that the young man is a cutout figure made of Camel packs. The ad advises that "this ad contains package tampering, self parole, and overdue books".[72] Another ad shows a jungle scene, with women and men in a large cauldron over a fire. The "Viewer Discretion Advised" box warns of "hungry women, hot guys, and man stew".[73] Another ad spoofs the latest resurgence of health warnings about large steaks and big drinks. It shows a street parade with floats. One float has a large golden Camel, a pyramid, an overweight sultan, and belly dancers. Another shows a huge dancing steak and butchers (one smoking a cigarette) holding sausages and hams. The "Viewer Discretion Advised" box notes the "politically incorrect parade, red meat, and moving violations".[74]

Marlboro's current ads for Marlboro Lights feature a two-page Marlboro cowboy, "Come to where the flavor is",[75] scenic cliffs with "Come to Marlboro Country",[76] and a deep blue riverside scene.[77] Marlboro Lights enjoy extensive popularity with women and girls, who may prefer their milder taste. Lucky Strike (Brown & Williamson) has a retro ad featuring a diner with a male smoker and a faceless waitress and the slogan "An American Original".[78] Newport's (Lorillard) "Alive with pleasure!" ad shows a man clowning with an umbrella, a woman at the beach, and a bright green sky.[79] Another menthol cigarette, Kool (Brown & Williamson), also features green prominently in its "B Kool" ad, showing a large man's arm with a chain-link bracelet, the hand holding a lit cigarette and a pack of Kools. Two non-white women are looking at the man, and an Afro-American man has his arm around one of the women.[80] In the United States, menthol cigarettes are used more frequently by non-whites than by whites.

Winston Lights (R. J. Reynolds) uses a red-and-white motif to promote its "No additives, no bull" theme. One ad proclaims, "Blue collar. White collar. How about no collar. No bull".[81] It shows two men and a woman in a recording studio. Another approach is used in an ad in which a woman looks disgusted as she says, "I wanted a light, not his life story. No additives. No bull".[82] An edgier ad for Regular Winston (R. J. Reynolds) is a two-page spread. One page has a grainy black-and-white photo of a flying-saucer spaceship. The copy on the

facing page reads, "If aliens are smart enough to travel through space, why do they keep abducting the dumbest people on earth? Winston. Straight up. No additives. True taste".[83] Interestingly, Asian models are starting to appear in tobacco ads. Two Virginia Slims ads mentioned previously[62] feature an Asian woman, and a Merit ad features a sumo wrestler.[69] The industry obviously sees great potential in marketing to women in Asia, since smoking prevalence among Asian women is low compared to prevalence among women in Western countries. In essence, advertising becomes globalized when the same ad is used in different countries.

Just as in the United States, marketing is a crucial component of the tobacco industry's expansion and is the primary method of competition in a highly concentrated industry dominated by a small number of relatively large firms.

Marketing Tobacco to Women and Girls in Asia

Women and girls in Asia constitute a vast untapped market for the tobacco industry. Despite the financial crises occurring throughout Asia, transnational tobacco companies continue to identify positive aspects of the Asian market. An editorial in *Tobacco Reporter* reinforces this optimism: "The situation does not fundamentally change the underlying strengths of the market. Rising per-capita consumption, a growing population, and an increasing acceptance of women smoking continue to generate new demand".[84] Changing gender norms and roles combined with increases in women's earning power may lead to increased marketing resources being directed towards tobacco consumption.

Just as in the United States, marketing is a crucial component of the tobacco industry's expansion and is the primary method of competition in a highly concentrated industry dominated by a small number of relatively large firms. The largest international tobacco company is Altria/Philip Morris, with 17% of the global market, 8.5% of which is accounted for by Marlboro, the world's most popular cigarette.[85] British American Tobacco (BAT), which has merged with Rothmans, has 16% of the global market share.[86] Japan Tobacco, which bought out R. J. Reynolds, has become the third largest tobacco company,[87] and China National Tobacco Corporation also has substantial shares in the global market.

Marketing expenditures in China are substantial: in 1994, Marlboro was the biggest advertiser (US$ 5.2 million), followed by 555-State Express (US$ 3.1 million), which is produced by PT BAT Indonesia. The absence of domestic cigarette advertising in China has allowed foreign tobacco companies to use their marketing expertise with great effect.

Industry documents reveal that in 1993, a BAT corporate strategy, code-named Project Battalion, was conceptualized. The strategy targeted marketing efforts at a hit list of the "top 50 cigarette markets". Asia was the largest target, with China at the top of the list, closely followed by India, Brazil, and Indonesia. Other Asian countries, including Thailand, Malaysia, and Viet Nam, were also on the list.[88] Multinational tobacco companies are already doing an impressive business in Asia, where almost half of the world's cigarettes are consumed.[89]

Cigarette sales, which fell by almost 5% in North America between 1990 and 1995, increased by 8% in the Asia Pacific region during the same time period.[90] In 1996, 70% of the cigarettes sold by Philip Morris and almost 60% of those sold by R. J. Reynolds were sold overseas, with exports totalling 11 billion packs.[91] In general,

tobacco consumption in Asia continued its upward trend between 2002 and 2007.[92,93] Cigarette consumption in China rose from 1643 billion sticks in 2002 to 2163 billion sticks in 2007.[92,93]

Tobacco companies rank among the 10 top marketers in several Asian countries. In Hong Kong Special Administrative Region, Philip Morris is the ninth largest marketer, spending US$ 12.9 million annually. In Malaysia, three tobacco companies rank among the top four marketers. Rothmans ranks first, with annual spending of US$ 36.2 million, BAT ranks second (US$ 19.7 million), and R. J. Reynolds is fourth (US$ 9.5 million). While it is not possible to determine what percentage of the overall marketing expenditures is spent on women and girls, tobacco advertising in Asia is so ubiquitous that it has a powerful effect on everyone, including young children. What can be said with some certainty is that women and girls are strategically important to the long-term growth of the industry. In the past five years, Philip Morris International and BAT have purchased the largest tobacco companies in Indonesia. The industry recognizes that there are strategic opportunities to enter the large and growing market of kreteks (locally manufactured clove cigarettes), which are smoked by over 90% of smokers in Indonesia. This market could include women in the future.

In a marketing strategy paper, BAT outlined details for transforming its staid, traditionally male Benson & Hedges brand to a woman's-appeal cigarette, as part of an "up-market socializing" strategy. Describing Benson & Hedges' present male smokers as loyal but "getting older", the paper reports that "in many ways, they [men] represent the cigarette world of yesterday, rather than the market of tomorrow".[93] It is to women and girls that they will turn for tomorrow's market. Women in China represent the largest potential market for the tobacco industry. As noted by a vice president of Philip Morris Asia some years ago, "No discussion of the tobacco industry in the year 2000 would be complete without addressing what may be the most important feature on the landscape, the China market. In every respect, China confounds the imagination".[94]

Marketing expenditures in China are substantial: In 1994, Marlboro was the biggest advertiser (US$ 5.2 million), followed by 555-State Express (US$ 3.1 million), which is produced by PT BAT Indonesia. The absence of domestic cigarette advertising in China has allowed foreign

World Health Organization

tobacco companies to use their marketing expertise with great effect. Intensive marketing efforts by transnationals seem to be paying off, as smoking is reported to be on the rise, particularly among men. Trade restrictions are still in place, however, so current sales of foreign cigarettes in China are somewhat limited.[95] Nevertheless, a former BAT executive with knowledge of the company's Chinese operations reported that in 1995, BAT sold 400 million cigarettes to the China National Tobacco Corporation, 3 billion to duty-free shops, 4 billion to special economic zones, and 38 billion to distributors who smuggle the goods into China.[96] In fact, there is evidence to suggest that smuggling is good for business, as it keeps the price of foreign cigarettes down (no taxes are levied) and eliminates the need for warning labels.[97]

Despite the fact that advertisements in China are not allowed to mention cigarettes or actually show people smoking, foreign cigarettes have become firmly entrenched and may influence brand preference and future buying patterns. Foreign brands are important status symbols in China.[98] A recent study of 1900 college students in three Chinese cities revealed that Marlboro was the most familiar brand of cigarette as well as the most preferred.[99] Importantly, non-smokers and smokers were equally familiar with tobacco products, suggesting that communal knowledge is a better predictor of familiarity with cigarette brands than is smoking status. It is disconcerting to consider that advertising effects may be amplified in such a market, where information gleaned from cigarette advertisements is effectively channelled into a shared pool of knowledge among women and men. Cigarette advertisements for products such as Marlboro and Salem may be a particularly potent force in China and other Asian countries, since their level of sophistication renders them visually distinct from indigenous advertising.

Global advertisements sometimes require "makeovers", as was the case with the Marlboro Man when he first appeared in Hong Kong SAR. During an interview, the advertising director for Hong Kong SAR's Leo Burnett, the advertising agency responsible for creating the Marlboro Man in the United States, explained how people in Hong Kong SAR did not identify with the worker image of the cowboy, although the Chinese consider the horse a very good symbol, representing health, success, vitality, and energy. The Marlboro Man had to be transformed and upgraded from a labourer to a leader.[100]

Consumer Culture

An understanding of consumer culture is critical to a discussion of the marketing of tobacco to women and girls in Asia. Consumer culture can best be characterized as a culture of mass consumption, wherein the consumption of goods carries with it the consumption of meaning and symbols. Consumer culture is visual, and images—often images of Western-styled modern women—play a dominant role in Asia. They imply that through the practice of consumption—i.e. by buying the advertised product—one can create a new identity. Consumer culture "holds out the promise of a beautiful and fulfilling life: the achievement of individuality through the transformation of self and lifestyle".[101] Tobacco advertising engages the consumer in a fantasy, inviting her or him to participate in a promise "that the product can do something for you that you cannot do for yourself".[102] Although only the elite in the developing world can consume in a truly Western manner, cigarettes promise to fulfil this fantasy inexpensively. In some countries, costly foreign brands can be purchased as single sticks, rendering them relatively more affordable.

> *Consumer culture is visual, and images—often images of Western-styled modern women—play a dominant role in Asia. Through the practice of consumption—i.e. by buying the advertised product—one can create a new identity.*

Three important points may be noted with regard to consumption in Asia, particularly in developing countries. First, regardless of whether an individual chooses to consume the product (the cigarette) or not, he or she can still observe and absorb the image. Like window-shopping, observing ads can be a vicarious form of consumption. Second, despite the fact that many people in Asia, particularly women and girls, are illiterate, most have visual literacy. That is, even those who cannot read are influenced by and understand the intent of image-based tobacco advertising. Third, pervasive, highly seductive images of what cigarettes can do for you exist in environments where little information is available about the negative health consequences of tobacco use.

Women's bodies have been used to sell tobacco, alcohol, and other products worldwide for many years, and tobacco advertising in the Philippines provides some excellent examples of this strategy.

In Western cultures, identity is not ascribed by or anchored in tradition or religion but is generally chosen by the individual. Asian youth, who are often caught between the traditional world of their family and the modern world they encounter in advertisements and the media, may be particularly susceptible to images of modernization that link products with feelings, emotions, and lifestyles. For young women, creating a new, fashionable identity is intricately linked to the body. Female college students interviewed in South India repeatedly stated that in order to wear Western clothes (e.g. jeans and short skirts) and look good in them, a girl *needed* to be thin. Whereas traditional dress, which is loose and unfitted, was viewed as complimentary to all women, Western dress required that one have the "right" body shape. In the global consumer culture, having the right body becomes central to a woman's identity. By using women's bodies to sell cigarettes, the tobacco industry reinforces a strong association between the two.

Women's Bodies and the Selling of Cigarettes

Women's bodies have been used to sell tobacco, alcohol, and other products worldwide for many years, and tobacco advertising in the Philippines provides some excellent examples of this strategy. Calendars produced and widely distributed by Fortune Tobacco Corporation, the largest tobacco company in the Philippines, are a prominent medium of cigarette advertising. One calendar that is posted in local provision shops throughout the islands shows a fair-skinned model seated with her legs wide apart, wearing a see-through, netted bra and silk boxers, gazing off into the distance. Behind her is a box of Hope cigarettes that is almost as large as she is. She clutches a pack of Hope in one hand, and in the other, she holds an unlit cigarette. Appearing to be absorbed in her daydreams, her image suggests that her cigarettes can help her relax and enjoy the experience. In fact, observational data suggest that Hope is the cigarette brand of choice for many young Filipinas.[103] The brand name itself reflects the dream of many Filipinas, that is, hope for a better life and a good marriage.

In another ad, a light-skinned model with pronounced cleavage is seated on a deck overlooking the ocean. She wears only an oversized men's shirt, unbuttoned to reveal most of her breasts, and a baseball cap with "Alaska" written across it. Her pose is provocative, and her eyes boldly stare at the viewer. In her hand, she holds an unlit cigarette. Pictured next to her are two cameras, leading one to imagine that she is a photographer. A carton of Champion cigarettes and two unopened packs lie next to her legs. The logo for Fortune Tobacco Company is visible in the corner of the calendar.

The model (the same one is featured on both calendars) embodies the characteristics of a Filipina beauty: She is a Euro-American mestiza, with white skin and a pronounced "American-style" nose. Her unbuttoned blouse reveals her "American-sized" breasts, referred to locally as *pakwan suso*, or watermelon breasts. Large breasts, such as those of Baywatch's Pamela Anderson, are discussed and admired by Filipino women, who refer to their breasts as small fruits (*calamansi suso*) in comparison with those of foreigners.[104] Not only is the Fortune calendar model endowed with a beautiful "Western" body, she is also daring enough to show it off in revealing attire. Typically, Filipino women are modest and do not go to the seashore in anything more revealing than a T-shirt and blue jeans, for fear of being labelled promiscuous.

Remarkably, these calendars find their ways into the homes of villagers in remote islands of the Philippines. They are tacked up in small, one-room thatched homes,

World Health Organization

where they represent images of beauty and whiteness, which serve as much-desired symbols of modernity and wealth. These images are typically hung near the family religious shrine, which consists of statues and candles, often side-by-side with Jesus and the Virgin Mary.[105] In fact, one Fortune calendar "ingeniously used the Filipino faith in Mother Mary"[105] to sell cigarettes. It featured the face of a very white Mary (sometimes called "American Mary"), bordered by all 17 brands of cigarettes distributed by Fortune Tobacco.

Similar to the advertising in the Philippines, advertisements in Viet Nam commonly use women's bodies to sell products, particularly on posters advertising beer and cigarettes. Such posters typically portray big-busted foreign women in scanty clothing. In real life as well, women's bodies become the medium by which cigarettes are distributed to men. On the streets of Hanoi, for example, attractive young women are employed to dress in the recognizable colours of cigarette brands and stand on street corners, smilingly giving away free samples to passers-by.[106]

In Tonga, multinational corporations such as Benson & Hedges and Royal Beer sponsor beauty contests, replacing the original sponsors who were the heads of extended families and the eiki (ruling class). The winners of the contests then become spokeswomen and promoters of the sponsors' products for the reigning year. The shift in sponsorship has also been marked by shifts in desired body shape. Increasingly, the body of choice is a more streamlined Western body, narrowing notions of diversity and promoting a global consensus of what constitutes beauty.[107]

Women's Brands in Asia

As in the United States, brands of cigarettes designed to appeal to women have been introduced in many Asian countries, typically with themes highlighting independence, sophistication, glamour, and sexuality.

These images hold particular appeal for young and impressionable women and girls who seek to emulate or acquire the attributes of the models in the ads. Not uncommonly, advertisements for women's brands in Asia feature Western models. For example, the model in advertisements for Capri Superslim cigarettes in

Japan is a blonde woman who is both an executive and an artist, while Salem's Pianissimo cigarettes similarly feature a Nordic blonde woman. Why, we might ask, are foreigners used in these ads? What do they lend to the visual image and say about the product that a local model would not? To put it most simply, Westerners function as symbols of the West. According to Japan's largest advertising agency, Dentsu, Caucasian models lend a sense of foreignness to Japanese products, serving as symbols of prestige, quality, and modernity.[108,109]

> *In Tonga, multinational corporations such as Benson & Hedges and Royal Beer sponsor beauty contests, replacing the original sponsors who were the heads of extended families and the eiki (ruling class). The winners of the contests then become spokeswomen and promoters of the sponsors' products for the reigning year.*

Remarkably, however, the Tobacco Institute of Japan, headed by the President of Philip Morris's Japan branch, insists that the ads that feature women are targeted at men.[110] The institute echoes the time-weary argument that advertising and marketing activities do not cause new segments of the population to initiate smoking, but rather are designed to influence existing smokers to switch their brand loyalty.

To emphasize the link between smoking and fashion, Vogue cigarettes in Japan feature a "whippet-thin, chiseled-cheek-boned model" who stares coolly into the distance as an adoring man nuzzles her neck. Floating in the corner of the ad is a pastel-coloured pack of cigarettes. In case her European features are not obvious enough, flowing Japanese script declares, "This woman is Vogue".[110] In the globalized context of consumer culture, a Western woman and her choice of cigarettes project a powerful symbol. Interestingly, the Vogue brand is described in the

European journal *Tobacco* as "a stylish type of cigarette with obvious feminine appeal, being slim and therefore highly distinctive".[111]

According to an advertising expert in Tokyo, "Tobacco companies are putting a great emphasis on advertising low-smoke cigarettes that are basically designed for women who hate to have their hair and dresses spoiled with the smell of tobacco smoke".[112] R. J. Reynolds has marketed Pianissimos as a low-smoke, reduced-smell version of Salem that has been popular among women.[113] Smoking among young Japanese women has been on an increase in recent years, although as recently as 1950, smoking was considered to be a habit of professionally promiscuous women, such as prostitutes and geisha. This is true in other Asian countries as well.[114] In a 1999 nationwide survey on smoking behaviour in Japan conducted by the Ministry of Health and Welfare, smoking prevalence among adult women was reported to be 13.4%. About 44% of current female smokers reported smoking their first cigarette while they were minors. Data from two nationwide surveys conducted in 1996 and 2000 among Japanese high-school adolescents showed that current and daily smoking rates for girls increased across all grades.[115]

To emphasize the link between smoking and fashion, Vogue cigarettes in Japan feature a "whippet-thin, chiseled-cheek-boned model" who stares coolly into the distance as an adoring man nuzzles her neck.

Foreign brands, like foreign models, are gaining in popularity in Japan. A Philip Morris executive, commenting on the increase in sales of the company's products in Japan, noted, "We have been relentless in the last few years. Our marketing is really good: I think we're feeling the pulse of the consumer as well as possible. For many years, Marlboro was a slow burner here, but now it's on fire. It's growing more than 25% year-to-year".[116] Although clearly not advertised as a woman's cigarette, Marlboro is the most popular brand among both male and female adolescent smokers in the United States, with 60% of the market share.[117]

Data from Thailand indicate that young smokers prefer foreign brands and that young women in particular show a marked preference for foreign cigarettes, especially Marlboro Lights. Little research to date has identified what underlies these preferences, although it is not difficult to imagine that there is a connection to weight control and concern with smoking what is perceived to be a "healthier" cigarette.[118]

In India, where smoking by women and girls is generally considered to be culturally inappropriate, a BAT subsidiary launched a women's cigarette named Ms in 1990. The launch involved large-scale promotion and the use of attractive female models who promoted Ms and gave away free samples. In response to protests by women activists about the direct targeting of women and girls in a culture where females traditionally do not smoke, company representatives rallied to the defence of Ms, explaining that "the brand was targeted towards emancipated women, that they were showing models only in Western rather than traditional Indian dress, and that the female models were not actually shown smoking".[119] Concerned that Indian women might be hesitant to purchase the cigarettes in shops, advertising copy proclaimed, "Just give us a call and we will deliver a carton at your address!"

In 1997, Just Black, a cigarette in an all-black box, was introduced in Goa, India. The advertisement for this product featured a young, fair-skinned woman sporting long braids, a tennis outfit, and a demure smile. She was shown leaning against a large black motorcycle, holding her tennis racket, seemingly waiting for her boyfriend, her tennis partner, to return. She appeared both innocent and sexy, and the reader was left to wonder whose cigarette it was—his or hers. The handwritten copy read, "Me and him and Just Black", implying that it was "their" mutual friend, something they shared. It is an interesting circumventing of cultural prohibitions on women's smoking: her smoking was implied, although not overtly spoken about. The advertisement also posited a spurious association between being athletic and being a smoker.

Industry documents reveal that the Just Black campaign arose out of a secret BAT project, code-named Project Kestrel, whose objective was to develop a brand that "breaks the rules", appeals to a new generation of youth, and shocks their parents.[120] The memo directly refers to the "literate youth of today, being very image-oriented" who require a unique brand of cigarettes, not like Marlboro, "but which are completely unconventional, which set new standards encouraging their rebellion, not necessarily just against parents". This new brand would be responsive to teens' individuality and have a totally distinct brand name "so that no preconceived ideas could be formed". The brand needed to reflect durable youth values such as rebellion and the glamour of danger. The packaging was to be distinctive, preferably black, a colour that was noted to be popular among youth.[120] Despite the obvious ramifications of increased marketing to youth, the industry adamantly denies that it has specifically targeted them. "We don't advertise to children…. First of all, we don't want young people to smoke. And we're running ads aimed specifically at young people advising them that we think smoking is strictly for adults. Kids just don't pay attention to cigarette ads, and that's how it should be".[121]

Although China already consumes 37% of the world's cigarettes,[92] this market might be substantially enlarged if women, who presently constitute only a small percentage of smokers, could be enticed to smoke. Attempts to lure women into smoking have been documented. In 1998, two new Chinese cigarette brands targeted at women smokers were introduced. Chahua and Yuren (literally, "pretty woman") are promoted as low-tar products, delivering 12 and 15 mg of tar, respectively, in contrast to the average 18-mg delivery of other domestic cigarettes. Yuren is described as slim, with a white filter and "mild" taste.[122] Cigarette advertising worldwide has persistently used images and language to reassure present and potential smokers that they can engage in "healthy smoking".[123] In actuality, smokers of lower-yield cigarettes puff more frequently or more intensely than those smoking higher-yield cigarettes to obtain their usual level of nicotine.[123]

Interviewed about Yuren, the manager of the Kunming Cigarette Factory was quoted as saying, "China has more than 30 million female smokers, and yet China made no cigarettes specially designed for women. In the past, women smokers had to rely on imported and smuggled cigarettes made for female smokers".[124] No data are available at present about the popularity of these products among Chinese women, and it will be important to monitor this, as well as the development of other wom-

en's brands. Throughout Asia, packaging is an important component of women's brands and promotional materials. The "feminine touch" is apparent: Brown & Williamson's Capri cigarettes are sold in slim white boxes and feature a floral design. In Viet Nam, feminine-style lighters that are slim and pink (imported from Japan) are available in the marketplace; other lighters for women resemble a perfume bottle or feature a romantic picture of a couple.[106]

Prominent Themes in Advertising to Women and Girls in Asia

Several key themes noted earlier in the section on marketing tobacco to women in the United States have been documented in cigarette ads targeted at women and girls in Asia. These themes are discussed below.

In India, where smoking by women and girls is generally considered to be culturally inappropriate, a BAT subsidiary launched a women's cigarette named Ms in 1990. The launch involved large-scale promotion and the use of attractive female models who promoted Ms and gave away free samples.

Independence

The woman who smokes is typically depicted as free and autonomous. Philip Morris advertised its Virginia Slims brand with the slogans "Be you" and "You're on your way". One Virginia Slims ad in Japan features a ballerina, with the caption "I want to dance to my own music without others' direction". A Japanese brand, Frontier Slims, echoes a similar theme of independence. It features

World Health Organization

a young-looking, slim Japanese woman with the copy stating, "I care for my feelings, not for others!".[125]

Research confirms that the theme of independence is important to women smokers. A study conducted among female airline cabin crew from 10 Asian countries found that when shown a Virginia Slims advertisement and asked to classify the woman featured, more smoking than non-smoking respondents viewed the woman as attractive, elegant, fit, and sociable. The authors of the study suggest that these women may smoke to enhance their images of independence.[126]

Stress Relief

Intensive market research conducted in the United States has enabled sophisticated segmentation of the female market, and these strategies are being transferred abroad. An industry document from Brown & Williamson shows a plan to market cigarettes for working women who have to juggle multiple roles. It states, "Keep it simple. Make them comfortable. To deal with the stress, complexity and speed, they will be looking for relief".[127]

Phillip Morris advertised its Virginia Slims brand with the slogans "Be you" and "You're on your way". One Virginia Slims ad in Japan features a ballerina, with the caption "I want to dance to my own music without others' direction".

Stress and tension relief are common themes discussed among youths in the United States and Asia with regard to smoking.[128] For example, when Hong Kong SAR youths were asked about the positive attributes of smoking, "smoking calms your nerves" was reported by more than one third of the male and female ever-smokers.[129] Similarly, the study of female airline cabin crew described above found that the most

common reasons these women gave for smoking were to control their mood, to gain control over their life, and to help cope with stress.[126]

Weight Control

As discussed earlier, the association between weight control and smoking has been documented in the marketing of cigarettes to women for many years. A study among Asian women that specifically asked about smoking and weight control found that almost 40% of the women sampled believed that smoking would help control body weight.[129]

Tobacco Use as a Gendered Experience

The increase in smoking among females in Asia is not the only issue of concern. Of equal importance is the question of why this shift is occurring. What role does smoking play in the lives of women and adolescent girls? If women and girls are beginning to smoke more and at younger ages, why are they doing so? Beyond the advertised image, what is women's experience with tobacco, and does it differ from the experience of men? In other words, from the layperson's perspective, does smoking confer distinct benefits for men and women? To answer these questions, it is necessary to consider the behaviour of females and males within specific cultural contexts. While few published studies have been conducted on gendered patterns of smoking, some anthropological accounts from fieldwork in the Philippines, India, Indonesia, Viet Nam, and China provide preliminary insights.

Trends in the Philippines

The 2003 World Health Survey on tobacco consumption in the Philippines reported that 58% of adult males and 12% of adult females were current tobacco smokers.[130] Data from the Global Youth Tobacco Survey showed that 28% of adolescent males and nearly 18% of adolescent females (13 to 15 years of age) were current tobacco smokers in 2007.[130] Little is known about the age of smoking initiation among women and girls. While there are no distinctive women's brands on the market, particular brands seem to be popular among women of different ages.

World Health Organization

Although about 12% of the women in the Philippines presently smoke,[130] smoking is a private habit for women rather than a public one.[131] While some women in their twenties do smoke when they go to bars or clubs, if they are seen smoking on the street, their behaviour may be misinterpreted. Men routinely discourage their girlfriends from smoking on the street, warning them overtly, "Don't smoke. It doesn't look good. You'll look like a prostitute".[131] Both smoking and drinking are commonplace among bar girls and among the foreign men who frequent bars.

Despite cultural restrictions on smoking by young women, smoking is acceptable among older women, who tend to smoke alone rather than in social situations. Observations of Filipinas who smoke indicate that cigarettes are often used as a substitute for expressing feelings, indicating sadness, anger, or depression. In a culture in which it is inappropriate to talk about one's feelings overtly, a woman can show displeasure or loneliness by smoking quietly while listening to evangelical music. Thus, smoking may serve as a form of self-medication in an environment where few other resources are available. When a woman smokes, she is rarely talkative. Men in her household who observe her smoking may choose to leave her alone, recognizing that she wants her own space. In contrast to women's patterns of smoking, Filipino men light up frequently and in multiple social settings—at work, while drinking beer, playing pool, killing time, etc. When a group of men are smoking, women smokers typically do not join them.[131]

Observational data and ethnographic interviews indicate that some girls in their late teens believe that smoking helps reduce hunger and appetite.[132] Young women in the Philippines are extremely conscious of their body shape and weight, and many wish to lose weight to increase their popularity with the opposite sex. Considering the ubiquitous cigarette advertising featuring nearly nude, thin women, it is not surprising that some girls associate weight control with smoking. However, cigarettes are not considered to be suitable (hiyang) for everyone, and both cigarettes and alcohol are discussed in relation to body type. Some women complain that cigarettes are not hiyang for their body and that smoking results in undesirable weight loss.[132] Research is needed to understand the changing pattern of smoking among young Filipino women and the complex association between dieting and smoking.

Trends in India

In India, the rate of cigarette smoking among females is low (3.1% in 2005[133]), and women's smoking of cigarettes is confined to the urban elite classes of such large cosmopolitan cities as Delhi, Pune, Mumbai, and Bangalore. In these cities, modern girls are reported to smoke in pubs and at colleges, with particular colleges having "reputations" for female smoking. A note of caution should be raised, however. While conducting focus groups on smoking with female students at a medical college in a small South Indian city (Mangalore), anthropologist Mimi Nichter was told, "If you come back to India in ten years, all the professional women will be smoking!" When asked why this would be so, responses included, "to be modern, to be free, to be like boys, for weight control, and for tension". "In the cinema," one girl explained, "a guy smokes when he is depressed, when he has tension. In Hindi movies, women also smoke—especially the modern wife".[133] Recently, the Hindi film *Godmother* featured smoking by the heroine throughout the film. The actress who plays the godmother, Shabana Azmi, is extremely popular and is known for her social activism. The depiction of such a well-known actress smoking may serve as a role model for other Indian women.

> *Observations of Filipinas who smoke indicate that cigarettes are often used as a substitute for expressing feelings, indicating sadness, anger, or depression.*

Further discussions with college students identified a strong association between stress relief and smoking, a connection clearly garnered from the media. One male college student noted, "We know from advertisements that we see in the newspaper and in the cinema that cigarettes help with tension. In the ads, you see businessmen preparing their accounts, and they always have a cigarette in one hand and a packet on the table. In Hindi films, when the hero loses his girlfriend, he smokes a cigarette. Films and advertisements give us the reason why we should do it, and we follow".[134]

World Health Organization

When female college students in India were asked what percentage of women their age in the United States were smokers, responses ranged from 50% to 75%. Further discussion substantiated that this impression was largely derived from watching imported Western movies and from satellite television. Satellite television, another important factor in Indian women's exposure to female smoking, is increasingly popular and is also influencing dress style and behaviour.[134]

With regard to gender differences, several Indian girls noted that boys smoked to impress girls and that some male college students believed that "a cigarette in hand makes you a man". One girl explained, "Boys feel great if they're smoking". When asked what image a young male smoker projects, responses were largely positive: smokers were seen as being modern, macho, confident, and fashion-minded. These depictions mirrored the images of men in cigarette advertisements and in the cinema. Although many of the young women interviewed actually disliked smoking, the majority thought it would be inappropriate to disclose those feelings to a male.[134]

Indonesia is the fourth largest market for tobacco in the world. Tobacco advertising literally saturates the landscape. The country can best be described as an "advertiser's paradise", as it provides a largely unrestricted regulatory environment.

Despite the positive features attributed to the image of a smoker, male and female college students in India know of the health risks of smoking. In a survey conducted among more than 1600 college students, over 80% stated that they believe tobacco use is a problem among youth in India, and 90% stated that students should receive more information about tobacco in school settings.[134] Many male students who smoked were interested in getting information on how to quit. Concern was expressed, however, that if one were accustomed to smoking, quitting would "shock" the

body and would be harmful. Cultural perceptions about tobacco were also revealed. For example, college students believe that more-expensive cigarettes are made of better tobacco, which they believe is less harmful to one's health. In addition, they believe that it is easier to become addicted to more-expensive cigarettes, because they are smoother and easier to smoke. This results in higher levels of smoking.[134]

It is important to emphasize that the vast majority of women in India do not smoke, and cultural restrictions continue to be in place throughout the subcontinent. While it is critical to understand changes that are occurring among some upper-class segments of the population, it is equally important to identify protective factors within specific cultural contexts that promote resiliency in women and girls and serve to inhibit the initiation of smoking.

Trends in Indonesia

Indonesia is the fourth largest market for tobacco in the world. Tobacco advertising literally saturates the landscape. The country can best be described as an "advertiser's paradise", as it provides a largely unrestricted regulatory environment.[135] Cigarette marketing in Indonesia is among the most aggressive and innovative marketing in the world. The ubiquity of tobacco advertising serves to normalize the behaviour of smoking. As of 2009, Indonesia was the only country in South-East Asia that had not signed the WHO FCTC, which would require implementation of a ban or, if constitutional limits precluded a ban, restriction on advertising, promotion, and sponsorship. According to a 2007 national survey, almost 60% of men and 5% of women in Indonesia smoke.[135]

Although it is considered culturally inappropriate for women to smoke, smoking appears to be on the increase among affluent and educated women in urban areas, such as Jakarta, and among women working in nongovernmental organizations (NGOs).[136] In recent years, women have begun to be featured in cigarette advertisements, sometimes alone—that is, without men accompanying them, as was more typical of earlier advertising. For example, ads for the Clas Mild brand, typically thought of as a starter product, show a young, wealthy, modern woman on a cell phone, wearing a mini dress. She is perched next to an expensive foreign convertible car and appears to be dressed for a night out on the town. The copy

World Health Organization

reads, "Yesterday is gone, Clas Mild is today". Although the attractive model in the ad is not holding a cigarette or smoking, the implication is that this is the type of woman who could be a smoker. Another Clas Mild ad shows a beautiful young woman, heavily made up and wearing a jacket with a fur collar, snuggling against her boyfriend, a Westerner. The tag line repeats the message "Clas Mild is today", suggesting changing possibilities for women. Indeed, most of the ads for this popular youth brand portray modern women, and the copy emphasizes "the new sensation, the new classy breed" that the cigarette promises. Ads for other youth brands, such as L.A. Lights, feature a lineup of cosmopolitan males and females dressed for a night out on the town.[137] It will be important to document the growing placement of women in tobacco advertising in Indonesia, as well as changes in smoking prevalence rates. In a recent study, young adults noted that women who smoke prefer brands such as Clas Mild, L.A. Menthol Lights, and Marlboro Lights. Of the three brands, the first two include women in their advertisements. In 2008, two new slim cigarettes (Djarum Black Slims and Surya Slims) were introduced into the Indonesian market. The billboards and banners advertising these brands do not carry a photo, but rather feature the slim, sleek package. Although women are not visibly connected to these new product lines, slim cigarettes are typically targeted at women.[137]

Trends in Viet Nam

In Viet Nam, nearly 50% of the men currently smoke, but only 2% of the women do.[138] Smoking among women is considered to be unfeminine and a sign of promiscuity. One study that asked Vietnamese women about their attitudes towards male smoking found that they considered smoking to be a strong, masculine behaviour. "When I was young," one woman explained, "I liked my boyfriend to know how to smoke because it made him seem more manly". Despite the associations between smoking and masculinity, another survey among Vietnamese women found that almost three quarters were bothered by men's smoking.[139] However, women expressed a feeling of powerlessness to object to their husbands' or other men's smoking. As one woman poignantly noted, "If you hate cigarette smoke, you'll still have to marry a man who's heavily addicted to tobacco. Out of 100 men, 99 smoke. If you're afraid of tobacco then you'll have to live alone; it will be very depressing".[138]

Trends in China

As noted earlier, smoking prevalence among Chinese women is low. Traditionally, it has been considered inappropriate for women to smoke or drink alcohol. Although few qualitative data exist on smoking among women, a recent ethnographic study of changing gender roles in China provides insights into this behaviour.[139] Some young working women who were interviewed expressed resentment at their social status compared with that of men. One 23-year-old woman explained her discontent in the following way: "It's not fair. Women must have children, they must do housework; women can't smoke, can't drink". Not only were smoking and drinking considered by the interviewees to be social activities that men could engage in with friends, these behaviours also appeared to be powerful coping devices for dealing with life's pressures. These "resources" are presently unavailable to women. It will be important to document how Chinese women of different ages view cultural restrictions on smoking and whether their perceptions change over time.

Brand-stretching, the use of tobacco brand names on non-tobacco merchandise or services, is a strategy that has been used worldwide by the tobacco industry.

Circumventing Legislation: Brand-Stretching

In the face of increasing bans and restrictions on tobacco advertising in electronic and print media throughout Asia, the transnational tobacco industry has been forced to become increasingly creative in designing new forms of advertising to circumvent existing legislation and procure the product exposure that is critical to sales. Brand-stretching, the use of tobacco brand names on non-tobacco merchandise or services, is a strategy that has been used worldwide by the tobacco industry. The explicit purpose of brand-stretching is "to find non-tobacco products and other services that can be used to communicate the brand", together with their essential visual identifiers. The principle is to ensure that tobacco can be effectively publicized when all direct lines of communication are denied.[140]

> *Three nights per week, one of Beijing's large discos literally becomes "transformed into a free-floating advertisement" for BAT's 555 brands of cigarettes. Entering the disco, one is greeted by "slim Chinese women in blue tops, miniskirts, and boots emblazoned with the 555 logo, handing out free cigarettes".*

Internal documents from R. J. Reynolds define a similar strategy for circumventing bans, recommending "a creative approach to legal matters" to achieve "a balance between legal risks and desired benefits". Specifically, they advocate the adoption of cigarette brand names for "lifestyle products" such as clothing, shoes, and watches. Brand-stretching has been practised in Asia for some years, and a recent study in Hong Kong SAR provides data on the impact of this strategy on youth. When asked whether they had recently seen cigarette logos on products, both male and female students overwhelmingly reported that they had. The products included cigarette lighters (50%), ashtrays (37%), T-shirts (28%), compact discs (26%), hats (21%), jeans (18%), backpacks (13%), and watches (12%), to name but a few.[141] Although such products were not considered tobacco "advertisements" by the industry, they clearly have the effect of normalizing cigarettes, bringing them into the everyday lives of school-age youths. Other brand-name-bearing items that have been observed are Marlboro packets of tissues and Marlboro disposable cameras.[106]

There are many examples of how brand-stretching is being implemented throughout Asia, with Malaysia some-

times regarded as a "showcase" country. Although direct advertising of tobacco was banned in Malaysia in 1993, and many tobacco control measures have been implemented (including raising taxes, banning smoking in many public places, and controlling the amount of tar and nicotine in cigarettes), indirect advertising is still permitted. In 1996, four of the top 10 advertisers in Malaysia had a cigarette brand in their name: Peter Stuyvesant Travel, Benson & Hedges Bistro, Dunhill Accessories, and Salem Cool Planet.[142]

Faced with a declining market share, Benson & Hedges opened bistros in Kuala Lumpur that were well advertised on television and in newspapers. At these bistros, customers are served a special blend of Benson & Hedges coffee by waiters whose uniforms are adorned with a gold-coloured cigarette package. Gold, a prominent colour in all of Benson & Hedges-sponsored "experience environments", was purposely selected to represent the company's "confidence in a bright future".[143] A spokesperson for one bistro explained, "Of course, this is all about keeping the Benson & Hedges brand name to the front. The idea is to be smoker friendly. Smokers associate a coffee with a cigarette. They are both drugs of a type".[144] The bistros provide a context in which smoking is both anticipated and encouraged. Looking beyond their bistros, BAT noted that it was also planning to sell Lucky Strike clothing and Kent travel.

The effect of this "indirect" advertising is noteworthy: The number of smokers in Malaysia is increasing by about 3% per year, with the incidence among girls reported to have increased nearly threefold in the past 10 years.[145]

Sponsoring Discos

Another form of brand-stretching has been the sponsoring of discos, which have an obvious appeal to young people. In China, BAT has aggressively and relentlessly pursued the youth market, including women. Three nights per week, one of Beijing's large discos literally becomes "transformed into a free-floating advertisement" for BAT's 555 brands of cigarettes. Entering the disco, one is greeted by "slim Chinese women in blue tops, miniskirts, and boots emblazoned with the 555 logo, handing out free cigarettes. Customers crowd the smoke-filled dance floor, writhing to rock music below two huge banners with the 555 logo that proclaim: 'Be free from worldly cares'".[146]

Similar enticements of young women have been reported in Sri Lanka, where less than 3% of women presently smoke, and there are strong cultural sanctions against women smoking.[130] While conducting fieldwork, researcher Tamsyn Seimon visited a disco sponsored by a BAT subsidiary, the Ceylon Tobacco Company. "Within a minute," Seimon writes, "a 'golden girl' approached me, holding out a box of Benson & Hedges: 'Here take one.' I took it—she encouraged me: 'Go ahead—I want to see you smoke it now.' I told her I thought it would make me cough. 'No, these are smoother, not so strong,' she reassured me. 'I want to see you smoke it now'".[147]

The golden girls, who were probably fashion models, were dressed in gold-coloured saris and matching gold platform shoes. Throughout the night, the words "Benson & Hedges" flashed onto the walls of the disco with a laser beam, as blaring music filled the room with the top 10 dance hits from the West. Benson & Hedges cigarettes and alcohol were freely available from the golden girls. Draws for prizes that included Benson & Hedges key rings, shirts, and caps were held repeatedly during the evening.[147]

To further popularize and normalize their product, Ceylon Tobacco Company hires young women to "hang out" at popular shopping malls, on university campuses, and on upscale commuter trains, where they distribute free cigarettes and merchandise. Young women are also employed as drivers of bright red Player's Gold Leaf-brand cars and jeeps, from which they distribute free cigarette samples and promotional items, including hats, T-shirts, and lighters.[147] Notably, these women are paid higher salaries than those typically earned by university graduates.[148]

In the inner world of the disco in China, Sri Lanka, and other Asian countries, young women are invited to participate in behaviours associated with being modern, fashionable, and Western. They are directly cajoled and challenged to smoke by glamorous, thin fashion models whose attire is at once traditional (the sari) and modern (gold and glittery). Fears of the cigarette's strength are assuaged—the women are told that these are mild cigarettes, suitable for a woman. In contrast to the direct encouragement to smoke that young women encounter in the protected world of the disco, in the outside world, where smoking remains culturally inappropriate, young women are used as vehicles for product promotion rather than as overt participants in it. Both inside and outside, however, the connection between women and cigarettes is normalized through widespread and repeated exposure.

One of the most prevalent methods of tobacco advertising in Asia is the prominent display of cigarettes in local shops. In effect, the shop itself becomes the advertisement.

Selling Fashion

Selling fashion accessories in shops has become a profitable way to advertise cigarettes indirectly, as well as a way to increase visibility of the products. For example, Marlboro Classics clothes, designed to capture the imagery of the "Wild West", are immensely popular—there are more than 1000 established Marlboro Classic Stores in Europe and Asia.[149] Similarly, R. J. Reynolds has designed Salem Attitude (clothing stores) in Asia in an effort "to extend their trademark beyond tobacco category restrictions". An internal document from the company unabashedly states, "The Salem Attitude image will circumvent marketing restrictions".[150] In Thailand, Camel Trophy clothing, including T-shirts, pants, and other adventure-style garments, has become very popular among young people. While many youths are unaware that the clothes are connected to cigarettes, Camel as a brand is becoming increasingly recognizable in the Thai market.[118]

Product Placement

One of the most prevalent methods of tobacco advertising in Asia is the prominent display of cigarettes in local shops. In effect, the shop itself becomes the advertisement. Throughout India, for example, even in states that have enacted advertising bans (such as Kerala), the tobacco industry has provided signage for shops. These signs, which bear the name of the cigarette, are attractive, modern, and painted in the signifying colour of the brand. Point-of-sale advertising is an excellent means by which new brands can get

World Health Organization

maximum exposure. Poor shopkeepers are more than willing to accept these signs that confer status to their shops. In Thailand and the Philippines, display cabinets with company and brand logos are common in almost every corner store. The cabinets, provided by the tobacco companies, ensure that cigarettes are highly visible.

A survey conducted among 6000 male and female secondary-school students in Hong Kong SAR found that more than one third of them had watched a tobacco-sponsored tennis tournament.

Sports Sponsorship

Sponsorship of sporting events, a long-established form of brand-stretching worldwide, has taken on a new intensity in Asia. In China, sports represent one of the most conspicuous examples of the commercialization of contemporary Chinese society. Philip Morris invests heavily in soccer and sponsors the national league known as the Marlboro Professional League. During the league's extremely popular, nationally broadcast games, ads for Marlboro are seen everywhere in the stadiums.[151] Basketball is also a popular sport, and in 1996, a spokesperson for Chinese basketball noted, "We are developing our commodity economy and professional basketball treats players as commodities—so this is our direction".[152] Not surprisingly, one year later, in 1997, Chinese basketball acquired its own professional league—the Hilton League—named after the cigarette brand of its sponsor.[153] Another popular event with cigarette sponsorship is the 555 Hong Kong SAR-to-Beijing motor rally, a nationally televised long-distance automobile race.[154] While one might think of these sports as traditionally male-oriented, women in many countries share in the excitement that such programming brings into their homes.

Tennis star Michael Chang, who was regarded as an idol of adolescent girls, regularly played in Marlboro and Salem tennis events in China, Japan, Hong Kong SAR,

and the Republic of Korea. A release of industry documents shows that Chang was paid US$ 80 000 to "maintain a good relationship" with the companies. In addition, the organizers of the Salem Open, Hong Kong SAR's leading tennis event, signed a contract stating that they would use their "best efforts" to prevent players from criticizing smoking. Marlboro executives described Chang's signing "as a coup" and proudly disclosed in a sales review, "We have been successful in drawing an unusually targeted audience to this otherwise fairly upscale sport in great part due to Michael Chang's enormous popularity".[155]

A survey conducted among 6000 male and female secondary-school students in Hong Kong SAR found that more than one third of them had watched a tobacco-sponsored tennis tournament.[156] In addition, children who were stopped on the street during a Salem tournament were asked what cigarette Michael Chang smoked, and they quickly responded, "Salem!" In 1995, Princess Diana attended the Salem Open Tennis Tournament in Hong Kong SAR and accepted a check from the sponsor, R. J. Reynolds, as a donation for the Hong Kong SAR Red Cross.[157] The linking of internationally regarded women with tobacco sponsorship serves to legitimize and valorize the industry, transferring attention from the selling of addiction to charitable works.

Although female athletes are less commonly sponsored by tobacco companies, one notable exception was a full-page ad that appeared in Malaysian newspapers featuring popular female climber Lum Yuet Mei suspended from a rock face. The copy read, "She took the challenge and realized her golden dream".[158] Displayed prominently on the page were the Benson & Hedges logo and the company's gold colours. In Viet Nam, the manufacturers of Dunhill cigarettes have given almost a half-million dollars to help develop professional soccer in the country.[159] They also sponsor television broadcasts of Saturday night soccer, circumventing the country's advertising ban by showing their logo with the slogan "The Best Taste in the World" without showing the actual cigarette.[160]

Cricket, a sport that enjoys immense popularity in Asia, has long had tobacco sponsorship. In Sri Lanka, BAT began marketing Benson & Hedges by introducing it on a televised cricket match from Australia, where the Sri Lankan team, the defending world champions, was playing. This allowed the company to circumvent Sri Lanka's ban on domestic cigarette advertising.[161] In India, Wills, a BAT subsidiary, is the official sponsor of the national cricket team, and its logo is prominently displayed on the outfits of the players. Cricket matches are widely televised, and both male and female audiences are ardent fans of the game. Child-size T-shirts bearing the Wills logo are available internationally. Wills' sponsorship of cricket has been contested in India by anti-tobacco activists, who insist that it be stopped. A spokesperson for the Voluntary Health Association of India stated, "It [Wills' sponsorship] is not popularizing cricket in India, but hooking young people to the deadly smoking habit. The playing fields of India must not be turned into mass graves where children lie buried. It is this realization that has to seep into the Board of Cricket Control in India who have been accepting tobacco sponsorships".[162]

Advertising for the Marlboro Tour in the Philippines, a 23-day cycle race on several islands, declares, "The Marlboro Tour is the biggest national summer sports spectacle held yearly in the Philippines". Internal documents, however, describe a far more insidious plan behind this event, particularly for low-income Filipinos: "The tour inspires poor young men. It gives them hope of making it big. It answers their dreams".[163]

Sponsorship of Music, Art, and Cultural Events

In Sri Lanka, BAT circumvents a ban on cigarette advertising on the radio by underwriting a "Golden Tones Contest" on the English-language radio station, which is especially popular with trendy, Western-influenced youth. BAT also publishes a weekly pop music supplement in an English-language newspaper, which features large, colourful advertisements for Benson & Hedges cigarettes with the motto "Turn to gold".[147]

In Malaysia, Rothmans' Peter Stuyvesant brand sponsored a nationwide tour by Malay singer Ziana Zain, who is very popular with adolescent girls. BAT's subsidiary, the Malaysian Tobacco Company, launched its Benson & Hedges Lights in Malaysia by organizing live concerts and subsequently releasing an album called Benson & Hedges Light Tones.[164] Jewel, an American teen star who is particularly popular among adolescent girls, toured Malaysia with Salem sponsorship. Of late, best-selling pop star and teen idol Robbie Williams expressed anger over his name being used to promote Benson &

Hedges in Asia. His publicist noted, "Although Robbie smokes, he would never endorse tobacco. He smokes but is desperate to give it up".[165]

In Sri Lanka, BAT circumvents a ban on cigarette advertising on the radio by underwriting a "Golden Tones Contest" on the English-language radio station, which is especially popular with trendy, Western-influenced youth.

The opening of music stores, such as the Salem Power Station in Kuala Lumpur, has also been used to reach youth and imprint a brand logo on their consciousness.[163] Obviously, the main customers for such businesses are teens, who leave the shop as walking advertisements for cigarettes. The Philip Morris Group has sponsored the prestigious ASEAN Art Awards, which it credits with building links for cooperation between art communities in ASEAN and bringing art to the public in South East Asia.[166] In 1994, an exhibition of finalists was held in Singapore, where the government gave Philip Morris special exemption to stage the event;[167] the next award ceremony was held in Hanoi, amid much fanfare and publicity. The Philip Morris Group has also donated US$ 100 000 for purchasing winning paintings from the contest that are kept in a permanent collection at the Singapore Art Museum.[166]

It is important to note that the ASEAN art awards are viewed with scepticism in some countries. Because of protests from anti-tobacco activists in Thailand, the event receives little coverage in the Thai media. Activists have discussed the difficulty of protesting this contest because, technically, Philip Morris is not in breach of Thailand's tobacco laws, and the activists do not want to appear "overzealous in the eyes of the public".[166] Such a perception might jeopardize the legitimacy of the position they have established in trying to prevent transnational tobacco companies from making further inroads into Thailand.

In 1999, a Gay Pride event in the Philippines benefited from sponsorship by Lucky Strike, which paid for the stage and the master of ceremonies and widely publicized its contribution to the event. Some activists participating in the event were angered by the commercialization of the gathering and the selling out to big tobacco and have vowed not to allow tobacco sponsorship of such activities in the future.[168]

Television and Movies

In the Philippines, where television advertisements of tobacco products are still permitted, commercials for Winston cigarettes show young adult American men and women happily partying. The message states that these young people (and their cigarettes) represent the "spirit of the USA", an image that further perpetuates the colonial mentality among Filipino youth.[168] In Japan, television commercials for Lark cigarettes have featured popular Western actors, including James Coburn, Pierce Brosnan, and Robert Wagner, starring in action vignettes.[169]

> *In 1999, a Gay Pride event in the Philippines benefited from sponsorship by Lucky Strike, which paid for the stage and the master of ceremonies and widely publicized its contribution to the event.*

India, which has the largest film industry in the world, produces more than 800 films per year. Tobacco use appears to be widespread in Indian films, although no formal studies have investigated this subject. Some popular actors are renowned for their individualistic smoking styles, and it is common for youth to attempt to emulate these styles in front of their friends. Increasingly, women in the developing world are being reached by satellite television and the Internet, which are practically unrestricted. Even countries that have comprehensive advertising bans on tobacco products are exposed to tobacco promotion in these media.

The Impact of Tobacco Marketing on Smoking Behaviour: United States and Asia

Individual Behaviour

A monograph published in the United States by the National Cancer Institute in 2008 found that the total weight of evidence, from multiple studies using data from many countries, demonstrates a causal relationship between tobacco advertising and promotion and increased tobacco use.[170] A study that looked at prevalence data from 1890 to 1997 found two historic periods of increases in smoking uptake among young women and not among young men: one from 1926 to 1939 and the other from 1968 to 1977. The first coincided with the early Chesterfield and Lucky Strike campaigns aimed at women, and the second followed the introduction of Virginia Slims and the proliferation of women's brands that began in 1967.[171,172]

Research in the United States has provided evidence of the effect of advertising on youth smoking. A study of the exposure of junior-high-school students to tobacco advertising in magazines found that adolescents with high exposure to advertising were more likely to be smokers than were students with low exposure.[173] A study that reviewed 20 years of cigarette advertising found that when the advertising of a brand increased, teen smoking of that brand was three times more likely to increase than adult smoking.[174]

A longitudinal study of adolescents in California who had never smoked provides evidence that advertising and promotional activities can influence them to start.[175] Although having a favourite advertisement predicted progression to use from non-use, the availability of a promotional item more effectively predicted progression to use. The authors attributed 34% of smoking initiation to advertising and promotion. Another longitudinal analysis of adolescent California never-smokers determined that tobacco marketing was a stronger influence on adolescents than was exposure to peer or family smokers or demographic variables.[176]

Other research has also shown a link between familiarity with advertising and brand preferences to

World Health Organization

smoking among adolescents in the United States.[177–180] Owning promotional items and willingness to possess a promotional item have been strongly associated with smoking experimentation.[175,178,181] In addition, two studies in the United States found that the three most heavily advertised brands—Marlboro, Camel, and Newport— have substantially higher market penetration among adolescents than among adults.[182,183]

Research conducted after the introduction of Joe Camel revealed that children 6 to 11 years of age identified the Camel brand of cigarettes with the new cartoon camel and that these advertisements made smoking more appealing to children.[184] After the introduction of Joe Camel, Camel cigarettes' market share of smokers under the age of 18 increased almost 650%, from virtually nothing to almost one third, with sales estimated at US$ 476 million per year.[184]

In Asia, cigarette advertising has had similar effects on smoking behaviour. In one study of 198 female nursing students in Japan, 95% of the respondents reported having exposure to advertising.[185] More than 50% of the students who had past or current smoking histories reported being "frequently" exposed to cigarette advertising via television and billboards, while 50% of the never-smokers reported only "occasional" exposure.

A study in three cities in China looked at brand familiarity, recall of advertising, attitudes towards advertising, and cigarette use among college students at 12 universities.[186] Eight brands were most familiar, four foreign and four domestic. The leading brand was Marlboro. Chinese students were more likely to have seen advertising for foreign brands than ads for domestic brands. Current smokers who reported having seen a Marlboro ad in the previous month were significantly more likely to prefer Marlboros.

Among adolescents 13 to 15 years of age in Hong Kong SAR, perceiving advertisements for cigarettes as attractive was more strongly associated with smoking than were 13 other factors (adjusted odds ratio (OR)= 2.68; OR = 2.62 in boys and 2.71 in girls).[187] Participation in a cigarette promotional activity was also positively related to use (adjusted OR = 1.24). Another study of more than 9500 Hong Kong SAR students 8 to 13 years of age found that ever-smokers were more successful than non-smokers in recognizing cigarette

brand names and logos (adjusted OR = 1.67).[188] The two brands most successfully identified (95%) were Salem and Marlboro.

A 1997 study of smoking in Viet Nam found that 73% of males were smokers, and where print, electronic, and outdoor advertising were banned, 38% recalled tobacco advertising.[189] Of these, 71% recalled a non-Vietnamese brand as the brand advertised. Only 16% smoked non-Vietnamese cigarettes, although 38% would have liked to if they could afford them.

After the 1995 India–New Zealand cricket series, a survey was conducted among youths in Goa to determine the effect of sports sponsorship on tobacco experimentation. Despite a high level of knowledge about the adverse effects of tobacco, both boys and girls were more likely to experiment with smoking as a result of cricket sponsorship by tobacco companies.[190] A majority of those surveyed believed that cricket players smoked, and some expressed the opinion that smoking improved athletic performance, including batting and fielding. The notion that cigarette smoking increases concentration and helps one think is widespread among college students in South India.[134]

Girls in both the industrialized and the developing world may be more vulnerable to advertisements than young men are. Studies based in the United States show that girls' sense of self-worth and perception of their appearance are lower than those of boys, that they fall with increasing age during adolescence, and that they are associated with regular smoking.[191] Young women may also be more concerned than young men about what is socially acceptable and may face gender-role conflicts different from those of their male peers.[192-194] Certainly, the developing world, with its much lower rates of smoking among women, is prime territory for targeted tobacco marketing that uses gender differences to create appeal. In addition to affecting individual behaviour, cigarette marketing affects organizational behaviour that influences women's preferences.

Women's Magazines

Cigarette advertising appears to affect the coverage of the risks of smoking in magazines, especially women's magazines. A study of magazines in the United States from 1959 to 1969 and 1973 to 1986 looked at the probability that magazines carrying cigarette advertisements would have articles on the risks of smoking.[195] The probability of including an article addressing health risks of smoking was 11.9% if the magazine did not carry cigarette advertising and 8.3% if it did. For women's magazines, the probabilities were 11.7% and 5%, respectively. An increase of 1% in the share of advertising revenue derived from cigarette ads decreased the probability of women's magazines covering the risks of smoking three times as much as it did in other magazines.[195] Studies in the United Kingdom similarly found that magazines that accepted cigarette advertising were less likely to cover the health consequences of tobacco use.[196]

A study of 13 popular women's magazines from 1997 and 1998 noted that the ratio of cigarette advertisements to antismoking messages increased from 6:1 in 1997 to 11:1 in 1998.[197] Between 1997 and 1998, anti-smoking messages declined 54%, and cigarette advertisements declined 13%. Articles about smoking made up 1% or less of all health-related articles. When tobacco was mentioned, it was often relegated to a mere reference. For example, a Redbook article on ways to prevent cancer mentioned quitting smoking in the introduction but did not list it as one of the "top nine ways".[197]

Marketing of tobacco, then, affects both individual and organizational behaviour. Individual women, both novice and experienced tobacco users, receive and act on marketing messages transmitted through brand name, packaging, advertising, and promotion strategies. Direct-advertising revenues affect the coverage of health concerns about smoking in media such as women's magazines. Sponsorships and the placement of tobacco within components of popular culture send additional signals that make tobacco use appear normal and re-inforce the marketing messages of more-direct forms of advertising and promotion. In some cases, such as sponsorship signage at televised motorsport racing events, sponsorship provides advertising exposure that circumvents advertising bans. Sponsorship of organizations with which women and their families interact (e.g. the arts, museums, and community fairs) associate tobacco with everyday life and the social fabric or infrastructure in which women live. Finally, tobacco support for advocacy organizations and political leadership groups limits the involvement of these organizations in protecting the health of women.

Actions Against Tobacco Marketing

There is increasing evidence that the tobacco industry is focusing its efforts on the marketing of tobacco to women globally. While the WHO FCTC provides tools to assist countries in enacting comprehensive tobacco control legislation, there remains an urgent need for global monitoring of how the industry fights and circumvents this legislation. As the Guidelines for Implementation of WHO FCTC Article 5.3 note, there is a fundamental and irreconcilable conflict between the tobacco industry's interests and public health policy interests. Among the countries that are Parties to the WHO FCTC, it will be critical to document delaying tactics of the industry, as well as emergent forms of advertising, promotion, and other marketing strategies being developed to specifically target women. In addition to the implementation of industry monitoring and controlling tobacco advertising, in accordance with Articles 5.3 and 13 of the treaty, respectively, it is important to ensure that gender-sensitive warnings are used on all tobacco products. The WHO FCTC's Article 11, *Packaging and labelling of tobacco products,* establishes an obligation for Parties to ensure that warning labels that clearly communicate the dangers of tobacco use in the principal national language constitute not less than 30% of the principal display areas on all tobacco products and that they rotate periodically.

Transnational tobacco companies use similar strategies at different times in different parts of the world, and domestic tobacco companies mimic the successful approaches. A gender-sensitive early warning system could advise tobacco activists about strategies likely to be used, especially new developments, enabling them to devise global responses.

Uniform, ongoing reporting on the acceptance of tobacco sponsorship funds is needed, similar to the reporting on political campaign financing in the United States. Women who belong to affinity or advocacy groups should be aware of which of these organizations accept tobacco funding and at what levels.

To promote women's active participation, tobacco control activists need to increase and strengthen their outreach to organizations concerned with children's and womens rights in order to involve them actively in this fundamental rights issue.

World Health Organization

Wider recognition is needed of the global health problem resulting from women's tobacco use and their exposure to second-hand smoke and of the need to develop women-centred programmes.[198] Non-traditional partners should be sought to organize women speaking out against predatory marketing practices. A global movement to find alternative sources of funding for women's organizations should be a priority. Corporate sponsors of women's products (i.e. non-tobacco products) should be approached for this funding.

Gender-specific approaches that focus on women are needed. Media literacy skills that teach women and girls to analyse the messages of tobacco advertising and how the industry targets them are essential to protect them from these messages. Media literacy should be included in health education in schools and should also be provided by women's rights and service organizations. The potential impact of tobacco use on health needs to become a part of basic education and must be incorporated in medical- and nursing-school curricula.[199] In countries in Asia where smoking among women is culturally inappropriate, it is important to actively involve women in heightening community awareness of the negative effects of passive smoking on women's and children's health, as well as to encourage their efforts at helping male family members quit smoking.

References

1. Rogers D. Overseas memo. *Tobacco Reporter*, February 1982.
2. Tennant RB. *The American cigarette industry: a study in economic analysis and public policy*. New Haven, CT, Yale University Press, 1950.
3. Ernster VL. Mixed messages for women: a social history of cigarette smoking and advertising. *New York State Journal of Medicine*, 1985, 85:335–340 (see also Amos A, Haglund M. From social taboo to "torch of freedom" – the marketing of cigarettes to women. *Tobacco Control*, 2000, 9:3–8.
4. Gunther J. *Taken at the flood: the story of Albert D. Lasker*. New York, NY, Harper and Brothers, 1960.
5. Bernays EL. *Biography of an idea: memoirs of public relations counsel Edward L. Bernays*. New York, NY, Simon and Schuster, 1965.
6. Tilley NM. *The R. J. Reynolds Tobacco Company*. Chapel Hill, NC, University of North Carolina Press, 1985.
7. Jones KE. *Women's brands: cigarette advertising explicitly directed toward women*. Cambridge, MA, Harvard University Press, 1987.
8. Breast cancer deaths and cigarettes advertising dollars rise. *Marketing to Women*, 1991, 4:8.
9. *American Tobacco Company*. Internal report by unknown author, 17 November 1983 (BW ATX040017950/7951).
10. Chapman S, Fitzgerald B. Brand preference and advertising recall in adolescent smokers: some implications for health promotion. *American Journal of Public Health*, 1982, 72:491–494.
11. Britt SH. *Psychological principles of marketing and consumer behavior*. Lexington, MA, Lexington Books/Heath & Co., 1978.
12. Beede P, Lawson R. The effect of plain packages on the perception of cigarette health warnings. *Public Health*, 1992, 106:315–322.
13. Health Canada. *When packages can't speak: possible impacts of generic packaging of tobacco products. Expert Panel report*. Ottawa, Canadian Ministry of Health, 1995.
14. Elkind AK. The social definition of women's smoking behavior. *Social Science & Medicine*, 1985, 20:1269–1278.
15. Leeming EJ. Letter from Executive Director, Marketing to Women, to Sharon Dean, Corporate Fact Finders, 12 April 1993.
16. Bissell J. How do you market an image brand when the image falls out of favor? *Brandweek*, 1994, 35:16.
17. Percy L, Rossiter JR. A model of brand awareness and brand advertising strategies. *Psychology and Marketing*, 1992, 9:263–274.
18. Opatow L. Packaging is most effective when it works in harmony with the positioning of a brand. *Marketing News*, 1984, 3:3–4.
19. Gordon A, Finlay K, Watts T. The psychological effects of colour in consumer product packaging. *Canadian Journal of Marketing Research*, 1994, 13:3–11.
20. *Federal Trade Commission report to Congress for 1996: pursuant to the Federal Cigarette Labeling and Advertising Act*. Washington, DC, Federal Trade Commission, 1998.
21. Kindra GS, Laroche M, Muller TE. *Consumer behavior: the Canadian perspective*, 2nd ed. Scarborough, Nelson Canada, 1994.
22. Solomon MR. The role of products as social stimuli: a symbolic interactionism perspective. *Journal of Consumer Research*, 1983, 10:319–329.
23. Trachtenburg JA. Here's one tough cowboy. *Forbes*, 1987, February 9:108–110.
24. Bearden WO, Etzel MJ. Reference group influence on product and brand purchase decisions. *Journal of Consumer Research*, 1982, 9:183–194.
25. Action on Smoking and Health. *Big tobacco and women*. November 1998 (see also Botvin GJ et al. Smoking behavior of adolescents exposed to cigarette advertising. *Public Health Reports*, 1993, 108:217–224).
26. Raj SP. Striking a balance between brand "popularity" and brand loyalty. *Journal of Marketing*, 1985, 49:53–59.
27. *Federal Trade Commission cigarette report for 2004 and 2005* (http://www.ftc.gov/reports/tobacco/2007cigarette2004–2005.pdf, accessed 21 May 2009).
28. Kotler P. *Marketing management: analysis, planning, implementation, and control*, 7th ed. Englewood Cliffs, NJ, Prentice Hall, 1991.
29. Ray ML. *Advertising and communication management*. Englewood Cliffs, NJ, Prentice Hall, 1982.
30. Kinnear TC, Bernhardt KL, Krentler KA. *Principles of marketing*, 4th ed. New York, NY, Harper Collins, 1995.
31. Zinn L. The smoke clears at Marlboro. *Business Week*, 1994, January 31:76–77.
32. Townsend J, Roderick P, Cooper J. Cigarette smoking by socioeconomic group, sex, and age: effect of price, income, and health publicity. *British Medical Journal*, 1994, 309:923–927.
33. Slade J. Why unbranded promos? *Tobacco Control*, 1994, 3:72.
34. Virginia Slims advertisement. *People*, 1995, 44:12.
35. *The tax burden on tobacco*. Washington, DC, The Tobacco Institute, 1998: 33.
36. Warner KE et al. Promotion of tobacco products: issues and policy options. *Journal of Health Politics, Policy and Law*, 1986, 11:367–392.
37. Pollay RW, Lavack AM. The targeting of youths by cigarette marketers: archival evidence on trial. *Advances in Consumer Research*, 1993, 20:266–271.
38. Lynch BS, Bonnie RJ. *Growing up tobacco free: preventing nicotine addiction in children and youths*. Washington, DC, National Academy Press, 1994.

39. *Preventing tobacco use among young people; a report of the Surgeon General.* Washington, DC: US Department of Health and Human Services, Public Health Service, Centers for Disease Control and Prevention, 1994.

40. *IEG intelligence report on tobacco company sponsorship for the Robert Wood Johnson Foundation: 1995 sponsorship.* Chicago, IL, IEG, 1995.

41. *IEG's Complete guide to sponsorship: everything you need to know about sports, arts, event, entertainment and cause marketing.* Chicago, IL, IEG, 1995.

42. Levin M. The tobacco industry's strange bedfellows. *Business and Society Review*, 1988, Spring, 65:11–17.

43. Williams M. Tobacco's hold on women's groups: anti-smokers charge leaders have sold out to industry money. *The Washington Post*, 14 November 1991, Sect A.

44. Ernster VL. Women, smoking, cigarette advertising, and cancer. *Women's Health*, 1986, 11:217–235.

45. *Virginia Slims Media Guide.* Philip Morris. 1995.

46. Ernster VL. Trends in smoking, cancer risk, and cigarette promotion: current priorities for reducing tobacco exposure. *Cancer*, 1988, 62:1702–1712.

47. Camel advertisement. *People*, various dates.

48. Novelli WD. Rock 'til they drop: tunes, teens, and tobacco. *The Washington Post*, 11 May 1997, Outlook, C02.

49. *Study for the Center for Tobacco-Free Kids.* Washington, DC, Simmons Market Research Bureau, 1996.

50. Slade J. Tobacco product advertising during motorsports broadcasts: a quantitative assessment. In: Slama K ed. *Tobacco and health.* New York, NY, Plenum Press, 1995, 939–941.

51. Schlabach M. Friday special inside NASCAR: did you know? *The Atlanta Journal Constitution*, 19 March 1999, Sect D:8.

52. Clarke L. To attract kids, stock car racing shifts gears. *The Washington Post*, 22 May 1998, Sect A, 1.

53. Kaufman NJ. Smoking and young women: the physician's role in stopping an equal opportunity killer. *Journal of the American Medical Association*, 1994, 271:629–630.

54. Stockwell TF, Glantz SA. Tobacco use is increasing in popular films. *Tobacco Control*, 1997, 6:282–284.

55. Everett SA, Schnuth RL, Tribble JL. Tobacco and alcohol use in top-grossing American films. *Journal of Community Health*, 1998, 23:317–324.

56. Thomas K. No waiting to inhale: cigarettes light up the movies. *USA Today*, 7 November 1996, Sect Life:1D.

57. Christenson PG, Henriksen L, Roberts DF. *Substance abuse in popular music and movies.* Washington, DC, Office of National Drug Control Policy, Department of Health and Human Services, Substance Abuse and Mental Health Services Administration, 1999.

58. Goldstein AO, Sobel RA, Newman GR. Tobacco and alcohol use in G-rated children's animated films. *Journal of the American Medical Association*, 1999, 281:1131–1136.

59. Cruz J, Wallack L. Trends in tobacco use on television. *American Journal of Public Health*, 1986, 76:698–699.

60. Hazan AR, Glantz SA. Current trends in tobacco use on prime-time fictional television. *American Journal of Public Health*, 1995, 35:116–117.

61. DuRant RH et al. Tobacco and alcohol use behaviors portrayed in music videos: a content analysis. *Journal of American Public Health*, 1997, 87:1131–1135.

62. Virginia Slims advertisement. *Marie Claire*, August 1999:157.

63. Virginia Slims advertisement. *In Style*, August 1999: back cover.

64. Virginia Slims advertisement. *US*, July 1999:39.

65. Capri advertisement. *Vogue*, July 1999:213.

66. Basic advertisement. *US*, July 1999:47.

67. GPC advertisement. *People*, 28 June 1999:126.

68. Doral advertisement. *People*, 28 June 1999:36–37.

69. Merit advertisement. *People*, 1999, June 14:inside back cover.

70. Merit advertisement. *Vogue*, July 1999:221.

71. Carlton advertisement. *People*, 5 July 1999:116.

72. Camel advertisement. *Rolling Stone*, 8 July 1999–22:45.

73. Camel advertisement. *US*, July 1999:12–13.

74. Camel advertisement. *In Style*, August 1999:86–87.

75. Marlboro advertisement. *Marie Claire*, August 1999:36–37.

76. Marlboro advertisement. *Vogue*, July 1999:44–45.

77. Marlboro Lights advertisement. *People*, 5 July 1999:10–11.

78. Stone. Lucky Strike advertisement. *Rolling Stone*, 8 July 1999–22:84.

79. Stone. Newport advertisement. *Rolling Stone*, 8 July 1999–22:112.

80. Kool advertisement. *Rolling Stone*, 8 July 1999–22:17.

81. Winston Lights advertisement. *In Style*, August 1999:66–7.

82. Winston Lights advertisement. *People*, 5 July 1999:60.

83. Winston advertisement. *Rolling Stone*, 8–22 July 1999:64–5.

84. Tunistra T. Editorial. *Tobacco Reporter*, Summer 1998.

85. Beck E. BAT takes aim at dominant Marlboro but may lack a killer brand for the job. *Wall Street Journal*, 21 October 1997.

86. World Health Organization. Combating the tobacco epidemic. In: *The world health report 1999 – Making a difference. Geneva,* World Health Organization, 1999: 65–79 (www.who.int/whr/1999/; see also Hammond R. *Addicted to profit: big tobacco's expanding global reach.* Washington, DC, Essential Action, 1998).

87. Hwang SL, Sherer PM. RJR Nabisco to spin off units and sell overseas operation. *Wall Street Journal*, 10 March 1999.

88. *Documents on Project Battalion,* San Francisco, CA, University of California, Legacy Tobacco Documents Library.

89. Sesser S. Opium war redux. *The New Yorker*, 13 September 1993:78–89.

90. *Tobacco giants target Asia to offset losses in US, Europe.* 21 October 1998. Interpress Service, (www.oneworld.org/ips2/oct98/21_00_094.html).

91. Exporting tobacco addiction from the USA. Editorial. *The Lancet*, 1998, 351:1597.

92. Shafey O et al. *The tobacco atlas*, 3rd ed. Atlanta, GA, American Cancer Society, 2009.

93. Mackay J, Eriksen M. *The tobacco atlas.* Geneva, World Health Organization, 2002.

94. Scull R. Bright future predicted for Asia Pacific. *World Tobacco*, 1986, 94:35.

95. Smith C. Western tobacco sales are booming in China, thanks to smuggling. *Wall Street Journal Europe*, 18 December 1996:1.

96. Cigarette production down: contraband and counterfeits flourish. *Tobacco Reporter*, 1997, 32.

97. Hammond R, ed. *Addicted to profit: big tobacco's expanding global reach.* Washington, DC, Essential Action, 1998.

98. Zhao B. Consumerism, Confucianism, communism: making sense of China today. *New Left Review*, 1997, 222:54.

99. Zhu S et al. Perception of foreign cigarettes and their advertising in China: a study of college students from 12 universities. *Tobacco Control*, 1998, 7:134–140.

100. Thomas H, Gagliardi J. The cigarette papers: a strategy of manipulation. *South China Morning Post*, 19 January 1999.

101. Featherstone M. Consumer culture, symbolic power and universalism. In: Stauth G, Zubaida S, eds. *Mass culture, popular culture, and social life in the Middle East.* Frankfurt am Main, Campus Verlag, 1987.

102. Comerford A, Slade J. *Selling cigarettes: a salesman's perspective.* Paper commissioned by the Committee on Preventing Nicotine Addiction on Children and Youths, 1994.

103. Nichter M. Personal communication, 1997.

104. Ratcliffe E. *"American noses and talented boobs": the discursive correlations of race, femininity and national identity in the Philippines.* 1998 (unpublished manuscript).

105. Villanueva WG. Nothing is sacred on the Philippines smoking front. *Tobacco Control*, 1997, 6:357–359.

106. Efroymson D. *Women and tobacco: cause for concern in Viet Nam.* Ottawa, International Development Research Centre, 1966 (unpublished report, May 1996).

107. Teilhet-Fisk J. The Miss Heilala beauty pageant: where beauty is more than skin deep. In: Cohen CB, Wilk R, Stoeltje B, eds. *Beauty queens on the global stage: gender, contests and power.* New York, NY, Routledge, 1996.

108. Mueller B. Standardization vs specialization: an examination of westernization in Japanese advertising. *Journal of Advertising Research*, 1992, January/February:18.

109. Lin CA. Cultural differences in message strategies: a comparison between American and Japanese TV commercials. *Journal of Advertising Research*, 1993, July/August:41.

110. Gaouette N. Despite ban Japan ads sell women on smoking. *Christian Science Monitor*, 9 March 1998:1.

111. Cole J. Women: a separate market? *Tobacco*, 1988, March:7–9.

112. Azuma N. Smoke and mirrors: Japanese women buying into sweet song of US tobacco companies. *Asia Times*, 18 July 1997.

113. John G. Japan: always something new. *Tobacco International*, 1996, August.

114. Waldron I et al. Gender differences in tobacco use in Africa, Asia, the Pacific and Latin America. *Social Science & Medicine*, 1988, 27:1269–1275.

115. Mochizuki-Kobayashi Y, Yamaguchi N, Samet JM, eds. *Tobacco free Japan: recommendations for tobacco control policy*. Baltimore, MD, Tobacco Free Japan and the Institute for Global Tobacco Control, Department of Epidemiology, Johns Hopkins Bloomberg School of Public Health, 2004.

116. Philip Morris tops import sales. *Tobacco Reporter*, February 1996:20.

117. Comparison of cigarette brand preferences of adult and teenaged smokers—United States, 1989, and 10 US Communities, 1988 and 1990. *Morbidity and Mortality Weekly Report*, 1992, 41:173.

118. Hughes B. Action on Smoking and Health, Bangkok, Thailand. Globalink communication, June 1999.

119. Prakash Gupta. Personal communication, 1990.

120. *Project Kestrel*. Unsigned, undated document from the files of the British American Tobacco Company (BAT), (www.gate.net/~jcannon/documents/kestrel.txt).

121. RJ Reynolds Tobacco Company. We don't advertise to children. Cited in *Tobacco explained: the truth about the tobacco industry...in its own words",* London, Action on Smoking and Health, 1998.

122. Hui L. Chinese smokers take to slim cigarettes. *World Tobacco*, 1998, July.

123. Lynch BS, Bonnie RJ, eds. *Growing up tobacco free: preventing nicotine addiction in children and youths*. Washington, DC, National Academy Press, 1994.

124. Zheng Tianyi (manager of Kunming cigarette factory). Quoted in Hui L. Chinese smokers take to slim cigarettes. *World Tobacco*, 1998, July.

125. *Frontier Slims*. 1996. (http://www.jtnet.ad.jp/FRONTIERslims).

126. Li C et al. Smoking behaviour among female airline cabin crew from ten Asian countries. *Tobacco Control*, 1994, 3:21–29.

127. Brown and Williamson. *Staying ahead of a moving target*. January 1989, B & W, 300120527–300120531 (Tobacco resolution).

128. Nichter M et al. Smoking experimentation and initiation among adolescent females: qualitative and quantitative findings. *Tobacco Control*, 1997, 6:285–295.

129. Lam TH et al. *Youth smoking: knowledge, attitudes, smoking in schools and families, and symptoms due to passive smoking*. Hong Kong, Hong Kong Council on Smoking and Health (COSH), 1994 (Report 2).

130. *WHO report on the global tobacco epidemic, 2009: implementing smoke-free environments*. Geneva, World Health Organization, 2009.

131. Nichter M. Personal communication, 1997.

132. Nichter M. Field notes, Mindoro, Philippines, 1992 (unpublished).

133. Nichter M. Field notes, Karnataka, India, April 1998 (unpublished; see also India: movie shoots at women. *Tobacco Control*, March 2000, 9:10).

134. Nichter M, Nichter M, Van Sickle D. Popular perceptions of tobacco products and patterns of use among male college students in India. *Social Science & Medicine*, 2004, 59:415–431.

135. Reynolds C. The fourth largest market in the world. *Tobacco Control*, 2000, 9:9–10

136. Barraclough S. Women and tobacco in Indonesia. *Tobacco Control*, 1999, 8:327–332.

137. Nichter M et al. Reading culture from tobacco advertisements in Indonesia. *Tobacco Control*, 2009, 18:98–107.

138. Hanoi Cancer Registry 1991–1992 and HCMC Cancer Center Statistics 1994. In: Efroymson D. *Women and tobacco: cause for concern in Vietnam*. International Development Research Centre (IDRC), 1996 (unpublished report, May 1996).

139. Coffee C. *"Strong women" and "weak men": gender paradoxes in urban Yunnan, China*. Tucson, AZ, University of Arizona, Department of Anthropology, 1999 (PhD dissertation).

140. BAT document, 1979. In: ASH briefing on "brand stretching". *Documents on Project Battalion*. London, Action on Smoking and Health, 1998 (http://www.ash.org.uk).

141. Lam TH et al. *Youth smoking: knowledge, attitudes, smoking in schools and families, and symptoms due to passive smoking*. Hong Kong, Hong Kong Council on Smoking and Health (COSH), March 1994, Report 2.

142. Malaysia tobacco companies find ways to skirt the bans. *New Straits Times*, 7 May 1996.

143. Tunistra T. A new face. *Tobacco Reporter*, 1998, January:20–22.

144. Nuki P. Tobacco firms brew up coffee to beat the ban. *The Sunday Times*, 18 January 1998.

145. ASH briefing on "brand-stretching". *Documents on Project Battalion*. London, Action on Smoking and Health, 1998 (http://www.ash.org.uk.

146. Frankel G, Mufson S. Vast China market key to smoking disputes. *The Washington Post*, 20 November 1996, Sect A:1.

147. Seimon T, Mehl G. Strategic marketing of cigarettes to young people in Sri Lanka: "Go ahead: I want to see you smoke it now". *Tobacco Control*, 1998, 7:429–433.

148. Garrett Mehl. Personal communication, 1999.

149. Malaysia tobacco companies find ways to skirt the bans. *New Straits Times*, 7 May 1996.

150. Warner F. Tobacco brands outmanoeuvre Asian advertising brands. *Wall Street Journal Europe*, 7 August 1996.

151. "Kick off, cash in": Asian sport is now big business. *Far Eastern Economic Review*, 1997, 160:4650.

152. Emerson T. Global ball. *Newsweek*, 1996, 1 April 127:47.

153. Forney M. Hoop nightmares. *Far Eastern Economic Review*, 19 December 1996:64.

154. Keenan F. Staying in the game—tobacco firms in China live with sponsorship limits. *Far Eastern Economic Review*, 1995, 158:167.

155. Manuel G. Tobacco, the real winner. *South China Morning Post*, 11 April 1999.

156. Lam TH et al. *Youth smoking, health and tobacco promotion*. Hong Kong, Hong Kong Council on Smoking and Health (COSH), 1994 (Report 1).

157. Harper M. Di's big haul for charity. *The Washington Post*, 24 April 1995, Sect A:3.

158. Benson & Hedges advertisement. *New Straits Times*, August 1995, 14:5.

159. *Cigarette firm financing soccer in Viet Nam*. Reuters. 19 December, 1994.

160. Jenkins CN et al. Tobacco use in Viet Nam: prevalence, predictors, and the role of the transnational tobacco corporations. *Journal of the American Medical Association*, 1997, 277:1726–1731.

161. Mehl G. In: Hammond R, ed. *Addicted to profit: big tobacco's expanding global reach*. Washington, DC, Essential Action, 1998.

162. *ASH challenges British tobacco company for using World Cup Cricket to market cigarettes to third world children*. London, Action on Smoking and Health, Globalink press release, 28 May 1999. (http://www.ash.org.uk).

163. Sesser S. Opium war redux. *The New Yorker*, 1993, September 13:78–89.

164. *BAT targets third world: secret documents reveal new evidence*, London, Action on Smoking and Health, Globalink press release, 11 May 1999.

165. Woolf M. Robbie Williams angry over B & H teen smoking campaign. *The Independent (London)*, 2 May1999.

166. Siytangco D. Philip Morris ASEAN Art Awards to open at Hanoi Opera House. *Manila Bulletin*, 21 November 1998.

167. Michael Tan. Personal communication, 1999.

168. Nina Castillo. Personal communication, 1999.

169. Frankel G, Mufson S. Vast China market key to smoking disputes. *The Washington Post*, 20 November 1996, Sect A:1.

170. National Cancer Institute. *The role of the media in promoting and reducing tobacco use*. Bethesda, MD, National Institutes of Health, 2008 (Tobacco Control Monograph No. 19).

171. Pierce JP, Gilpin EA. A historical analysis of tobacco marketing and the uptake of smoking by youth in the United States: 1890–1977. *Health Psychology*, 1995, 14:500–508.

172. Pierce JP, Lee L, Gilpin EA. Smoking initiation by adolescent girls, 1944 through 1988: an association with targeted advertising. *Journal of the American Medical Association*, 1994, 271:608–611.

173. Botvin GJ et al. Smoking behavior of adolescents exposed to cigarette advertising. *Public Health Reports*, 1993, 108:217–223.

174. Pollay RW et al. The last straw? Cigarette advertising and realized market shares among youths and adults, 1979–1993. *Journal of Marketing*, 1996, 60:1–16.

175. Pierce JP et al. Tobacco industry promotion of cigarettes and adolescent smoking. *Journal of the American Medical Association*, 1998, 279:511–515.

176. Evans N et al. Influence of tobacco marketing and exposure to smokers on adolescent susceptibility to smoking. *Journal of the National Cancer Institute*, 1995, 87:1538–1545.

177. Volk RJ, Edwards DW, Schulenberg J. Smoking and preference for brand of cigarette among adolescents. *Journal of Substance Abuse*, 1996, 8:347–359.

178. Schooler C, Feighery E, Flora JA. Seventh graders' self-reported exposure to cigarette marketing and its relationship to their smoking behavior. *American Journal of Public Health*, 1996, 86:1216–1221.

179. Klitzner M, Gruenewald PJ, Bamberger E. Cigarette advertising and adolescent experimentation with smoking. *British Journal of Addiction*, 1991, 86:287–298.

180. Pierce JP et al. Does tobacco advertising target young people to start smoking? *Journal of the American Medical Association*, 1991, 266:3154–3158.

181. Sargent JD et al. Cigarette promotional items in public schools. *Archives of Pediatric Adolescent Medicine*, 1997, 151:1189–1196.

182. Cummings KM et al. Comparison of recent trends in adolescent and adult cigarette smoking behaviour and brand preferences. *Tobacco Control*, 1997, 6 (Suppl.):S31–S37.

183. Barker D. Changes in the cigarette brand preferences of adolescent smokers—United States, 1989–1993. *Morbidity and Mortality Weekly Report*, 1994, 43:577–581.

184. DiFranza JR et al. RJR Nabisco's cartoon camel promotes cigarettes to children. *Journal of the American Medical Association*, 1991, 266:3149–3153.

185. Sone T. Frequency of contact with cigarette advertising and smoking experience among young women in Japan. *Journal of Epidemiology*, 1997, 7:43–47.

186. Zhu S et al. Perception of foreign cigarettes and their advertising in China: a study of college students from 12 universities. *Tobacco Control*, 1998, 7:134–140.

187. Lam TH et al. Tobacco advertisements: one of the strongest risk factors for smoking in Hong Kong students. *American Journal of Preventive Medicine*, 1998, 14:217–223.

188. Peters J et al. A comprehensive study of smoking in primary schoolchildren in Hong Kong: implications for prevention. *Journal of Epidemiology and Community Health*, 1997, 51:239–245.

189. Jenkins CNH et al. Tobacco use in Viet Nam: prevalence, predictors, and the role of transnational tobacco corporations. *Journal of the American Medical Association*, 1997, 277:1726–1731.

190. Vaidya S. Effect of sport sponsorship by tobacco companies on children's experimentation with tobacco. *British Medical Journal*, 1996, 313:400.

191. Minigawa K, While D, Charlton A. Smoking and self-perception in secondary school students. *Tobacco Control*, 1993, 2:215–221.

192. Waldron I. Patterns and causes of gender differences in smoking. *Social Science & Medicine*, 1991, 82:989–1005.

193. Nichter M. *Fat talk: what girls and their parents say about dieting.* Cambridge, MA, Harvard University Press, 2000.

194. Nichter M et al. Gendered dimensions of smoking among college students. *Journal of Adolescence Research*, May 2006, 21:215–243.

195. Warner KE, Goldenhar LM, McLaughlin CG. Cigarette advertising and magazine coverage of the hazards of smoking. *New England Journal of Medicine*, 1992, 326:305–309.

196. Amos A, Jacobson B, White P. Cigarette advertising policy and coverage of smoking and health in British women's magazines. *The Lancet*, 1992, 337:93–96 (see also Amos A, Bostock C, Bostock Y. Women's magazines and tobacco in Europe. *The Lancet*, 1995, 352:786–787).

197. Luckachko A, Whelan EM. *You've come a long way baby, or have you?* New York, NY, The American Council on Science and Health, March 1999.

198. Mackay J, Amos A. Women and tobacco. *Respirology*, 2003, 8:123–130.

199. Nichter M for the Project Quit Tobacco International Group. Introducing tobacco cessation in developing countries: an overview of Project Quit Tobacco International. *Tobacco Control*, 2006, 15 (Suppl. 1):i12–i17.

7. Addiction to Nicotine

Introduction

Addiction to tobacco kills one person prematurely every six seconds. One in two long-term smokers—largely in low- and middle-income countries—will die from tobacco addiction.[1,2] This epidemic reflects the highly addictive nature of tobacco, and specifically of nicotine, its principal addicting component. It is imperative to effectively implement Article 12 of the WHO Framework Convention on Tobacco Control (WHO FCTC), *Education, communication, training and public awareness,* which calls for Parties to promote access to information about the dangers of tobacco consumption and the benefits of cessation.

Forms of Tobacco

Nicotine's effects on a user vary depending on how the nicotine enters the body. Thus, before discussing the critera for addiction or how nicotine addiction develops, it is useful to understand different forms of tobacco. People have used tobacco in various forms for centuries. Historically, tobacco was most often chewed or smoked in pipes. Today, the most common method of using tobacco is in manufactured cigarettes.[3] Tobacco products are generally categorized as combustible (tobacco that is smoked) or non-combustible (primarily various forms of chewing tobacco and snuff).

Combustible Tobacco (Smoked)

Manufactured Cigarettes

Manufactured cigarettes contain shredded and/or reconstituted tobacco combined with hundreds of chemical additives. The contents are wrapped in paper and may have a filter tip. According to the second edition of the American Cancer Society's *Tobacco Atlas,*[4] "cigarettes account for the largest share of manufactured tobacco products in the world—96% of total sales". Although cigarettes are the most common way to consume tobacco, other products predominate in a few countries (e.g. chewing tobacco and bidis in India and kreteks in Indonesia[4]).

Roll-Your-Own Cigarettes

Roll-your-own (RYO) cigarettes are hand-filled cigarettes made from loose tobacco and rolling papers (i.e. cigarette paper). RYO cigarettes can be hand-rolled by the user or made with a hand-held rolling machine.[4] A common misconception is that RYO cigarettes are more natural and therefore "safer" than manufactured cigarettes; however, both contain the same ingredients. Additionally, in all combustible tobacco products, it is the actual burning of the tobacco that produces many of the toxic chemical components in tobacco smoke.

Cigars

Cigars consist of tightly rolled dried and fermented tobaccos wrapped in tobacco leaf. The user draws the smoke into his or her mouth but typically does not inhale it.[5] However, cigar smokers who also smoke cigarettes or are ex-smokers of cigarettes are significantly more likely to inhale the smoke than are users of cigars only.[5] Cigars come in a variety of shapes and sizes (e.g. cigarillos, double coronas, cheroots, stumpen, chuttas, and dhumtis), and they can also be "reverse smoked," which means that the ignited end of the cigar (chutta and dhumti) is placed inside the mouth. Cigars have regained some popularity with both men and women in some parts of the world.[4] In the United States, cigar smoking among women increased fivefold in a six-year period in the 1990s.[6,7]

Pipes and Water Pipes

Pipes are made of a variety of substances, including wood, briar, slate, and clay. Tobacco is placed in the bowl of the pipe, and the smoke is inhaled through the stem. Clay pipes are used throughout South-East Asia.[4] The water pipe (also known as narghile, shisha, hookah, or hubble-bubble) is widely used to smoke tobacco in the Middle East, Northern Africa, and some parts of Asia, and it has gained popularity in some Western countries.[4,8] In some regions, use of the water pipe is more prevalent than use of cigarettes, and in some Arab countries, there is less stigma associated with women's use of the water pipe than with cigarette smoking.[9]

Hookahs vary widely in shape and size, but the basic design includes a head, consisting of a ceramic bowl with a conical cap; a metal body that is attached to a glass bottle partially filled with water; and a flexible tube with a mouthpiece affixed to the neck of the bottle. The tobacco (shisha, maassel, tumbâk, or jurâk) is moist, shredded, and mixed with sweeteners such as honey, molasses, or fruit. It is placed in the head of the hookah with a heating apparatus (usually charcoal). Combustion begins in the head, and the smoke then passes through the water in the body of the pipe, where it is cooled and diluted before travelling through the hose from which the smoker inhales it.

Approximately three quarters (74.1%) of female university students in Egypt reported preferring smoking tobacco via a water pipe to smoking cigarettes because they believed it to be less harmful.

Many smokers believe that the water in the hookah filters out any harmful toxins, making it a safer alternative than cigarettes or cigars. But as Dr Christopher Loffredo, Director of the Cancer Genetics and Epidemiology programme at Georgetown University, states, "People who use these devices don't realize that they could be inhaling what is believed to be the equivalent of a pack of cigarettes in one typical 30- to 60-minute session with a water pipe because such a large quantity of pure, shredded tobacco is used".[10] Approximately three quarters (74.1%) of female university students in Egypt reported preferring smoking tobacco via a water pipe to smoking cigarettes because they believed it to be less harmful.[11] While the water filtration in a hookah does reduce some toxins, it does not reduce the level of tar in the smoke, which contains the most carcinogens (cancer-causing chemicals). Thus hookah smokers may be at greater risk for harm than cigarette smokers, since water-pipe smokers are exposed to greater overall amounts of nicotine, carbon monoxide, and other toxins.[9]

Bidis

Bidis (pronounced "bee-dees") are thin, hand-rolled, filterless cigarettes consisting of flavoured or unflavoured tobacco wrapped in a tendu or temburni leaf (plants indigenous to India and South-East Asian countries). They may be tied with a coloured string at either end, and they come in a wide variety of flavours (e.g. vanilla, strawberry, mango). Bidis may be perceived as less harmful or more natural than conventional cigarettes; however, bidi smoke contains higher concentrations of nicotine, tar, and carbon monoxide than conventional cigarettes sold in the United States. Tar and carbon monoxide levels of bidi smoke can be higher than those of manufactured cigarettes because the user needs to puff harder to keep a bidi lit.[4] Bidis are India's most used type of tobacco.[4] Jha and colleagues[12] examined prevalence data from India and Sri Lanka and estimate that about half of the male smokers and roughly 80% of the female smokers smoke bidis.

Kreteks

Kreteks are clove-flavoured cigarettes widely smoked in Indonesia.[4] They contain a mixture of shredded clove buds and tobacco, which produces a distinct, pungent smell. Kreteks often contain eugenol, which has an anaesthetic effect and thus allows for deeper inhalation. Clove cigarette smoke contains more nicotine, tar, and carbon monoxide than smoke from conventional cigarettes.[13]

Smokeless Tobacco

Smokeless tobacco comes in two main forms: chewing tobacco and snuff (moist or dry).

Chewing Tobacco

Chewing tobacco is used orally by placing a pinch between the gum and cheek and gently sucking and chewing. According to the *Tobacco Atlas*,[4] "Chewing tobacco is also known as plug, loose-leaf, chimo, toobak, gutkha, and twist. Pan masala or betel quid consists of tobacco, areca nuts and slaked lime wrapped in a betel leaf. These products also contain sweetening and flavouring agents. Varieties of pan include kaddipudi, hogesoppu,

World Health Organization

gundi, kadapam, zarda, pattiwala, kiwam and mishri". Chewing tobacco is used throughout the world but primarily in South-East Asia.[4] In Mumbai, India, more than half of the women (56%) chew tobacco.[4]

Moist and Dry Snuff

Snuff users place a small amount of snuff (ground or powdered tobacco) in the mouth between the cheek and gum. Snuff may be either moist or dry. One type of moist snuff is snus. Used primarily in Sweden and Norway—and currently being test-marketed in the United States—snus can be rolled by the user or purchased in porous packs which are placed under the upper lip. Snus that comes in prepackaged pouches does not require the user to spit out the tobacco juice. Dry snuff is powdered tobacco that is inhaled through the nose or taken orally. Once widespread, its use in now in decline.[8] There are a variety of other types of smokeless tobacco products, which are used throughout the world, including khaini, shammaah, nass, and naswa.[4]

Potentially Reduced Exposure Products

The best way to reduce the harm caused by smoking is to quit. But while the adverse effects of smoking are well documented, not all smokers are ready to quit. For decades, tobacco companies have recognized a market of individuals wanting to reduce harm without giving up nicotine and have introduced several potentially reduced exposure products (PREPs)—tobacco-based products that are marketed with the claim of reduced exposure to and harm from the toxins found in tobacco.[14]

The addition of filters to cigarettes in the 1950s to reduce tar intake is an early example of an attempt to reduce exposure to disease-causing agents. Today, in the United States and many other countries, most cigarettes have filters. Some of the new PREPs (e.g. Eclipse, Accord) are lit the same way as a cigarette, but they heat rather than burn the tobacco, theoretically reducing the concentration of toxic combustion products. Other products, such as Omni and Advance cigarettes, are claimed to reduce levels of toxins through different tobacco curing or fermentation processes or by adding chemicals (such as palladium) to the tobacco leaves. Still others are claimed to reduce nicotine levels by using genetically engineered tobacco leaves (e.g.

Quest). Finally, there are several oral non-combustible tobacco products. Hard tobacco lozenges, or "cigaletts" (e.g. Ariva and Stonewall) and tobacco packets (e.g. Revel and Exalt) are currently marketed as tobacco alternatives to smoking, but not as cessation products.

A cigarette is an efficient, well-engineered nicotine delivery device that has proved to be deadly when smoked regularly. Nicotine from a smoked cigarette will reach the brain in as little as 7 seconds after inhalation.

There has been much debate about whether these PREPs promote harm reduction or are just another marketing ploy by the tobacco industry to keep people "hooked". The evidence of whether PREPs are associated with reduced risk has been inconclusive. A recent study found the levels of tobacco-specific nitrosamines (TSNAs, the cancer-causing chemicals found in tobacco) in PREPs to be low for some brands and as high as levels found in conventional cigarettes for other brands.[15] More studies are needed to settle this debate.

Nicotine Content

A cigarette is an efficient, well-engineered nicotine delivery device that has proved to be deadly when smoked regularly. Nicotine from a smoked cigarette will reach the brain in as little as 7 seconds after inhalation.[16] A typical cigarette contains approximately 0.5 to 1.0 g of tobacco and, on average, 10 mg of nicotine.[8,17] A cigarette is typically smoked in 10 puffs and within 5 minutes.[17] A typical smoker will absorb 1 to 2 mg of nicotine, but absorption can range from 0.5 to 3 mg.[18,19] The elimination half-life of nicotine is 2 to 3 hours, meaning that the level of nicotine in the blood decreases by one half after a smoker stops smoking for that length of time.[19]

Cigars vary in size, as does their nicotine content. Cigars commonly have from 5 to 17 g of tobacco,[5] and

World Health Organization

the tobacco contains from 10 mg to more than 300 mg of nicotine.[20] Most cigars do not have filters and take an hour or more to smoke.

Nicotine concentrations in the tobacco of bidis (21.2 mg/g) have been found to be significantly higher than the concentrations in manufactured filtered (16.3 mg/g) and unfiltered cigarettes (13.5 mg/g).[21]

A typical pipe (e.g. a clay bowl filled with tobacco, with smoke inhaled through a stem) will use 3–4 g of tobacco.[8] Much more tobacco is used in a typical water-pipe (e.g. hookah) session—on average, 20 g.[8] Nicotine levels after smoking a water pipe for 45 minutes are reported to be higher than those measured after smoking a cigarette.[8]

Smokeless tobacco products vary considerably in nicotine content, pH, and levels of various carcinogens. Since nicotine is absorbed through the buccal mucosa of the smokeless tobacco user's mouth, uptake is affected by both the pH of the tobacco product and the pH of the mouth.[8,22] The rate of absorption and action for nicotine from smokeless tobacco is thus slower than that from tobacco that enters the body via the lungs when smoked. The delayed effect may make smokeless products less addictive than cigarettes.[23] However, some smokeless tobacco users report that quitting cigarettes is easier than quitting smokeless tobacco.

A study of six popular brands of moist snuff found that nicotine content ranged from 3.4 mg/g to 11.5 mg/g.[24] The highest concentrations of nicotine are in dry snuff, which has an average of 16.8 mg/g, followed by moist snuff (12.6 mg/g) and chewing tobacco (9.9 mg/g).[24] Use of smokeless tobacco is associated with cancer of the pharynx, larynx, and oesophagus.[25,26] The process of fermenting and curing smokeless tobacco increases the levels of TSNAs, which exist in relatively low concentrations in green tobacco.[27] Content of TSNAs varies widely among different forms of smokeless tobacco. Swedish snuff (snus) contains the lowest levels of TSNAs (2.8 µg/g of dried tobacco),[28] whereas Skoal® and Copenhagen®, two popular brands in the United States, contain high levels: 64.0 µg per gram of dried tobacco and 41.1 µg per gram of dried tobacco, respectively.[29]

Creation and Maintenance of Addiction

Nicotine's Effects

The role of nicotine in addiction has been extensively reviewed and reported (see, for example, the Royal College of Physicians' 2007 report on harm reduction;[8] Matta et al.'s 2007 review of the guidelines on nicotine dose selection for in vivo research;[30] and Brigham on the addiction model[31]). The following is a brief overview of nicotine's role in the development and maintenance of addiction.

The active ingredient for addiction is nicotine, a naturally occurring drug found in all the different forms of tobacco. Nicotine is highly addictive, as addictive as heroin and cocaine.[25,32] All leading authorities, including WHO, the Royal College of Physicians, and the American Psychiatric Association (APA),[33-35] have supported the three major conclusions of a 1988 report by the Surgeon General of the United States[32] regarding nicotine and tobacco:

1. Cigarettes and other forms of tobacco are addictive.

2. Nicotine is the drug in tobacco that causes addiction.

3. The physiological and behavioural processes that determine tobacco addiction are similar to those that determine heroin and cocaine addiction.

All forms of tobacco have the potential to be addictive because they all contain nicotine, but cigarettes are the most efficient for delivering nicotine into the body.[33]

The tobacco industry has long understood the role of nicotine. A leading Philip Morris nicotine researcher, William L. Dunn, concluded in 1972:

> *The cigarette should be conceived not as a product but as a package. The product is nicotine … Think of the cigarette pack as a storage container for a day's supply of nicotine … Think of the cigarette as a dispenser of a dose unit of nicotine … Think of a puff of smoke as the vehicle of nicotine … Smoke is beyond question the most optimized vehicle of nicotine and the cigarette the most optimized dispenser of smoke.*
> (quoted in Hurt & Robertston[36])

 World Health Organization

Nicotine is an alkaloid found in abundance in the tobacco plant and to a much lesser degree in potatoes, eggplants, and tomatoes.[8] Nicotine's effects on the brain and on body systems have been reviewed extensively (see, again, Royal College of Physicians,[8] Matta[30]).

Nicotine is classified as a stimulant drug, but many people who use it report decreased arousal. Nicotine produces paradoxical effects, acting as both a stimulant and a depressant. As a stimulant, it has been shown to increase attention, memory, information processing, and learning.[30,37] It has also been shown to alleviate anxiety, depression, and pain. For these reasons, smokers often report that smoking is a stress reliever and that they are more apt to smoke in response to stressful situations or negative moods.[38]

As noted above, inhalation of nicotine in the form of smoke provides the quickest delivery,[30,37] with nicotine reaching the brain in approximately 7 seconds.[16] Nicotine stimulates the dopaminergic pathways of the mesolimbic system in the brain, an area that is involved in reinforcement for other drugs of abuse.[39] Nicotine binds to the nicotinic acetylcholine receptors in the brain (nAchRs), causing the release of dopamine in the nucleus accumbens[40] and the subsequent release of neurotransmitters, resulting in a variety of physiological effects, including behavioural arousal and neural activation.[19] Release of dopamine, norepinephrine, and serotonin is associated with pleasurable feelings and also with appetite suppression. The excess release of acetylcholine associated with nicotine consumption is related to improved attention,[41] increased vigilance in the performance of repetitive tasks, and memory improvements.[19,41] These pharmacological effects play a large role in maintaining smoking behaviour in the addicted smoker.

Nicotine improves mood. Smokers commonly report increased pleasure and reduced anger, tension, depression, and stress after smoking a cigarette. It is unclear whether these effects are due to the effect of nicotine on the brain or to the alleviation of withdrawal symptoms. The perceived calming effect from the reduction of withdrawal symptoms may be what nicotine users find reinforcing. Some of these effects may be pharmacological, but some of the sedating psychological effect of smoking comes from the smoker's perception of coping with stress successfully while smoking.[16]

Nicotine also affects metabolism by decreasing appetite and increasing metabolic rate.[38] Evidence of this metabolic effect can be found in the weight gain by ex-smokers, an average of 4 kg of body weight after quitting.[42] Increased appetite can persist for several months upon quitting.[40] Weight control and reduction of appetite are critical aspects of the appeal of smoking for many women and girls. Further, weight gain and fear of weight gain can be important deterrents to smoking cessation, particularly among women.[43,44] Both girls and women are more likely to smoke to control their weight than males are.[6] Studies have shown that girls and women are more fearful of weight gain than boys and men are and may use smoking as a method of weight control.[45] Additionally, some studies have found that women gain more weight after quitting than men do.[45,46] Research suggests that women who quit smoking may also be at a greater risk of resuming smoking in order to avoid weight gain.

Weight control and reduction of appetite are critical aspects of the appeal of smoking for many women and girls.

Women experience greater subjective pleasurable effects from tobacco smoke than men do.[47] Research has also shown that male and female smokers differ in their intake of nicotine. Women do not take in as much nicotine as men do and appear to have greater sensitivity to nicotine's effects on reducing both negative affect and body weight.[42] Rates of nicotine metabolism are also significantly higher in women smokers who use oral contraceptives[30] and those who are pregnant.[48]

Criteria for Addiction

Addiction is a term commonly applied to maladaptive drug-seeking behaviour, often performed despite knowledge of negative health consequences. Nicotine meets the established criteria for a drug that produces addiction, specifically, dependence and withdrawal. Both WHO in its *International Classification of Diseases (ICD)*[49] and the APA in its *Diagnostic and Statistical Manual (DSM-IV &*

DSM-IV-TR)[34,50] have issued diagnostic criteria to assess dependence and withdrawal. Both WHO and APA recognize dependence as, in essence, the repetitive and compulsive use of a drug. Withdrawal is a syndrome of symptoms that occur when a regular user abruptly stops use (e.g. following or during a quit attempt). Nicotine withdrawal and dependence are viewed as separate, albeit related, disorders, each with its own specific diagnostic criteria.[34]

Addiction and dependence are often used synonymously by both WHO and APA. With dependence, tolerance to a drug—i.e. a decreased response to a repeated dose of the drug—can often occur. In essence, more nicotine is needed to produce the same effects that were once produced by lower doses. Neuroadaptation occurs when the brain has adapted to the presence of nicotine and needs nicotine in order to function normally.[19] When nicotine is not available (such as when a smoker stops smoking), the brain function becomes disturbed, resulting in withdrawal.

The diagnostic criteria for dependence-producing drugs are given in Table 7.1.

Greater nicotine dependence has been shown to be associated with lower motivation to quit, difficulty in trying to quit, and failure to quit,[51] as well as with smoking the first cigarette earlier in the day and smoking more cigarettes per day.[32,52]

Withdrawal produces a constellation of symptoms that tobacco users may experience when they stop tobacco use abruptly (see Table 7.2 for a list of the criteria for nicotine withdrawal). Withdrawal symptoms vary but include a craving for nicotine, irritability, frustration or anger, anxiety, depression, difficulty concentrating, restlessness, and increased appetite (which can lead to weight gain). Most symptoms reach maximum intensity 24 to 48 hours after cessation and then gradually diminish over a period of a few weeks.[19] Some withdrawal symptoms, such as dysphoria,[18] mild depression,[18] anhedonia,[18] and increased appetite,[6,40,33] may persist for months.

It is important to note that withdrawal is neither necessary nor sufficient for the development of dependence.[34,49] For instance, intermittent smokers (e.g. "chippers"), social smokers, and non-daily smokers may meet the criteria for nicotine dependence but may not meet the criteria for withdrawal disorder.[8] Shiffman and Paty found that chippers do not appear to smoke to avoid nicotine withdrawal symptoms; rather, smoking by these low-level smokers was associated with more "indulgent" activities such as socializing, eating, and drinking alcohol.[53]

Withdrawal and dependence can be associated; persons who show signs of dependence (e.g. high tolerance to nicotine and difficulty quitting smoking) are more likely to experience withdrawal symptoms if they discontinue smoking. Withdrawal symptoms are also related to the severity of dependence, and they may increase temptations to smoke and alleviate the withdrawal, especially within the first 30 days after cessation. Withdrawal symptoms can be present, albeit in a milder form, when a smoker

Table 7.1. Diagnostic Criteria for Nicotine Dependence

Dependence is a maladaptive pattern of substance use, leading to clinically significant impairment or distress, as manifested by three (or more) of the following, occurring at any time in the same 12-month period:

1. Tolerance, as defined by either
   - a need for markedly increased amounts of the substance to achieve the desired effect, or
   - markedly diminished effect with continued use of the same amount of substance.

2. Withdrawal, as manifested by either
   - the characteristic withdrawal syndrome for the substance, or
   - the substance being taken to relieve or avoid withdrawal symptoms.

3. Taking larger amounts of the substance or over a longer period than was intended.

4. A persistent desire for or unsuccessful efforts to cut down on substance use.

5. A great deal of time being spent in activities necessary to obtain or use a substance.

6. Abandonment or reduction of important social, occupational, or recreational activities because of substance abuse.

Source: Ref. 50.

reduces the number of cigarettes smoked or switches to a low-nicotine cigarette.[54]

Withdrawal can begin within hours of smoking the last cigarette, and symptoms typically peak within one to three weeks after stopping use,[46] reaching maximal intensity during the first week.[40] Cravings can persist for months, especially if triggered by situational cues.[40] Hendricks and colleagues[55] found that nicotine withdrawal occurs quickly after abstaining from smoking, with nicotine-dependent study participants who abstained from smoking reporting greater cravings (a symptom of withdrawal) for cigarettes after 30 minutes than non-abstaining nicotine-dependent participants.

Cessation Rates

As discussed in greater detail in the chapter of this monograph on quitting smoking, dependent smokers have low rates of smoking cessation and total abstinence from cigarettes. Research suggests that cessation may be more difficult for women than for men.[44,56] Examination of cessation rates provides some insight into the addictive nature of nicotine and the difficulty associated with stopping. In the United States and some other countries, most cigarette smokers (70%) report wanting to quit smoking; however, it is estimated that each year less than 1% of self-quitters (i.e. smokers who quit without any formal treatment intervention) will actually succeed.[57] SRI International[58] reported that the US Centers for Disease Control and Prevention (CDC) found only a 5% abstinence rate after three months for people who quit "cold turkey" (i.e. abruptly and without assistance). Hughes and colleagues[59] found that only one third of the smokers who quit on their own remained abstinent after two days, only one quarter after seven days, and less than one in five (19%) after one month.

Further evidence of the addictive nature of nicotine is the high rate of relapse (i.e. return to smoking), even among people faced with life-threatening illnesses. A recent study of more than 5000 patients receiving treatment for coronary heart disease in 15 European countries revealed that only half of them quit smoking after suffering a heart attack.[60] Even more compelling, Walker and colleagues[61] found that more than 40% of patients smoked at some point after having surgery to remove non-small-cell lung cancer, and more than one third (36.9%) of them were

smoking one year post-surgery. Resumption of smoking was related to shorter quit duration prior to the surgery and more-intense cravings.

It is not uncommon for smokers to "slip" or even relapse after a quit attempt. Most smokers who manage to quit will make 8 to 11 attempts before actually succeeding.[6] For most smokers, quitting represents stopping an addiction they have had for many years. Aside from breaking the addiction to nicotine, smokers have to break the many associations they have with smoking (e.g. smoking while relaxing, talking on the phone, or in a car). It is not difficult to understand why so many smokers who have quit slip or relapse when these triggers are present.

Slips can be defined as the re-engagement of some smoking behaviour (e.g. smoking less than a whole cigarette

---

Table 7.2. **Diagnostic Criteria for Nicotine Withdrawal**

A. Daily use of nicotine for at least several weeks.

B. Abrupt cessation of nicotine use or reduction in the amount of nicotine used, followed by four (or more) of the following signs within 24 hours:

1. dysphoric or depressed mood
2. insomnia
3. irritability, frustration, or anger
4. anxiety
5. difficulty concentrating
6. restlessness
7. decreased heart rate
8. increased appetite or weight gain.

C. Clinically significant distress or impairment in social, occupational, or other important areas of functioning.

D. Symptoms not due to a general medical condition and not better accounted for by a mental disorder.

Source: Refs. 34, 50.

on one or more occasions) that does not progress into a full-blown relapse (i.e. resumption of a regular smoking pattern). But a slip is often viewed as a failure, which can be very demoralizing and can lead to relapse. Both slips and relapse should be viewed as learning experiences[62] and part of the process of recovery from addiction.[63] Failed quit attempts should be reframed as learning experiences of what to do and what not to do in future quit attempts.[62] Smokers are most likely to relapse in the first three months but can be vulnerable to relapse through the first year following a quit attempt.[62]

Evidence shows that around 50% of those who start smoking in the adolescent years continue to smoke for 15 to 20 years.

How Nicotine Addiction Develops

Addiction to nicotine does not happen quickly, after using tobacco once or twice; it develops over time. Most smokers go through a series of steps from experimentation to regular use on their way to becoming addicted. Particularly in the industrialized countries, most people addicted to nicotine initiated smoking during adolescence. As many as one third to one half of adolescents who experiment with smoking go on to become regular smokers.[64] In the United States, more than 90% of current adult smokers began smoking before the age of 18.[65] The younger an individual is when he or she experiments with smoking, the more likely he or she is to become a regular or daily smoker. For example, two thirds of children who begin smoking in the sixth grade become regular adult smokers, and almost half (46%) of those who initiate smoking in the eleventh grade become regular adult smokers.[66] Evidence shows that around 50% of those who start smoking in the adolescent years continue to smoke for 15 to 20 years.[67] Unfortunately, sales to minors (addressed in Article 16 of the WHO FCTC, *Sales to and by minors*) often go unregulated. The following brief overview of smoking initiation in industrialized countries such as the United

States is elaborated further in the chapter on initiation and maintenance of tobacco use.

It can take from months to three years for a person to become addicted to tobacco.[25] The Surgeon General of the United States[25] reported that children and adolescents progress through the following stages in developing an addiction to tobacco:

1. Forming attitudes and beliefs about tobacco

2. Trying tobacco

3. Experimenting with tobacco

4. Regularly using tobacco

5. Becoming addicted to tobacco.

A more recent stage-based conceptualization of smoking initiation uses the framework of the Transtheoretical Model of Intentional Behaviour Change (TTM).[63,68,69]

The TTM describes the process as one in which individuals move through the following five stages on the road to developing a well-maintained pattern of behaviour: precontemplation, contemplation, preparation, action, and maintenance.[69] The stages of smoking initiation are similar to but distinct from those of cessation or recovery.[63,68]

Figure 7.1 presents an overview of the stages of addiction as well as the stages of recovery. The top set of arrows (addiction) represents the stage progression of individuals who are in the process of adopting a new behaviour (e.g. smoking) moving from non-use (precontemplation, PC) to dependence (maintenance, M). The bottom set of arrows (cessation) represents the stage progression of individuals who are in the process of recovering from an addiction, moving from precontemplation (PC, unwilling or unable to stop the behaviour) to maintenance (M, sustained cessation). Movement through the stages (both addiction and cessation) is affected by the processes of change (behavioural and experiential), the individual's context (e.g. current life situation, beliefs and attitudes, interpersonal relationships), and markers of change (e.g. self-efficacy, decisional balance). Although the process is represented as linear, individuals can move backwards and forwards through the stages and often have to recycle through them before maintaining change.

Precontemplation is the stage in which individuals who are not considering adopting or changing a particular behaviour have become interested in acquiring a new one. This first stage would be experienced by youth who have never smoked cigarettes but are beginning to form or have already formed attitudes and beliefs about smoking. Beliefs at this stage are often negative but can be affected by media exposure or role modelling (i.e. parental smoking). In terms of initiation of smoking behaviour, a youth in precontemplation would be a non-smoker who is not considering smoking at any time in the foreseeable future.

As the adolescent enters *contemplation*, he or she becomes more aware of smoking, is open to considering smoking, and/or experiences some desire to experiment with smoking. Typically, the environmental pressures to smoke (e.g. media messages or peer pressure) are more salient to young people in this stage. They may think about trying smoking, but they are not fully committed to adopting the new behaviour. Experimentation can be considered part of this process, as the first few attempts produce important information that influences the decision to continue.

Youth in the *preparation* stage not only are interested in smoking but also have some intention to smoke in the near future, typically within the next 30 days. A youth in this stage of smoking initiation might seek out individuals who smoke and may begin to experiment with cigarette smoking. The initial reaction to experimentation with cigarettes (e.g. dizziness and/or positive reinforcement from friends) may determine the youth's progression through the stages. In addition, tobacco advertising may become more influential at this stage, and the person experimenting with smoking may begin to find more pros than cons with regard to the practice.

The *action* stage is defined by some pattern of regular smoking behaviour. As youths progress through this stage, they begin to change their environment so that the behaviour is more likely to occur. The action stage typically consists of up to six months of a regular pattern of smoking. An adolescent in action will repeatedly, but usually irregularly, smoke cigarettes. Smoking behaviour in this stage tends to occur in certain situations, such as at parties. If smoking behaviour is not viewed as sufficiently reinforcing, individuals may move back into one of the earlier stages of smoking initiation.

The fifth stage, *maintenance*, firmly establishes the addiction and consists of ongoing integration of cigarette smoking into the individual's life. An adolescent who is regularly using cigarettes will do so in many different contexts, such as before and after school, while driving a

Figure 7.1. Overview of the Stages of Addiction and Recovery

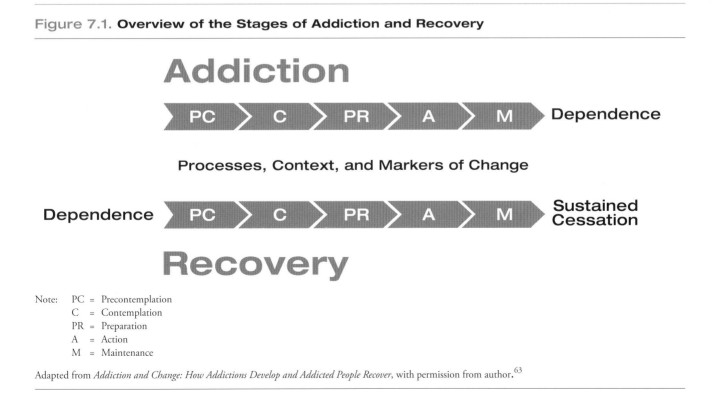

Note: PC = Precontemplation
C = Contemplation
PR = Preparation
A = Action
M = Maintenance

Adapted from *Addiction and Change: How Addictions Develop and Addicted People Recover*, with permission from author.[63]

car, or while alone, in a regular pattern of use. Individuals in this stage have an established pattern of regular smoking that has lasted for more than six months.

Psychosocial Risk Factors for Initiating Tobacco Use

Numerous factors are associated with an adolescent's progression through the stages of tobacco use. These factors include being in a lower-SES group;[70,71] owning promotional smoking merchandise;[72] overestimating peer smoking prevalence;[73] the adolescent's environment, including attitudes and behaviours of friends, siblings, and/or parents;[74] underestimating the addictive properties of smoking;[75] lack of parental monitoring;[76] low levels of academic achievement;[74,77] and previous experimentation with tobacco products.[78]

These factors appear to be related to an increase in risk for both boys and girls; however, some factors have more influence on girls than on boys in their progression through the process of initiation. For instance, available research indicates that girls who use tobacco tend to have stronger attachments to peers and friends than boys have; they also tend to overestimate smoking prevalence in their environment, are less committed to school, are less knowledgeable about nicotine and addiction, and usually have parents or friends who smoke.[6] Like women, girls are more likely than boys to believe that smoking can be a way of controlling weight.[6]

Behavioural and Psychological Factors of Nicotine Addiction

As discussed earlier, nicotine is a key and necessary component in the development of smoking addiction; however, behavioural, psychological, environmental, and social factors also contribute to the development and maintenance of addiction.

Since a typical smoker takes 10 puffs on each cigarette, a person who smokes a pack of cigarettes a day (20 cigarettes per pack) will receive 200 doses of nicotine daily.[18] No other drug is dosed at such a high frequency. This conditioning, in addition to the presence of nicotine, is critical to the addiction process. A pack-a-day smoker who smokes for 14 years will have over 1 million dosing opportunities. This repeated dosing, coupled with the fact that withdrawal symptoms are often averted with each cigarette, makes nicotine one of the most addictive drugs.

In addition to the repeated dosing of actual nicotine, certain behaviours, such as bringing the cigarette from hand to mouth at the same frequency, co-occur with the dosing. Other behaviours, such as smoking the first cigarette of the day or smoking after a meal, while on the phone, or driving a car, also become associated with smoking and reinforce continued use. As people progress from the action to the maintenance stage, smoking becomes conditioned and connected to more and more behaviours or becomes more firmly connected to specific times, events, and experiences. Behavioural factors, such as the hand-to-mouth motion, may be more critical and reinforcing for women than for men and more important than nicotine.[42,47]

Smokers often identify one of the main benefits of smoking as its calming effects. As mentioned previously, smokers begin to experience impairment of mood and performance within hours of their last cigarette, and certainly overnight, as they begin to experience withdrawal symptoms. These effects are completely alleviated by smoking a cigarette. According to Jarvis,[40] "smokers go through this process thousands of times over the course of their smoking career, and this may lead them to identify cigarettes as effective self-medication, even if the effect is the negative one of withdrawal relief rather than any absolute improvement". As any former smoker will tell you, it takes months or even years to achieve the extinction of these conditioned cues.

Social and Environmental Influences and Marketing

Social and environmental influences can both discourage and encourage tobacco use. For instance, enactment and enforcement of smoke-free policies, taxes, and social sanctions can discourage use and affect rates of initiation and progression to addiction; being surrounded by smokers (e.g. peer group or family members) can encourage smoking.[8,40] Marketing, portrayal in the media, and brand preference of specific populations (such as women and youth) can influence the progression to regular use and addiction.[8] The guidelines for the implementation of Article 13 of the WHO FCTC, *Tobacco advertising, promotion and sponsorship,* developed and adopted by Parties to the treaty, review a number of different forms of tobacco advertising, promotion, and sponsorship and make recommendations to effectively ban each of them.

The tobacco industry developed "light", or "low-tar", cigarettes in a misleading attempt to address concerns of smokers about the health effects of smoking. Smokers may smoke "light" cigarettes as an alternative to quitting, believing they are reducing their risks by smoking a lower-tar cigarette. A 2006 study[79] found that use of "light" cigarettes was common, and more than one third of the users reported using those cigarettes to reduce health risks. These smokers were about 50% less likely to quit than those who smoked non-"light" cigarettes.

More women than men smoke "light" or "ultra-light" cigarettes—almost two thirds of women smokers (63%) and less than half of men smokers (46%).[80] A common misconception is that "low tar" or "light" means low risk. "Light" cigarettes are not less harmful than regular cigarettes. "Light" cigarettes have that designation because when measured on standard smoking machines, they produce lower levels of nicotine and tar. However, most people do not smoke in the same manner as smoking machines. "Light" cigarettes are as dangerous as regular cigarettes because of the increased ventilation in the "light" cigarettes' filters. Smokers engage in compensatory smoking, meaning they inhale deeper in an effort to achieve the same amount of nicotine, which leads to inhaling the same amount of tar. Smokers of "light" cigarettes tend to smoke a higher number of cigarettes, inhale deeper, hold the smoke in their lungs longer, and/or take more-frequent puffs in an effort to satisfy their nicotine craving.[8,81] Additionally, smokers often cover the holes in the filter with their lips and/or fingers, which allows them to get as much nicotine as they would get from smoking a regular cigarette.[18,82]

In the United States in August 2006, US District Court Judge Gladys Kessler ruled that the use of descriptive labels of "low-tar" or "light" on tobacco products is false and misleading, because it implies a more healthful product and should not be used.[83] This ruling, made in a lawsuit of the US government against the tobacco industry, is currently on appeal, and the tobacco companies continue to market

"lights" and "low-tar" cigarettes. The WHO FCTC obligates its Parties to eliminate misleading descriptors from tobacco packaging in Article 11, *Packaging and labelling of tobacco products.*

Conclusion

It is critical to remember that all tobacco products can be deadly and addictive, regardless of their form or disguise.[84] Women and girls are beginning to follow the same trajectory of initiation into smoking as men, with variable patterns depending on sociocultural and economic status. All users of tobacco are at risk for increased morbidity and mortality. However, women face unique challenges such as greater difficulty in quitting and differences in tobacco-related health risks, including nicotine metabolism, weight issues, osteoporosis and increased risk of fracture, early menopause, and effects on sexual and reproductive health.

Nicotine is a powerful drug that meets all established criteria for a drug that produces addiction—specifically, dependence and withdrawal. Nicotine is as addictive as heroin and cocaine, and it has the paradoxical effects of being a stimulant and a depressant. No other drug doses at such a high frequency: a pack-a-day smoker who smokes for 14 years will have more than 1 million dosing opportunities.

Girls and women are more likely to smoke to control their weight than males are, and they tend to gain more weight after quitting smoking. Female smokers also derive greater subjective pleasurable effects from nicotine than males who smoke. They are at increased risk for female-specific reproductive issues, including painful, irregular periods; earlier menopause; and increased risks among those who use certain birth-control methods.

WHO and APA have issued diagnostic criteria for assessing dependence and withdrawal, the key components of addiction. Dependence is a maladaptive pattern of substance use in which tolerance develops (in the case of smoking, more nicotine is needed to produce the same effects that were once produced by lower doses). Withdrawal is a constellation of symptoms that a tobacco user may experience when he or she abruptly stops tobacco use (including irritability, anxiety, and increased appetite).

Smoking initiation by young people can be conceptualized as a series of five stages: precontemplation, contemplation, preparation, action, and maintenance. Female-specific issues with smoking initiation include concern about weight, less commitment to school, and stronger ties with peers.

Increasing effort should be devoted to developing better prevention strategies and investigating methods of cessation that are gender-specific. More research is needed on the addiction process in all types of tobacco use, as well as in the various subtypes of tobacco users (e.g. non-dependent "chippers"). In addition, more research is needed on the initiation process into smoking and the transitions from experimentation to addiction, as well as on identifying specific risk and protective factors for girls and women. Prevention and intervention strategies should be tailored to these factors.

References

1. Jha P et al. Tobacco addiction. In: Jamison DT et al., eds. *Disease control priorities in developing countries* 2nd ed. New York, NY, Oxford University Press, 2006, 869–886.

2. *WHO report on the global tobacco epidemic: implementing smoke-free environments,* Geneva, World Health Organization, 2009.

3. Brandt AM. *The cigarette century: the rise, fall, and the deadly persistence of the product that defined America.* New York, NY, Basic Books, 2007.

4. Mackay J, Eriksen M, Shafey O. *The tobacco atlas,* 2nd ed. Atlanta, GA, American Cancer Society, 2006.

5. Burns DM. Cigar smoking: overview and current state of the science. In: National Cancer Institute, *Cigars: health effects and trends.* Bethesda, MD, National Cancer Institute, 1998:1–20 (Smoking and Tobacco Control Monograph 9).

6. *Women and smoking: a report of the Surgeon General.* Rockville, MD, US Department of Health and Human Services, 2001.

7. Gerlach KK et al. Trends in cigar consumption and smoking prevalence. In: *Cigars: health effects and trends.* Bethesda, MD, National Cancer Institute, 1998:37–70 (Smoking and Tobacco Control Monograph 9).

8. *Harm reduction in nicotine addiction: helping people who can't quit. A report by the Tobacco Advisory Group of the Royal College of Physicians.* London, Royal College of Physicians, 2007.

9. Knishkowy B, Amitai Y. Water-pipe (narghile) smoking: an emerging health risk behaviour. *Pediatrics,* 2005, 116:e113–119.

10. Loffredo C. *Hold the hookah: research warns against trendy tobacco use.* 2006 (http://explore.georgetown.edu/news/?ID=18216, accessed 15 March 2008).

11. Labib N et al. Comparison of cigarette and water pipe smoking among female university students in Egypt. *Nicotine & tobacco research,* 2007, 9:591–596.

12. Jha P et al. Estimates of global and regional smoking prevalence in 1995, by age and sex. *American Journal of Public Health,* 2002, 92:1002–1006.

13. Malson JL et al. Clove cigarette smoking: biochemical, physiological, and subjective effects. *Pharmacology, Biochemistry, and Behaviour,* 2003, 74:739–745.

14. Hatsukami DK, Zeller M. *Tobacco harm reduction: the need for research to inform policy.* Washington, DC, American Psychological Association, 2004. (http://www.apa.org/science/psa/sb-hatsukami.html, accessed 15 February 2008).

15. Stepanov I et al. Tobacco-specific nitrosamines in new tobacco products. *Nicotine & Tobacco Research,* 2006, 8:309–313.

16. Maisto SA, Galizio M, Connors GJ, eds. *Drug use and abuse,* 4th ed. Belmont, CA, Wadsworth/Thompson Learning, 2004.

17. *Nicotine addiction.* Bethesda, MD, National Institute on Drug Abuse, 2001, rev. 2006 (http://www.drugabuse.gov/PDF/RRTobacco.pdf, accessed 15 February 2008).

18. Karan LD, Dani JA, Benowitz NL. The pharmacology of nicotine dependence. In: *Principles of addiction medicine,* 3rd ed. Washington, DC, American Society of Addiction Medicine, 2003:225–248.

19. Lynch B, Bonnie RJ, eds. *Growing up tobacco free: preventing nicotine addiction in children and youths.* Institute of Medicine Committee on Preventing Nicotine Addiction on Children and Youths. Washington, DC, National Academy Press, 1994.

20. Henningfield JE et al. Nicotine concentration, smoke pH and whole tobacco aqueous pH of some cigar brands and types popular in the United States. *Informa Healthcare,* 1999, 163–168.

21. Malson JL et al. Comparison of the nicotine content of tobacco used in bidis and conventional cigarettes. *Tobacco Control,* 2001, 10:181–183.

22. Hatsukami DK, Severson HH. Oral spit tobacco: addiction, prevention and treatment. *Nicotine & Tobacco Research,* 1999, 1:21–44.

23. Severson HH. What have we learned from 20 years of research on smokeless tobacco cessation? *The American Journal of the Medical Sciences,* 2003, 326:206–211.

24. Centers for Disease Control and Prevention. Determination of nicotine, pH, and moisture content of six US commercial moist snuff products—Florida, January-February 1999. *Morbidity and Mortality Weekly Report,* 1999, 48:398–401.

25. *Preventing tobacco use among young people: a report of the Surgeon General.* Atlanta, GA, Centers for Disease Control and Prevention, National Center for Chronic Disease Prevention and Health Promotion, 1994.

26. *The health consequences of using smokeless tobacco: a report of the Advisory Committee to the Surgeon General.* Bethesda, MD, US Department of Health and Human Services, Public Health Service, 1986.

27. *Reducing the health consequences of smoking: 25 years of progress. A report of the Surgeon General.* Rockville, MD, Centers for Disease Control, Center for Chronic Disease Prevention and Health Promotion, 1989.

28. Brunnemann KD, Qi J, Hoffmann D. *Aging of oral moist snuff and the yields of tobacco specific n-nitrosamines (TSNA).* Progress report prepared for the Massachusetts Tobacco Control Program, Boston, MA, 2001.

29. Hoffmann D et al. Five leading US commercial brands of moist snuff in 1994: assessment of carcinogenic N-nitrosamines. *Journal of the National Cancer Institute,* 1995, 87:1862–1869.

30. Matta SG et al. Guidelines on nicotine dose selection for in vivo research. *Psychopharmacology,* 2007, 190:269–319.

31. Brigham J. Addiction model. In: Samet JM, Yoon S, eds. *Women and the tobacco epidemic: challenges for the 21st century.* Geneva, World Health Organization, 2001.

32. US Department of Health and Human Services. *The health consequences of smoking: nicotine addiction: a report of the Surgeon General.* Washington, DC, US Government Printing Office, 1988.

33. Tobacco smoking in Britain: an overview. In: *Nicotine addiction in Britain: report of the Tobacco Advisory Group of the Royal College of Physicians.* London, Royal College of Physicians, 2000.

34. *Diagnostic and statistical manual of mental disorders,* 4th ed. Washington, DC, American Psychiatric Association, 1994.

35. *Advancing knowledge on regulating tobacco products.* Geneva, World Health Organization, 2001.

36. Hurt RD, Robertson CR. Prying open the door to the tobacco industry's secrets about nicotine: the Minnesota Tobacco Trial. *The Journal of the American Medical Association,* 1998, 280:1173–1181.

37. Benowitz NL. Pharmacology of nicotine: addiction and therapeutics. *Annual Review of Pharmacology and Toxicology,* 1996, 36:597–613.

38. Goldstein MG. Pharmacotherapy for smoking cessation. In: Abrams DB et al., eds. *The tobacco dependence treatment handbook: a guide to best practice.* New York, NY, The Guilford Press, 2003:230–248.

39. Benowitz NL. Cardiovascular toxicity of nicotine: pharmacokinetic and pharmacodynamic considerations. In: Benowitz NL, ed. *Nicotine safety and toxicity.* New York, NY, Oxford University Press, 1998, 19–28.

40. Jarvis MJ. ABC of smoking cessation: why people smoke. *British Medical Journal,* 2004, 328:277–279.

41. Rezvani AH, Levin ED. Cognitive effects of nicotine. *Biological Psychiatry,* 2001, 49:258–267.

42. Benowitz NL, ed. Gender differences in the pharmacology of nicotine addiction. *Addiction Biology,* 1998, 3:383–404.

World Health Organization

43. Borrelli B et al. Influences of gender and weight gain on short-term relapse to smoking in a cessation trial. *Journal of Consulting and Clinical Psychology*, 2001, 69:511–515.

44. Perkins KA. Smoking cessation in women: special considerations. *CNS Drugs*, 2001, 15:391–411.

45. *Gender, health and tobacco*. Geneva, World Health Organization, 2003. (http://www.who.int/gender/documents/Gender_Tobacco_2.pdf, accessed 7 March 2008).

46. Fiore MC et al. *Treating tobacco use and dependence; a clinical practice guideline*. Rockville, MD, US Department of Health and Human Services, Public Health Service, 2000.

47. Perkins KA, Donny E, Caggiula AR. Sex differences in nicotine effects and self-administration: review of human and animal evidence. *Nicotine & Tobacco Research*, 1999, 1:301–315.

48. Dempsey D, Jacob P III, Benowitz NL. Accelerated metabolism of nicotine and cotinine in pregnant smokers. *Pharmacology and Experimental Therapeutics*, 2002, 301:594–598.

49. *The ICD-10 classification of mental and behavioural disorders: clinical descriptions and diagnostic guidelines*. Geneva, World Health Organization, 1992.

50. *Diagnostic and statistical manual of mental disorders*, 4th ed., text revision. Washington, DC, American Psychiatric Association, 2000.

51. Bonnie RJ, Stratton K, Wallace RB, eds. *Ending the tobacco problem: a blueprint for the nation*. Washington DC, The National Academies Press, 2007.

52. Hymowitz N et al. Predictors of smoking cessation in a cohort of adult smokers followed for five years. *Tobacco Control*, 1997, 6 (Suppl. 2):S57–S62.

53. Shiffman S, Paty J. Smoking patterns and dependence: contrasting chippers and heavy smokers. *Journal of Abnormal Psychology*, 2006, 115:509–523.

54. Anderson JE et al. Treating tobacco use and dependence: an evidence-based clinical practice guideline for tobacco cessation. *Chest*, 2002, 121:932–941.

55. Hendricks S et al. The early time course of smoking withdrawal effects. *Psychopharmacology*, 2006, 187:385–396.

56. Mackay J, Amos A. Women and tobacco. *Respirology*, 2003, 8:123–130.

57. Jones RT, Benowitz NL. Therapeutics for nicotine addiction. In: Davis KL et al., eds. *Neuropsychopharmacology: the fifth generation of progress*, Philadelphia, PA, Lippincott, Williams & Wilkins, 2002, 1533–1544.

58. *Want to quit smoking? Study says success can improve significantly when drug therapy is combined with behavioural counseling*. Menlo Park, CA, SRI International, 2003. (http://www.sri.com/news/releases/10-28-03.html).

59. Hughes JR. Tobacco withdrawal in self-quitters. *Journal of Consulting and Clinical Psychology*, 1992, 60:689–697.

60. Scholte OP, Reimer W et al. Smoking behaviour in European patients with established coronary heart disease. *European Heart Journal*, 2006, 27:35–41.

61. Walker MS et al. Smoking relapse during the first year after treatment for early-stage non-small-cell lung cancer. *Cancer Epidemiology, Biomarkers & Prevention*, 2006, 15:2370–2377.

62. Abrams DB, Niaura R. Planning evidence-based treatment of tobacco dependence. In: *The tobacco dependence treatment handbook: a guide to best practices*. New York, NY, Guilford Press, 2003.

63. DiClemente CC. *Addiction and change: how addictions develop and addicted people recover*. New York, NY, Guilford Press, 2003.

64. Davis KL et al., eds. *Neuropsychopharmacology: the fifth generation of progress*. Philadelphia, PA, Lippincott, Williams & Wilkins, 2002.

65. Kessler DA et al. Nicotine addiction: a pediatric disease. *The Journal of Pediatrics*, 1997, 130:518–524.

66. Chassin L et al. The natural history of cigarette smoking: predicting young-adult smoking outcomes from adolescent smoking patterns. *Health Psychology*, 1990, 9:701–716.

67. *Smoking statistics fact sheet*. Manila, World Health Organization Regional Office for the Western Pacific, 2002 (http://www.wpro.who.int/media_centre/fact_sheets/fs_20020528.htm, accessed 5 March, 2008).

68. DiClemente CC et al. *Adolescent smoking in Maryland 2000-2002: an analysis of the stages of smoking initiation by county with suggestions for prevention strategies*, Baltimore, MD, University of Maryland, Baltimore County, 2004.

69. Prochaska JO, DiClemente CC, Norcross JC. In search of how people change: applications to addictive behaviors. *The American Psychologist*, 1992, 47:1102–1114.

70. Conrad KM, Flay BR, Hill D. Why children start smoking cigarettes: predictors of onset. *British Journal of Addiction*, 1992, 87:1711–1724.

71. Tyas SL, Pederson LL. Psychosocial factors related to adolescent smoking: a critical review of the literature. *Tobacco Control*, 1998, 7:409–420.

72. Sargent JD et al. Effect of cigarette promotions on smoking uptake among adolescents. *Preventive Medicine*, 2000, 30:320–327.

73. Chassin L et al. Predicting the onset of cigarette smoking in adolescents: a longitudinal study. *Journal of Applied Social Psychology*, 1984, 14:224–243.

74. Pederson LL, Koval JJ, O'Connor K. Are psychological factors related to smoking in grade 6 students? *Addictive Behaviors*, 1997, 22:169–181.

75. Bush T et al. Preteen attitudes about smoking and parental factors associated with favourable attitudes. *American Journal of Health Promotion*, 2005, 19:410–417.

76. Forrester K et al. Predictors of smoking onset over two years. *Nicotine & Tobacco Research*, 2007, 9:1259–1267.

77. Ellickson L, McGuigan KA, Klein DJ. Predictors of late-onset smoking and cessation over 10 years. *Journal of Adolescent Health*, 2001, 29:101–108.

78. Miller CH et al. Identifying principal risk factors for the initiation of adolescent smoking behaviors: the significance of psychological reactance. *Health Communication*, 2006, 19:241–252.

79. Tindle HA et al. Cessation among smokers of 'light' cigarettes: results from the 2000 National Health Interview Survey. *American Journal of Public Health*, 2006, 96:1498–1504.

80. Shiffman S et al. Smokers' beliefs about "light" and "ultra light" cigarettes. *Tobacco Control*, 2001, 10 (Suppl. 1):i17–i23.

81. *The truth about "light" cigarettes: questions and answers*. National Cancer Institute, 2004 (http://www.cancer.gov/cancertopics/factsheet/Tobacco/light-cigarettes, accessed 15 March 2008).

82. Kozlowski LT, O'Connor TJ. Cigarette filter ventilation is a defective design because of misleading taste, bigger puffs, and blocked vents. *Tobacco Control*, 2002, 11 (Suppl. 1):I40–50.

83. *Tobacco industry targeting of women and girls*. Campaign for Tobacco-Free Kids, 2007 (http://tobaccofreekids.org/research/factsheets/pdf/0138.pdf, accessed 12 February 2008).

84. *Tobacco: deadly in any form or disguise*. Geneva, World Health Organization, 2006 (http://www.who.int/tobacco/communications/events/wntd/2006/Tfi_Rapport.pdf, accessed 12 February 2008).

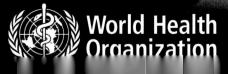

Tobacco-free: it's a woman's right.

SMOKING IS UGLY

WWW.WHO.INT/TOBACCO

31**MAY:**WORLD**NO**TOBACCO**DAY**

World Health Organization

© WORLD HEALTH ORGANIZATION 2010. DESIGNED BY NOVA S/B.

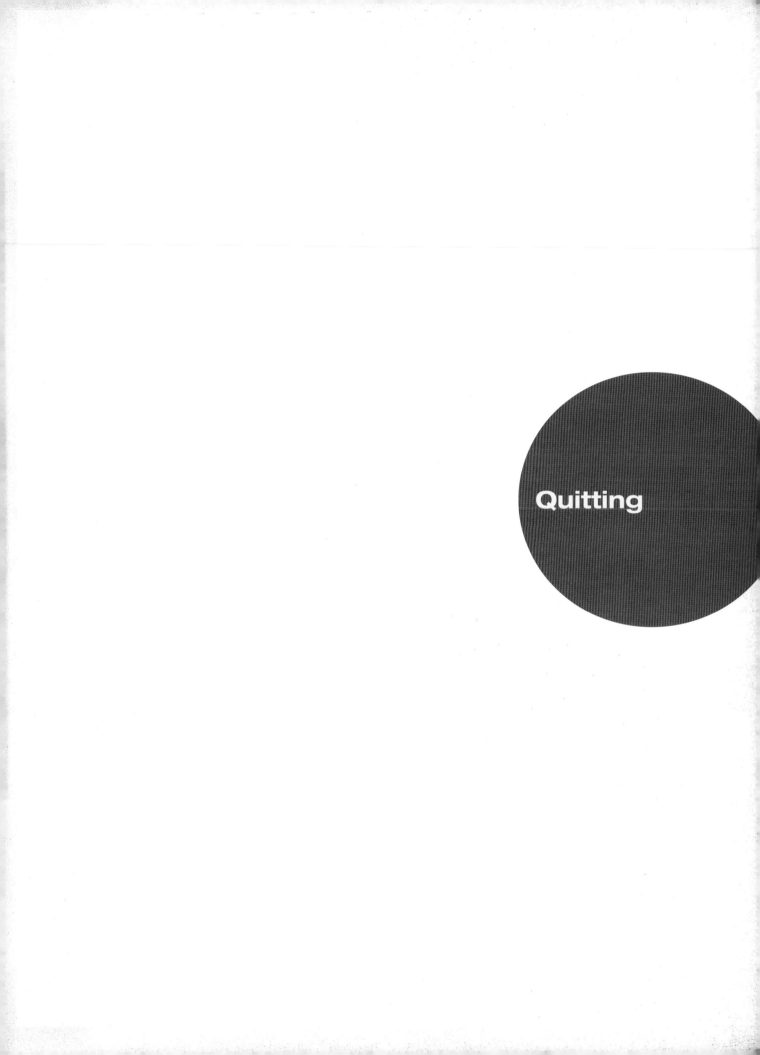

Quitting

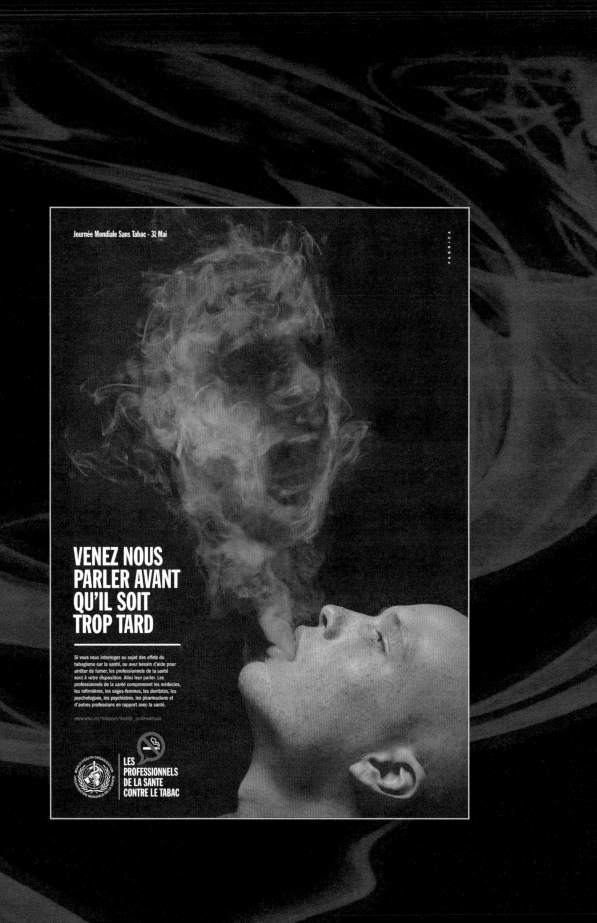

8. Quitting Smoking and Beating Nicotine Addiction

Introduction

Cessation of tobacco use by women worldwide must become an urgent priority to reduce the devastating effects of tobacco on the health of women and their children. Despite the warnings and known dangers of cigarette smoking and use of other tobacco products, over 5 million deaths annually are attributable to tobacco, according to the World Health Organization (WHO).[1] When tobacco use was predominantly a male behaviour, most of the burden of death and disability attributable to smoking fell on male smokers, as large numbers of men died of lung cancer, pulmonary and cardiovascular disease, and other tobacco-related diseases. However, the increase in women smokers over the past 30 years has made the long-term health consequences of smoking for women increasingly evident. As noted already in this monograph, lung cancer has become a significant cause of death for women worldwide and has become the leading cause of cancer death for women in the United States.[2]

In many countries, the majority of smokers want to quit. In a representative survey of 1750 smokers in Germany, Greece, Poland, Sweden, and the United Kingdom, 73.5% of the participants reported wanting to stop smoking.[3] In the United States, the demand for effective ways to reduce smoking is high: more than 70%[4] of smokers have expressed a desire to quit, and nearly 40% report an attempt to quit each year.[5] Most smokers are addicted tobacco consumers, not satisfied customers. Nearly 9 out of 10 smokers in four countries—Canada, the United Kingdom, Australia, and the United States— say they regret smoking. Women are more likely to express regret about smoking than men, and they find quitting more difficult.[6] The psychological, behavioural, and physical aspects of nicotine addiction make cessation difficult, leading to low rates of successful attempts to quit, despite the desire to do so and the discomfort of smoking. Policy changes and effective implementation of prevention and intervention programmes that address the needs of women smokers will be needed to increase successful and sustained cessation by women.

The importance of cessation is recognized in the WHO Framework Convention on Tobacco Control (WHO FCTC).[7] Article 14 of the WHO FCTC encourages Parties to implement demand-reduction measures concerning tobacco dependence and cessation, including implementing effective cessation programmes and providing counselling services.

Nearly 9 out of 10 smokers in four countries—Canada, the United Kingdom, Australia, and the United States—say they regret smoking.

Tobacco use worldwide differs by gender in important ways. Prevalence rates of smoking among men have remained steady or have declined, while rates among women and girls have increased.[4,8–10] Thus, smoking cessation among women is a major target of tobacco control and needs to be an essential component of a comprehensive tobacco control programme in every country. Programmes addressed to women should determine whether gender-specific considerations and programming are needed.[11] WHO has reported that tobacco control efforts increase cessation rates. In countries of all income levels, the most cost-effective ways to decrease tobacco use are increasing tobacco taxes and creating smoke-free environments.[11] Other methods that have proven effective globally include bans on tobacco company advertising and sponsorship, requiring tobacco containers to have warning labels, and publicizing policy interventions. Although gender differences regarding policy efforts have not been extensively studied, WHO recommends a gendered perspective in tobacco control measures. This would mean banning tobacco companies from sponsoring events such as female-dominated fashion shows, concerts, sporting events, and social events. Because in some countries women are more likely than men to be illiterate, the use of illustrated warning labels on tobacco containers is also recommended.[11] This chapter offers a view of tobacco cessation with a special focus on women and their needs. Factors affecting the process of quitting for women, such as depression and weight gain, are addressed, and recommendations are provided for achieving cessation of tobacco use by women.

Trends

The majority of smokers initiate tobacco use in their youth.[12] Cessation usually occurs later in life, after extensive exposure to nicotine and the injurious carcinogens and chemicals in tobacco smoke. Sustained smoking, genetic susceptibilities, exposure to other harmful substances, multiple life stresses and struggles, and social support for smoking contribute to creating and sustaining nicotine dependence. The addiction to nicotine is rooted in both physiological and psychological factors and is maintained by an environment that makes cessation difficult for both men and women. Nevertheless, quitting smoking as early as possible remains the single most effective method for decreasing risk from tobacco exposure and nicotine addiction. Surveys in many countries show that smokers can quit. In the United States, the 2006 National Health Interview Survey (NHIS) indicated that approximately 20.8% of adults (45.3 million) were classified as current cigarette smokers,[13] a significant decrease from the 42% rate in 1964. The majority of smokers in 1964 were males, whereas today the percentages of male and female smokers are almost equal. Most (80.1%) are daily smokers. However, the NHIS highlights the finding that more than half (50.2%, or 45.7 million individuals) of the 91 million individuals who have smoked at least 100 cigarettes in their lifetimes are now classified as former smokers. While the decline in prevalence for both men and women is encouraging, almost half of the ever-smokers in the United States continue to smoke, and approximately half of those smokers are women.

Many of the women who continue to smoke are disadvantaged from the standpoint of socioeconomic status (SES). International research has found that the SES of women smokers is relevant to quit rates. In three birth cohorts that included nearly 30 000 Italian women, those who had less than a high-school education were significantly less likely to quit smoking than those with a high-school education or more,[14] despite the fact that in the two older cohorts—those born between 1940 and 1959—rates of initiation were higher for women with more education. Similar inequalities have been found among women in other European countries, although shifts in the trend towards increased smoking among lower-SES groups have occurred during different decades.[15–17]

The inequality in cessation rates among women of different SES demonstrates a need to create specific approaches for reaching women who lack the resources to obtain traditional treatments. Federico et al. suggest that the failure to disseminate information regarding the harms of smoking in a timely and effective manner for all socioeconomic groups was one significant reason for that inequality.[14] In addition, tobacco companies target low-SES women with messages of achieving independence, weight loss, and stress relief through smoking.[18] These marketing messages are particularly effective because low-SES women often lack strong support systems and must cope with stressful or difficult living circumstances on a daily basis.

Although smoking is on the decline in many industrialized countries as a result of aggressive and comprehensive tobacco control efforts, smoking rates among women and girls are on the rise in developing countries,[19,20] and females in these countries have lower cessation rates.[21] Despite the efforts of organizations such as the Fogarty International Center (www.fic.nih.gov), the Institute for Global Tobacco Control (www.jhsph.edu/IGTC), the Pan American Health Association (www.paho.org), and Research for International Tobacco Control (www.idrc.ca/ritc), little research has addressed women's quitting patterns in many of these countries, partly because of limited and uncertain funding.[22] Therefore, most of our information is from studies in industrialized countries, although we recognize that information on women smokers in developing countries could be significantly different.

Perspectives on Change

Determining the best way to help smokers quit is a difficult task. Recently, researchers have begun to view smokers as consumers of cessation services and are actively investigating what smokers most want when they seek help to quit. The needs and wants appear to differ among different subgroups of smokers. Weber et al.[23] categorized 431 smokers in a medical-care setting into three subgroups, according to demand for smoking cessation services. Those who had the highest demand for smoking cessation were more likely to report being heavy smokers, but they also had some confidence in their ability to quit and considered quitting a high priority. Interest in cessation counselling seemed to be most related to age, cigarettes smoked per month, whether smokers were currently trying to quit, and whether they were ever told to quit smoking by a health-care provider. Successful marketing of cessation products and services requires knowledge of what would be most useful to current smokers.

The concept of consumer demand is also central to understanding the economics of the use of cessation aids. Tauras and Chaloupka[24] demonstrated that the demand for two types of nicotine replacement therapy (NRT) is elastic. They note that sales of NRT would increase substantially if NRT became less expensive and cigarettes more expensive. They report that a higher price for NRT reduces its use, while an increased price for cigarettes increases the demand for it, stating that a "10% decrease in the real price of NRT will increase average Nicoderm CQ and Nicorette demand by approximately 23% and 24% respectively".

Consumer demand for tobacco products and services also differs among subgroups of smokers. Ussher, West, and Hibbs[25] reported that 82% of 206 pregnant women in one study wanted behavioural support, and 77% wanted self-help materials. Those wanting behavioural support strongly preferred individual sessions over group therapy. Ussher, West, and Hibbs also found differences based on employment status and race. Smokers in professional or managerial positions were less likely to prefer a "buddy" system of quitting than those in other occupations, and non-Caucasians were more likely than Caucasians to be interested in behavioural support.

It is important to note that there are strategies or treatments that lack consistent evidence, and smokers are not encouraged to use them for cessation of tobacco use. For example, there is insufficient evidence about the long-term benefit of interventions that help smokers reduce but not quit tobacco use.[26]

Smokers are a minority of the population, and their basic demographics and characteristics are used by the tobacco companies to target advertising programmes and promotions.[27,28] Tobacco control advocates and providers also need to understand how to "market" their services and products to current smokers, since smokers in many countries begin or continue to smoke despite counter-advertising and anti-smoking campaigns. Although many may want to quit, their success rates are low, and improving the sophistication of outreach and connection with current smokers is critical for successfully reducing smoking.[29]

While the decline in prevalence for both men and women is encouraging, almost half of the ever-smokers in the United States continue to smoke, and approximately half of those smokers are women.

The dimensions of the process by which women quit using tobacco deserves special attention, as several factors make women's tobacco use and the process of quitting different from those of men. For example, evidence suggests that it is more difficult for women to quit smoking and that some cessation methods are less effective for women.[30] Weight-gain considerations often play a greater role in the initiation and maintenance of smoking in women than they do in men. Emotional and psychological reactions, such as anxiety and depressed moods, are more likely to be related to smoking in women, and effective social support during cessation may be more relevant for women. Physiologically, women seem to have lower tolerance and an increased sensitivity to nicotine than men do, and the potential effects of the menstrual cycle on quitting success are a topic of special concern for women. This is further elaborated in the chapter in this monograph on addiction to nicotine. In addition to the direct effects of smoking on women's health, smoking presents special health concerns for the fetus during pregnancy and for infants and children postpartum, as discussed in the chapter on pregnancy and postpartum smoking cessation.

Models of Behavioural Change

How do individuals go about changing health behaviours? A number of theories and models have been described in the literature. These models propose that several important dimensions can be used to understand smokers and intervene with them. It is important to note that almost all theories of addiction, behavioural-change theories, and models can be used for smoking cessation.

World Health Organization

Many of them focus on perceptions and attitudes, behaviours, intentions, and tasks that influence the modification of health behaviours. Models of change that address smoking behaviour include the widely accepted interpersonal-level behavioural-change theory—Social Cognitive Theory/Social Learning Theory—used in many group counselling programmes. The models that are reviewed below include the Health Belief Model (HBM), the Theory of Planned Behaviour (TPB), and the Transtheoretical Model (TTM).

Health Belief Model

In the HBM, changing a health behaviour is assumed to be related to the individual's beliefs and perceptions about engaging in adopting or stopping the behaviour.[31] Key elements that determine whether a smoker will quit include perceived susceptibility to the consequences of smoking behaviour, perceived severity of those consequences, and perceived and actual barriers to change (e.g. costs of quitting, beliefs about efficacy of treatment), as well as perceived benefits (decreased risk, better health). In addition, cues to action that stimulate motivation and increase readiness to change must be present to initiate a change in smoking behaviour.

Tobacco treatment based on the HBM requires appropriate assessment of the smoker's susceptibility to tobacco dependency and perceived severity of smoking outcomes. *Susceptibility* includes the perceived risk of developing a health condition as a result of smoking and, if illness does develop, includes acceptance of the diagnosis and beliefs about remission and re-emergence of disease. Accurate information about risks is usually highlighted in the material provided to smokers, and education is provided to correct misconceptions. *Perceived severity* refers to a smoker's belief that smoking will cause harm and bring medical and social consequences. The combination of susceptibility and severity is often called *perceived threat*. According to this model, the probability of quitting smoking increases as perceived threat increases.

A personal cost/benefit analysis is also central to the HBM and influences the decision to quit. Chances of a quit attempt increase as the smoker's perception of the negative aspects of quitting and the personally relevant benefits increase. Maximum treatment impact requires the smoker's belief that the intervention will be efficacious and the benefits are worth the cost of treatment. Cues to action that favour changing tobacco use, which can be internal (e.g. the presence of an illness) or external (e.g. pressure from others to quit), also motivate and may be necessary for change. Finally, confidence in the ability to abstain from smoking is viewed as essential for change.

Interventions that employ the HBM include open discussion of barriers to quitting tobacco use and attempts to develop realistic strategies for overcoming such barriers, along with help in identifying the perceived benefits of quitting, which are used as reinforcement for quitting.[32] Brief interventions in medical or other settings can increase perceived susceptibility and threat and also provide cues to action that are compatible with this model, as are various group and individual treatments. There are no indications of sex differences in the efficacy of using this model in cessation treatment. However, perceptions and decision considerations could be expected to differ between men and women. In one study, women perceived more risks of smoking than men but also perceived less benefit and more problems with cessation.[33] In another study, women reported more positive aspects of smoking, but also more negative aspects of continuing to smoke.[34]

Smoking is a complex behaviour, the determinants of which are often influenced by both internal factors and beliefs and external factors. The HBM focuses largely on internal determinants and may not sufficiently address all components of quitting[35] or the need for comprehensive cessation programming. Important factors that can be overlooked include nicotine dependence, environmental and economic factors, social norms, and peer influence. The Theory of Reasoned Action, discussed below, takes more of these factors into account.[35]

Theory of Planned Behaviour

Ajzen's TPB[36] is a later version of the Theory of Reasoned Action first presented by Fishbein and Ajzen.[37] The TPB adds the variable of perceived behavioural control. It posits that three types of cognitions—behavioural beliefs, normative beliefs (subjective norms), and control beliefs (perceived behavioural control)—interact to determine an individual's intent (i.e. motivation) to initiate, and ultimately complete, a particular behaviour change.

Behavioural beliefs consist of an individual's subjective assessment of whether a desired outcome will follow a behaviour change. These beliefs, along with the subjective value of the outcomes (i.e. how desirable the outcomes are), determine the individual's attitude to the behaviour. Thus, smoking is likely to continue if smoking is perceived as having benefits and the benefits are positively valued. Change would require an increase in negative perceptions of smoking and realization of its negative outcomes (e.g. risk for illness).

Normative beliefs are smokers' perceptions of the expectations that others have regarding their behaviour. The extent to which the smoker desires to comply with the wishes of others and the strength of the desire for change determine the effect of normative beliefs on change. These beliefs form the subjective norm, i.e. the perceived social pressure to engage (or not engage) in a behaviour. If the perceived pressure from friends and family to quit is high and there are increasing environmental restrictions (e.g. implementation of clean-indoor-air laws), individuals are more likely to quit smoking, especially if they are motivated to comply with the expectations of others.

Control beliefs reflect the degree of perceived behavioural control over factors that will either facilitate or impede progress in behaviour change. If individuals' perceived behaviour control is high and their perceptions are accurate, they have the resources and skills to perform the behaviour. Thus, identifying and addressing barriers to behavioural control is likely to be useful for successful change. Smokers can increase perceived control by seeking the encouragement and resources needed to increase their sense of control. These can be obtained from behavioural interventions, self-help materials, or quit lines. Possible strategies to increase perceptions of control, described by Bandura,[38] include setting smaller, realistic goals on the path to the desired change. For smokers, a realistic goal might be reducing the number of cigarettes smoked per day. The goal of this strategy is to increase the sense of mastery. Other ways to increase perceived control include observing the successes of others and using relaxation techniques to manage negative feelings related to quitting or symptoms of withdrawal.

Behavioural, normative, and control beliefs interact to produce the construct of intention, which reflects a person's readiness to perform a given behaviour. Intention,

in addition to actual behavioural control, can then predict the desired behaviour. Thus, if an individual has a positive attitude to the change (e.g. I think that quitting smoking is a good idea), a subjective norm that endorses a behaviour (e.g. others will be happy if I quit), and high perceived control (e.g. I have the necessary resources to quit), then the intent and motivation to quit smoking is expected to be strong, and the likelihood of success is high.

Smokers can increase perceived control by seeking the encouragement and resources needed to increase their sense of control.

Research on smoking behaviour using the TPB has focused on whether the model can predict intention to smoke. Hanson[39] found that among Afro-American adolescent females, attitude, subjective norms, and perceived behavioural control predicted their intention to smoke, with perceived behavioural control the strongest predictor. Among Puerto Rican and non-Hispanic white adolescent girls, attitude was the strongest predictor of smoking behaviour; attitude and perceived behavioural control were also predictors, but subjective norms were not. Of the three groups, non-Hispanic white girls had the strongest intention to smoke, which would hinder quitting. In another study, the TPB predicted intention to quit and actually attempting to quit among adults in a primary-care setting. However, it did not predict the length of abstinence.[40] In a consumer demand study, Weber[23] found that attitudes towards smoking and quitting, in addition to perceived effectiveness of cessation counselling, increased the ability to predict demand for cessation services better than other predictors (e.g. age or cigarettes smoked per month).

The TPB's focus on behavioural control and norms offers additional variables for use in media and cessation-focused interventions. However, the model does not include other variables that may be important in quitting, such as personality or cultural and demographic factors. And unlike the HBM, it does not consider perceived risk or susceptibility.[40] Nevertheless, some studies have shown that components of the TPB predict behaviour and behaviour change.

Transtheoretical Model of Intentional Behaviour Change

As the chapter on addiction to nicotine noted, the TTM[41–46] is a multidimensional model that attempts to integrate various behaviour-change theories. The discussion that follows focuses on its relevance to understanding the gender and sex factors influencing quitting. Research supports the notion that cessation success can be predicted by the stage of change, as advancement through the stages increases the likelihood of quitting.[47,48] Gender is generally not predictive of stage of change.[41,47,49] However, a few studies have reported sex differences in the proportion of smokers in a particular stage of change. O'Hea et al.[34] found that in a sample of 274 predominantly low-income Afro-American current and former smokers, significantly fewer women (37.1%) than men (51.4%) were in the maintenance stage. In addition, significantly more women than men (22.8% vs 9.7%) were in the precontemplation stage.

> *Relapse back to smoking after a period of abstinence and recycling through the stages are expected, because of the addictive nature of nicotine and the difficulty of adequately completing all the tasks in an attempt to quit.*

Each stage of change includes tasks that, if completed adequately, can increase the likelihood of success.[50,51] Completing these tasks requires active coping and using experiential and behavioural processes of change. Experiential processes include consciousness raising, dramatic relief, environmental re-evaluation, self-re-evaluation, and social liberation. Behavioural processes include reinforcement management, building helping relationships, counterconditioning, stimulus control, and self-liberation. These processes are related to completion

of the tasks of the stages. Experiential processes have been found to occur more frequently during precontemplation and contemplation, while an effective transition into the action stage is associated with increased use of behavioural processes. There is some evidence that those who do not use the "right" processes at the "right" time, particularly those who do not transition from using experiential to behavioural processes when they move to the action stage, may be more prone to relapse.[50] A study of gender differences in these processes demonstrated that women in the contemplation stage used more experiential processes than men did. However, in other stages, process use was very similar for males and females. Differences, when found, were small and may not be clinically meaningful.[52]

Relapse back to smoking after a period of abstinence and recycling through the stages are expected, because of the addictive nature of nicotine and the difficulty of adequately completing all the tasks in an attempt to quit.[46] The stage-based approach has been used to help providers determine clients' readiness for change and the processes that may be helpful at particular points as they move through the stages of quitting smoking and breaking the nicotine addiction. Understanding recycling puts the process of cessation into a social learning perspective that can decrease unrealistic expectations and offer long-term hope for success.

Several measures have been used as markers of progress through the stages, including decisional considerations of the pros and cons of smoking (similar to those of the HBM) and self-efficacy (the smoker's level of confidence that he or she can abstain from smoking in a variety of situations). As was true of the experiential processes, decisional balance considerations appear to be more important in the earlier stages of change, and self-efficacy is more important in action and maintenance. One study of sex differences on these markers found that women identified significantly more favourable aspects of smoking than men did ($P < 0.0001$). They also identified significantly more unfavourable aspects, but the size of the effect was smaller ($P < 0.05$).[34] Some research has found that women score significantly lower on measures of self-efficacy.[34,47]

Models provide useful frameworks for designing interventions and offer views of the process of change. However, some people see them as too rational to explain the process, which they view as chaotic, and some believe that the models underestimate the population dynamics of smoking cessation.[53,54]

Interventions

In some industrialized countries, smokers have many options among programmes, products, and techniques to choose from when planning to quit smoking. This abundance allows the individual to choose methods that seem helpful and efficacious. However, an informed decision is necessary, because some treatments are empirically supported and some are not. While some smokers seem to be able to quit with self-help materials or "cold turkey" (often used to mean completely and on one's own), others require or opt for more-intensive interventions such as group or individual behavioural therapy. NRT and non-nicotine pharmacotherapy are also available and helpful for some smokers. Combining behavioural and pharmacological treatments may increase quitting success, particularly for heavier smokers, because they address both physiological and psychological aspects of tobacco addiction. Alternative means of quitting, such as hypnosis and acupuncture, are used by some smokers, although there is no consistent evidence to support these interventions. Finally, some cultures emphasize seeking help from professionals in tobacco cessation, while others may promote obtaining help from spiritual leaders or faith healers.

A number of empirically supported treatments and products, including the tobacco cessation interventions described below, are available to women to help them quit smoking. Different individuals are likely to have different responses to these interventions, and there is always more than one path to successful cessation. Each individual must find the way that works best for her or him to accomplish the key tasks needed to successfully change smoking behaviour. It is also important to recognize that all of the interventions may need to be adapted for particular subgroups of smokers and specific cultures or countries.

Smoking cessation requires a combination of motivation and skills. Brief interventions that use simple advice and/or motivational enhancement strategies may be sufficient to address the issue of motivation, but some smokers lack the skills or ability to manage the actual quitting and maintenance of cessation or to deal with the various cues for smoking. These individuals may need more-intensive interventions, and significant support may be needed for them to be successful in quitting smoking. However, large numbers of smokers have been able to quit smoking on their own or with minimal assistance.[55] Thus, tobacco control efforts need to be multidimensional.[7] Although some health professionals believe and some studies indicate that women smokers who want to quit may need more support or skills-based interventions,[30] the data do not allow for a clear conclusion at the present time.

Less-Intensive and Motivational Interventions

Brief Opportunistic Interventions

One of the early smoking cessation strategies was based on findings that smokers who received physician advice to quit had significantly better outcomes than those who did not get such advice. The Public Health Service and the Agency for Healthcare Research and Quality (AHRQ) created a protocol that established the key dimensions for addressing tobacco cessation in health-care settings. The protocol was published in the AHRQ's Treating Tobacco Use and Dependence (TTUD) clinical practice guideline [56,57] and has been recommended for all health-care providers who have the opportunity to address a patient's tobacco use. It has five components, known as the 5 As:

1. **Ask** the client about his or her tobacco use at every visit.

2. **Advise** the client to quit, using strong, clear, and concise language.

3. **Assess** the client's willingness or readiness to quit, particularly in the next 30 days.

4. **Assist** the client in the quit attempt with either a brief or an intensive intervention or by referring him or her to an appropriate treatment provider.

5. **Arrange** for follow-up contact or relapse prevention.

This protocol has been disseminated widely, in part because it can be implemented in 3 minutes or less, making it attractive to busy health professionals. Although health-care providers have a general knowledge of the 5 As, adoption of the entire protocol has been sporadic.

Nevertheless, the number of smokers screened and offered at least one or two of the As (*ask* and *advise*) has increased dramatically over the past 10 years in the United States.

> *It has been estimated that physician interventions have the potential to raise long-term cessation rates from 7% to 30% among smokers trying to quit on their own.*

AHRQ has produced another brief motivational intervention, called the 5 Rs, for clients who are ambivalent or not ready to quit:[57]

1. **Relevance:** Provide information that is relevant to the client's situation, environment, and individual needs (e.g. health status, culture, and gender). Ask the client to identify how quitting is personally relevant and important for loved ones and encourage her or him to be as specific as possible.

2. **Risks:** Ask the client to identify the short- and long-term negative effects of tobacco use, focusing on those that are personally relevant.

3. **Rewards:** Ask the client to identify the benefits of quitting tobacco use, highlighting those that are most personally relevant (e.g. better health for self and family, money saved, improved self-esteem).

4. **Roadblocks:** Help the client identify obstacles to quitting, such as withdrawal symptoms, weight gain, friends and family who smoke, fear of failure, or lack of support. Discuss how to problem-solve or overcome these barriers.

5. **Repetition:** At every contact with smoking clients, address the 5 Rs. Remind them that many smokers need to make several quit attempts before they succeed. This information can be reassuring and can motivate them to try again.

The use of these protocols has been adopted and encouraged by practitioners in the United States and around the world in internal and family medicine, obstetrics and gynaecology, cardiology, pulmonology, and other subspecialties.[56–59] A Cochrane review of 39 studies found that brief physician advice to quit smoking produced cessation rates statistically significantly higher than those of smokers who received no advice (odds ratio (OR)= 1.74, 95% confidence interval (CI) = 1.48, 2.05).[58,60] Such advice has been shown to achieve double or triple the success rate of smokers who receive no assistance from a provider.[56,57] Orleans and Alper[61] estimate that physician interventions have the potential to raise long-term cessation rates from 7% to 30% among smokers trying to quit on their own. In the United States, limited coverage for cessation interventions, limited reimbursement for physician time, and limited understanding of billing codes for smoking cessation are three of the top six barriers to providing cessation services. Limited coverage has been cited by 54% of physicians, limited reimbursement has been cited by 52%, and lack of billing-code knowledge has been cited by 36%. Although it has been difficult to increase health-care providers' participation in cessation interventions, the recent trend of health insurance companies to reimburse for smoking interventions may encourage providers to integrate these services into standard care.[62]

Motivational Interviewing and Enhancement Protocols

Enhancing an individual's desire to change smoking behaviour can be a daunting task. Intensive group treatment is seen as the primary way to help smokers quit, and both the American Cancer Society and the American Lung Association have created group programmes that use cognitive and behavioural principles and strategies to promote smoking cessation. Brief motivational approaches began to be used in the late 1980s and early 1990s in the United States. Spurred on by the development of motivational interviewing (MI) by William Miller and Stephen Rollnick,[63] use of brief motivational interventions became more acknowledged and widespread. For smokers in the early stages of change, MI may be a particularly helpful approach to increasing readiness to change, or tipping the decisional balance to favour changing behaviour.[64]

MI is a directive, client-centred approach that guides and encourages clients to think about and resolve their ambivalence about quitting smoking or changing any behaviour. It derives from motivational psychology and is based on the belief that many individuals are ambivalent in the early stages of change. In MI, the responsibility for changing smoking is placed on the client, and the fact that the choice to change is a personal one is stressed, while confrontation and argumentation are avoided. The approach has five central principles: [62,64]

1. Express empathy.

2. Develop a discrepancy between the current behaviour of smoking and the desired behaviour (quitting smoking).

3. Avoid argumentation.

4. Roll with resistance.

5. Support self-efficacy.

In MI, ambivalence is described as a normal experience in quitting. Personalized feedback, reflective listening, exploring the pros and cons of change, and eliciting motivational statements such as problem recognition and concern are central to the process. Although most MI interventions are brief, not all are single-session.

Motivational-enhancement therapy[65] is a four-session, more-intensive intervention that uses feedback from an assessment battery to determine readiness to change, stage of change, and smoking status. It was developed for use with alcohol abusers and dependent patients, but it has also been used with smokers. Although the data on its use with smokers are limited, a number of studies have demonstrated efficacy.[66] Other studies, however, have shown no increase in cessation rates over those of controls, especially among women who have multiple problems, including drug abuse.[67,68]

Self-Help Materials and Internet Interventions

Distributing self-help materials without any other intervention is only minimally effective for helping smokers change their behaviour.[69] In fact, clinical guidelines for treating tobacco use and dependence recommend treatments other than self-help options.[56,57] Data from a decade ago showed that about 1% to 5% of smokers in the United States were "self-changers", quitting without any formal treatment.[46] More-recent studies have found that about 3% to 5% of smokers who quit unaided remain

abstinent six months later.[70] Research on this group indicates that quitting smoking is a slow process, with movement back and forth between stages and a variety of patterns of change over time.[71] Those who attempt to quit on their own are likely to use publicly available self-help materials on quitting, such as brochures, pamphlets, books, and videos.[72]

In recent years, a number of Internet smoking cessation sites have been developed to provide cessation information and support.

In recent years, a number of Internet smoking cessation sites have been developed to provide cessation information and support. Web sites allow smokers to enter personal information and receive messages and materials tailored to their particular needs and wants. QuitNet, for example, provides smokers with "quitting buddies" and 24-hour live discussions with other users via chat rooms, instant messaging, and message boards. A study of the QuitNet programme[73] found that those who logged on more often, spent more time online, visited more web pages, and used the social support options more frequently were more likely to be successful quitters than those who did none of these things. At the 3-month follow-up, the 7-day point prevalence abstinence rate was 7% when non-responders and bounced e-mails were counted as smokers. A 7-day point prevalence abstinence rate of 30% was reported for responders only. Among this group, 5.9% reported being abstinent for 30 days or more. Benefits were also observed for those who continued to smoke; for example, those smokers significantly reduced the number of cigarettes they smoked per day. Other preliminary studies have investigated the potential effectiveness of web-based cessation programmes, but Internet research is complex, and much work remains to be done. One such study measured cessation among European smokers who purchased nicotine patches, logged onto an Internet programme, and consented to participate in a study.[74] Those who received a tailored web-based programme had significantly higher cessation rates than those who did not (22.8% vs 18.1%). Other pilot and uncontrolled studies also show some positive results.[73] In addition to web sites that attempt to provide cessation

World Health Organization

programmes, the American Cancer Society's *Guide to Quitting Smoking*[3] and the CDC's *You Can Quit Smoking*[4] are available online. Sites that are dedicated to women include Smoke-Free Families, which provides online self-help materials for pregnant smokers and those wanting to help pregnant smokers quit, and the American Legacy Foundation's Legacy for Longer Healthier Lives, which provides fact sheets specific to the history of women's smoking and the effects of smoking on women.

Feedback and Tailored Messages

In many interventions, the strategy of gathering personal or group data and offering some type of feedback has been used to individualize the smoker's experience of the advice and materials. Providing feedback to those who want to quit smoking can be very useful, especially if the messages are tailored to incorporate personally relevant information and needs.[75] Feedback can be provided through many different formats (mail, e-mail, online) and can be given repeatedly to advise about progress and to support continued efforts to quit. Feedback can be used to compare current smoking to levels of smoking in a comparison group, indicating what is normative for an individual of similar age, sex, culture, and risk. Feedback also encourages self-monitoring, which can act as a mechanism for behaviour change. The intensity of feedback can vary significantly, from simple advice to quit smoking to the provision of intensive normative and comparative information that extends over a period of several months.[75,76] Such interventions have proved successful with smokers.[77–80] Among individuals who received three feedback reports at baseline, 6, and 12 months regarding changing multiple health behaviours, 25.4% moved into the action or maintenance stage for smoking cessation.[77] However, not all studies have found improvements in outcomes[81] (e.g. for pregnant women in the contemplation and action stages[82]).

Intensive and Skills-Based Interventions

Group Treatment

Group therapy can be an effective and efficient way to deliver cessation counselling. According to a recent Cochrane review of group smoking cessation, group treatment is more than twice as effective as self-help-only interventions.[60] Group treatments are usually led by trained smoking cessation counsellors and typically last four to eight weeks. While the number of participants in group therapy varies, all members should have the opportunity to share personal experiences during a session. Programmes that have been created for use in the group setting by nonprofit and other organizations include the American Cancer Society's Freshstart® and the American Lung Association's Freedom from Smoking.

Group therapy provides the opportunity to learn cognitive and behavioural techniques, such as coping skills for cravings and withdrawal, how to set a quit date, how to seek out social support, and how to control environmental exposure to smoke. For the many women who report that stress and frustration are reasons for relapse, the cognitive techniques taught during group sessions may help increase coping skills to manage these triggers.[56,57]

In general, women are more likely than men to seek treatment or support for both physical and mental health issues,[83] and this seems to generalize to smoking cessation. For example, women in Copenhagen, Denmark, were more likely than men to accept invitations to participate in cessation groups (OR = 1.24, 95% CI = 1.0, 1.5).[84] The group intervention format offers women the opportunity to provide mutual support to one another while learning effective techniques for smoking cessation. Since women are often more comfortable and willing to share opinions and advice in a group setting than men are,[85] some tobacco control professionals recommend offering women-only groups.[85]

Individual Counselling and Therapy

Individual counselling can produce smoking cessation rates twice those of smokers using self-help methods.[60] A Cochrane review found that when individual counselling is provided by a trained therapist, the odds ratio for successful cessation was 1.56 (95% CI = 1.32, 1.84). However, it indicated no difference between brief and intensive models of counselling.[86] The information and skills learned in individual counselling are similar to those learned in group treatment, but the content of sessions can more easily be tailored, allowing the counsellor to identify and address the client's personal stressors, effective cues and triggers, and specific withdrawal symptoms related to tobacco use. Individual counselling may also be particularly helpful for individuals suffering from co-occurring psychological symptoms or disorders (e.g. depression, post-traumatic stress, and other anxiety disorders). Those with multiple problems may need assistance with both tobacco dependence and psychological issues. Such psychological difficulties have been shown to make abstinence more difficult and to lead to relapse.[87,88] Populations with various types of mental illness, particularly serious mental illness, generally have higher rates of smoking than those without such illness, and depression and anxiety disorders are more likely to be reported by women, leading to the use of tobacco as a coping mechanism.[89]

Women whose work or child-care schedules do not permit them to attend scheduled group meetings may also require individual counselling. Others may prefer to have one-on-one sessions for other reasons. For example, many women desire individual counselling when they are pregnant,[25] especially if they are hesitant to attend groups because of actual or perceived disapproval of their smoking by other members of the group.

Quit Lines and Telephone Counselling

Quit lines and telephone counselling are becoming the largest providers of cessation services in many countries, as many local and national organizations now offer quit-line services for their citizens. Smokers who call a quit line may be offered a range of intervention options, from self-help materials and Internet support to multiple counselling sessions and pharmacotherapy. Quit lines, also known as help lines, provide free telephone support for individuals who are considering quitting tobacco use or are ready to quit; the support is easy to access and can provide contact with trained counsellors. A 2007 review of quit lines in Canada, the United States, and the United Kingdom[90] demonstrated their efficacy for smoking cessation. Services offered by quit lines include motivational counselling, follow-up calls from counsellors, mailed self-help materials and quit kits, recorded messages, access to pharmacotherapy, referrals to local resources for cessation, and combinations of these services. The review reported that in several studies, follow-up calls led to longer-term success rates than those achieved by single-call interventions (OR = 1.41, 95% CI = 1.27, 1.57). The number of follow-up calls necessary for maximum benefit has also begun to be studied. A Cochrane review suggested that three or more calls produce significantly better quit rates

than one or two calls, self-help materials, brief advice, or pharmacotherapy alone.[91] Studies in a recent meta-analysis showed minimally significant increases with additional calls (i.e. increases in quit rates of 2% or less). Another study demonstrated significant differences between groups that received three counselling calls without booster calls (8.5% quit rate) and groups that received five counselling calls with two boosters (14.1% quit rate).[92] Two large groups, the European Network of Quitlines (ENQ) and the North American Quitline Consortium (NAQC), are dedicated to evaluating and increasing the efficacy of quit lines.[93]

Telephone counselling is convenient in that it does not require the client to leave home. This is particularly useful for stay-at-home mothers and women who work while raising children.

When clients contact a quit line, trained cessation counsellors provide counselling that is tailored to the needs of the individual. During calls, clients may be helped to select a quit date and asked to think about barriers to quitting and methods of overcoming obstacles. They may also receive education about relapse prevention. Telephone counselling can be used as a stand-alone treatment or in addition to other ongoing interventions. Telephone counselling is convenient in that it does not require the client to leave home. This is particularly useful for stay-at-home mothers and women who work while raising children. A study of 1992–2006 data from the California Smokers Helpline showed that, except in 1993, significantly more callers 18 to 24 years of age were women than men. Thus, this may be a particularly appealing intervention for young adult women.

In addition to telephone conversations, text messaging on cellular phones is being used to provide cessation services.[94] In a New Zealand study, 1075 participants received personalized text messages on days near their quit date. Six weeks after quitting, the quit rate was 28% among those receiving the messages, but only 13% in the control group.[95]

World Health Organization

Pharmacological Interventions

The use of pharmacological aids for smoking cessation has been approved in many countries. In the United States, first-line therapies for tobacco cessation approved by the US Food and Drug Administration (FDA) include five forms of NRT, as well as the non-nicotine medications bupropion and varenicline. First-line interventions are those that have been shown to produce reliable increases in abstinence without excessive side-effects; second-line therapies include medications such as nortriptyline and clonidine. Since nicotine addiction has both physiological and behavioural components, a combination of pharmacotherapy and behavioural interventions is usually recommended, particularly for heavy smokers or smokers who have made several unsuccessful attempts to quit. Newer medications under investigation include nicotine vaccines and rimonabant, which is approved in European countries and the United States for treatment of obesity.

> *Since nicotine addiction has both physiological and behavioural components, a combination of pharmacotherapy and behavioural interventions is usually recommended.*

Nicotine Replacement Therapy

In NRT, nicotine is provided to the smoker in a manner other than smoking to reduce the physiological effects of withdrawal and enable the individual to break the smoking habit. A Cochrane report calculated the risk ratios from 132 studies that compared NRT to placebo or non-NRT control groups.[96] In 111 studies, the risk ratio of abstinence for any type of NRT was 1.58 (95% CI = 1.50, 1.66). Rates of quitting were increased by 50% to 70% when NRT was used. NRT can be delivered in transdermal patches, gum, lozenges, inhalers, nasal sprays, and sublingual tablets (not available in the United States). If one approach seems to be ineffective, there are alternatives that can fit the needs of the smoker.

When used appropriately, NRT products effectively decrease nicotine withdrawal symptoms such as irritability, anxiety, dysphoria, and restlessness. Patches provide a steady, constant amount of nicotine to the body throughout the day. Other types of NRT are delivered on an as-needed basis and, ideally, should be administered before cravings occur. Long-term use of NRT has been proposed as a relapse prevention strategy for individuals who have difficulty with cravings long after they have quit.

In an examination of whether responses to nicotine were gender-specific,[97] Evans and colleagues provided smokers with four different doses of nicotine patches (i.e. 0, 7, 21, or 42 mg) in four laboratory sessions. Both men and women experienced significant reductions in withdrawal after the patches were applied, and positive effects increased with higher doses. At the moment, there does not appear to be sufficient evidence of clinically important differences between men and women to guide treatment matching.[96]

Non-Nicotine Medications

Originally marketed as an antidepressant, bupropion is the non-nicotine medication most commonly prescribed for tobacco cessation. According to a Cochrane review,[98] bupropion can nearly double smoking cessation rates. Smokers begin by taking 150 mg a day, and the dose is then increased to 150 mg twice a day. Bupropion blocks the re-uptake of dopamine, serotonin, and norepinephrine,[99] neurotransmitters involved with the reinforcing effects of nicotine. Since it has some antidepressant effects, bupropion is also believed to help with depressive symptoms and to prevent negative reactions to quitting and withdrawal triggering a depressive episode. This is a particularly important benefit for women, who are at increased risk for depression and frequently give depressive symptoms as a reason for relapse.[100,101]

Smith and colleagues[100] used data from a study comparing bupropion to another non-nicotine medication, varenicline,[102] to investigate whether bupropion was particularly helpful for women smokers in general and those who had been previously depressed. Logistic regression showed that one year after quitting smoking, men and women who received bupropion had similar abstinence rates (30.8% and 35.1%, respectively); however,

World Health Organization

women who had been given a placebo quit at significantly lower rates than men did (10.0% and 23.4%, respectively). Gender differences were also not found in a 24-month evaluation of bupropion that was provided for 52 weeks.[103] Scharf and Shiffman[104] conducted both pooled analyses and meta-analyses of clinical trials using bupropion and found no significant gender differences regarding its effectiveness. Successful cessation was twice as likely for those taking the medication (OR = 2.49, 95% CI = 2.06, 3.00), but women smokers consistently had more difficulty quitting smoking (OR = 0.77, 95% CI = 0.66, 0.89).

Swan and colleagues[105] found that women given 150 mg of bupropion were far more likely to relapse within 12 months than were women given 300 mg or men given 150 mg. Risk factors for relapse for these women included not having a quit attempt that lasted longer than six months, higher perceived stress, and receipt of tailored mailings instead of telephone counselling. Persistent smoking during the follow-up period was predicted by lower doses (150 mg instead of 300 mg), younger age, smoking more cigarettes per day before treatment, the absence of a 24-hour quit attempt in the past year, and prior use of NRT. Overall, women were more likely to smoke during the first year after treatment (OR = 1.43, 95% CI = 1.13, 1.80). Similarly, Dale and colleagues[106] found that women were 67% more likely than men to return to smoking after they completed treatment with bupropion. Though this could lead to assumptions about the lack of effectiveness of bupropion for women, it could also simply reflect the greater difficulty women have quitting. Gender differences in predictors of relapse for women may indicate specific domains to target in relapse prevention interventions for women.

Despite the challenges to helping women abstain from smoking, bupropion may be particularly effective for women who are concerned about weight gain due to cessation. Some studies have indicated that bupropion may attenuate the weight gain associated with quitting smoking, at least in the short term.[107]

Varenicline provides a new option for smokers. It is an α4β2 nicotinic acetylcholine receptor (nAChR) partial agonist, and its efficacy is thought to be related to the way it binds to such receptors, causing the release of neurotransmitters (e.g. dopamine, norepinephrine, acetylcholine, and glutamate) and thereby reducing withdrawal symptoms.[99] In addition, it blocks the ability of nicotine to bind to the receptors, preventing the reinforcing effects of smoking. The usual protocol calls for patients to take varenicline 7 days before their quit date, titrating up to 1 mg twice a day for up to 12 weeks. The most common side-effects, nausea and vomiting, can be reduced by taking the medication with a full glass of water and food. Other side-effects include headaches, insomnia, and abnormal and vivid dreams. In the United States, Pfizer offers individuals taking its varenicline product one year of support through its GETQUIT™ online programme (www.get-quit.com).

Studies comparing the efficacy of bupropion, varenicline, and placebos found that varenicline produced somewhat higher short-term abstinence rates (9 to 12 weeks), though bupropion was also effective. Jorenby and colleagues[102] found abstinence rates of 43.9% for individuals taking varenicline, 29.8% for those taking bupropion, and 10.5% for those given a placebo (*P* < 0.001). The increased benefits of varenicline continued into weeks 9 through 24, with 29.7% of subjects remaining abstinent, compared with 20.2% for bupropion (*P* = 0.003) and 13.2% for placebo (*P* < 0.001). Gonzales et al.[108] found abstinence rates of 44%, 29.5%, and 10.5% for those on varenicline, bupropion, and placebo, respectively, at weeks 9 through 12 (*P* < 0.001).

Abstinence rates at or beyond 52 weeks showed that varenicline worked significantly better than placebo, but there were no consistently significant differences between varenicline and bupropion. While the Jorenby study showed continued superiority of varenicline over bupropion at week 52, Gonzales did not find a statistically significant difference between the two medications, though results favoured varenicline.[102,108]

Combination Pharmacological Therapy

Though still considered a second-line approach to quitting smoking, combining pharmacological aids has been shown in some studies to be helpful, particularly for smokers who have failed to quit when using monotherapy. Combination therapy typically involves adding nicotine gum, lozenge, inhaler, or nasal spray to either the nicotine patch or bupropion.[109] As with all pharmacological aids, providers need to be aware of problematic side-effects and potential complications.

Pharmacological Aids on the Horizon

Currently, three vaccines to help smokers quit are in development. The vaccines cause the body to produce antibodies, which bind to nicotine, preventing it from crossing the blood–brain barrier and thus reducing its reinforcing effects. One known drawback to the vaccines is that frequent injections are necessary to produce enough antibodies to create and maintain effectiveness. Four to 6 weeks of injections are needed to reach sufficient titers. In trials, the vaccines have performed significantly better than placebos in achieving 12-month continuous abstinence rates. The CYT002-NicQb vaccine resulted in 21% to 42% abstinence rates (placebos resulted in 21% abstinence); the TA-NIC 250–1000µg vaccine resulted in 19% to 38% abstinence rates (vs 8% for placebos); and NicVAX, which was fast-tracked by the FDA, resulted in 38% quit rates (vs 9% for placebos) in experimental trials.[109]

> *Using behavioural treatment in conjunction with pharmacological cessation aids has been shown to maximize success in quitting and is recommended in the Clinical Practice Guideline 2008 Update*

Rimonabant is a medication that works by blocking the cannabinoid receptor 1 (CB1), which reduces appetite and may therefore aid in smoking cessation. The FDA has approved rimonabant as a weight-loss drug but has not approved its use for smoking cessation in the United States. A review suggests that smokers taking a 20-mg dose of rimonabant were 1.5 times more likely to quit smoking than those in a placebo group. However, rimonabant's effectiveness for maintaining abstinence is unclear. Side-effects include nausea and upper respiratory tract infections, but serious adverse effects are reportedly rare. The STRATUS-US study (of nearly 800 participants at 11 sites in the United States) reported that smokers of normal weight who quit smoking on the 20-mg dose of rimonabant did not gain the typical postcessation weight.

Additionally, obese or overweight smokers who quit tended to lose weight. However, there are recent concerns regarding increases in suicidal thoughts and depression in people taking rimonabant for weight control.[110]

Combining Behavioural Therapy with Pharmacological Aids

Using behavioural treatment in conjunction with pharmacological cessation aids has been shown to maximize success in quitting and is recommended in the *Clinical Practice Guideline 2008 Update* published by the US Department of Health and Human Services.[56,57,111] In behavioural treatment, problems or concerns regarding treatment can be addressed with a knowledgeable professional, and compliance with the treatment regimen can be monitored to ensure that the medication is being used appropriately and the interventions are personally relevant and useful to the client. Barriers preventing the patient from successfully quitting can be addressed by making adjustments to the quit plan.

In a study of Brazilian smokers,[112] those receiving counselling, bupropion, and NRT had success rates at 12 months (38.5% abstinence) that surpassed the rates of those in groups with only counselling (14.5%) or counselling plus either bupropion or NRT interventions (22.8% and 25.4%, respectively). While the rates differed significantly ($P < 0.001$) by intervention, there were no gender differences in cessation success rates, although a higher level of nicotine dependence was predictive of failure to quit (OR = 1.63, 95% CI = 1.13, 2.35, $P = 0.009$).

Women are especially likely to benefit from combination therapy, because NRT seems to be less effective for them and psychosocial support seems to offer benefits. A multi-component approach is expected to be particularly helpful for women using NRT or those who are pregnant.[111,113]

Barriers to Cessation for Women

Tobacco cessation interventions for women should be designed with particular attention to the unique barriers faced by women smokers, including depression and

World Health Organization

depressive symptoms, fear of weight gain, hormonal and menstrual cycles, the need for social support, and increased vulnerability to relapse.

Depression

Research has established a relationship between depression and smoking in both men and women. Smokers in general are more likely than non-smokers to have a lifetime history of depression,[114,115] and those with a history of depression generally smoke more and report higher levels of nicotine dependence than those who are not depressed.[116–118] Moreover, they have poorer abstinence rates than smokers with no history of depression.[119,120] Depression occurring as early as adolescence has been linked with heavy smoking in adulthood.[121] Because women are twice as likely as men to experience affective disorders,[122] negative mood and depression may be more relevant to smoking cessation in women.[123] A link between depression and smoking has been found in many cultures. A national study in Australia demonstrated that current smokers were nearly twice as likely as non-smokers to have had a depressive episode in the past month (OR = 1.78, 95% CI = 1.18, 2.68). Previous smokers also had a higher risk of having a depressive episode than non-smokers (OR = 1.52, 95% CI = 1.05, 2.20).[87] Studies have also found a link between smoking and suicide risk. In one study, smoking was associated with a twofold increase in suicide risk for smokers of more than 7 cigarettes a day. For women specifically, the risk of suicide was doubled for smokers of 1 to 24 cigarettes a day. The risk of suicide for those who smoked 25 or more cigarettes a day was four times that for non-smokers.[124]

Approximately 30% of individuals entering treatment for smoking cessation have a history of major depressive disorder (MDD).[125] Findings on the influence of MDD on smoking cessation vary, depending on the nature of the study. Cross-sectional studies have found that a history of MDD predicts lower rates of cessation,[126] while the findings of prospective studies of differences in cessation rates based on MDD history have been inconsistent.[101,127] However, one consistent finding is that a history of MDD is associated with high negative affect at treatment initiation and higher levels of negative affect while quitting.[128]

Levine et al.[101] studied women smokers with a mean age of 44.5 years and found that 52.5% met criteria for MDD at some point in their lives, a rate significantly higher than the 30% estimated to experience MDD in the general population. Participants in the study were at least moderately ready to quit smoking and moderately concerned about postcessation weight gain (i.e. ratings of 50 or higher on a scale of 1 to 100). The women who met criteria for lifetime MDD had higher levels of depressive symptoms at treatment entry, reported higher levels of nicotine dependence, and were more likely to score above 10 on the Beck Depression Inventory (34.8%% with MDD vs 23.1% without MDD). However, abstinence at 3, 6, and 12 months after treatment did not differ significantly between groups. Although differences between overall rates of relapse were not significant, women with a history of MDD were more likely to relapse before treatment ended or to drop out of the study before attempting to quit (OR = 2.9, 95% CI = 0.99, 8.5). Depressive symptoms were related to abstinence after treatment—women with an increase in Beck Depression Inventory scores were significantly less likely to remain abstinent (OR = 0.80, 95% CI = 0.82–0.96). Depressive symptoms and MDD history were not related to weight changes among women who remained abstinent for 12 months.

Postcessation weight gain has been linked with an increase in caloric intake and a decrease in metabolic rate associated with quitting smoking.

Although Levine et al.[100] and others[128,129] show that a history of MDD and/or being female does not necessarily predict failure to quit smoking, other studies strongly suggest that these factors will predict greater difficulty in successfully abstaining from smoking.[30,130] Moreover, women with multiple episodes of MDD have been shown to have lower rates of successful cessation than women with only one MDD episode,[130] and NRT may not be as effective for depressed smokers.[128]

Women smokers with depressive symptoms as well as serious depressive disorders seem to require more extensive and intensive treatment and support, as would be true for any dual disorder. Hall and colleagues found that treatment lasting more than a year that included weekly sessions for a significant period of time[131] resulted in impressive success rates among women smokers who have serious depressive conditions.

Weight Gain

For women, smoking initiation[132] and maintenance, as well as relapse to smoking,[133] are often related to concerns about expected or actual weight gain.[30,134,135] Smoking to influence weight begins in adolescence. A study of dieting adolescent Irish girls found that they were more than twice as likely to be smokers as those who were not dieting or attempting to lose weight.[136] Tomeo and Field[137] and French et al.[138] reported that smoking among adolescent girls was associated with a nearly twofold probability of dieting. Concerns about weight gain during cessation are valid, since weight gain after quitting is common among both men and women. Postcessation weight gain has been linked with an increase in caloric intake and a decrease in metabolic rate associated with quitting smoking.[139] Women, however, report being more concerned than men about weight gain due to quitting,[133] and women have been found to gain more weight than men do when they quit. Both male and female smokers in the general population who quit while participating in the Denmark Inter99 study experienced significant increases in waist circumference, body-mass index (BMI), and weight between baseline and one-year follow-up.[84] However, the women's increases were significantly higher than the men's. Mean changes for women in waist circumference, BMI, and weight were 4.50 cm (±6.1), 1.73 kg (±1.7), and 4.86 kg (±4.9), respectively. Women who quit smoking had more than double the chance of substantial weight gain (OR = 2.36, 95% CI = 1.3, 4.3), and the risk increased as baseline levels of tobacco consumption increased. The chance of gaining 5 kg or more increased by 5% for every additional gram of tobacco consumed. However, some studies have failed to find significant relationships between concerns about or actual weight gain and smoking outcomes among women.[140,141]

Ethnic and cultural considerations are important when addressing weight concerns. While women typically gain an average of 6 to 8 pounds after quitting smoking, Afro-American women tend to gain significantly more than women of other ethnicities. This is an important public health concern, as more non-Hispanic Afro-American women (35.9%) are obese than Hispanic (31.0%) or white (21.7%) women, regardless of smoking status.[142] Thus, Afro-American women are at higher risk of the health complications associated with smoking and obesity (e.g. cardiovascular disease), regardless of the level of smoking or psychological concerns about weight.[143]

Hormonal Influences and Menstrual Cycles

Some research suggests that a woman's menstrual cycle may influence quitting. During certain phases of the cycle, symptoms of withdrawal and craving may be exacerbated. A recent review of studies of this relationship produced mixed results.[144] Three studies examined women who smoked ad libitum throughout the menstrual cycle, six investigated symptoms during experimental smoking abstinence, and four compared non-abstinent to abstinent women smokers. In the first group, phase of the menstrual cycle was related to increased symptoms of withdrawal, craving, or both. Symptom increases most often occurred during the luteal or late luteal phase (i.e. post-ovulation through the start of menses). In one study, irritability, restlessness, appetite change, and depressed mood—all withdrawal symptoms—were highest in the late luteal phase and were highly correlated with premenstrual symptoms, especially in this phase (r = 0.79).[145] Craving was not significantly related to phase in this study, but another study found that cue-induced craving was higher for women in the luteal phase than for those in the follicular phase (i.e. start of menses to ovulation).[146] The findings of studies comparing abstinent and non-abstinent women smokers are fairly mixed. However, the data tend to indicate less craving or withdrawal during the follicular phase than during the luteal phase.

It is important to note that many of the studies examining the effects of the menstrual cycle on abstinence and smoking have used small samples, followed participants for a relatively brief period of time, and could have done a better job of separating out withdrawal and craving symptoms from typical experiences during menstruation. In addition, many of the studies did not have a consistent protocol concerning whether to include women with premenstrual dysphoric disorder (PMDD). In fact, a number of the studies that did not find a significant connection between craving and withdrawal and menstrual phase excluded women with a diagnosis of PMDD.

Need for Social Support

Some research suggests that social support for quitting increases the probability of success.[147] This may be particularly relevant for women, as research, including a meta-analysis of 55 studies,[148] has shown that social support is more closely related to health in women than it is in men.

World Health Organization

Women also seek out and use more social support when making behaviour changes.[149] It is not certain whether social support while trying to quit smoking affects cessation success in men and women differently, although some studies have shown that social support may be more important for women.[150] Pregnant women have received the most attention in this area. Two thirds of the women in one study of pregnant smokers felt that if their partner, family, or friends quit smoking, it would be easier for them to quit.[146] Nearly 20% of these women reported that this would be the most important contributor to their quitting while pregnant.[151] Another study found that the strongest predictor of relapse for pregnant women was having a partner who smoked.[152] Turner et al.[153] reported that for women of low SES who completed a brief smoking cessation intervention, the effects of depression on cessation were moderated by social support. Women who were depressed but had more social support for quitting and not smoking achieved quit at levels similar to those of women who were not recently depressed. However, some studies have found no significant differences regarding the role of social support on cessation rates for men and women,[52] while others have found that the effects of support are more beneficial for men.[154]

Relapse

The psychological, behavioural, and physical components of tobacco dependence make relapse to smoking very common among all smokers. Relapse most often occurs within the first week of quitting,[70] when the symptoms of withdrawal typically peak. Those symptoms can last for weeks or months[155,156] and can be consistent with any of the components (psychological, behavioural, or physical) of dependence. Psychological withdrawal includes symptoms of irritability and frustration, depressed mood, anxiety, and difficulty concentrating; physical symptoms include cravings and increased appetite; behavioural difficulties include disassociating smoking from cues for smoking, such as places where one usually smoked, seeing others smoke, and times when one usually smoked.

Summary and Recommendations

As described throughout this chapter, women seem to be less successful at quitting smoking than men. Because

women are also more prone to depression, and depression increases the risk of relapse,[157] this is a special concern for women. In addition, women report finding smoking more pleasurable than men do[158] and are more sensitive to the effects of nicotine.[159] Finally, women are more concerned about weight gain than men and may resume smoking to avoid it.[30,132] These and other, yet-undefined causes seem to be important factors that contribute to higher relapse rates among women.

Comprehensive approaches to smoking cessation, such as including family and partners in treatment, encouraging increases in healthy behaviours such as physical activity and healthy diets, and paying attention to the emotional and psychological needs of clients would be particularly helpful for female smokers.

The literature indicates that all forms of smoking cessation treatment may be effective in helping women smokers quit, but they are often less effective for women than for men. Thus, treatment that addresses topics specific to the needs of women appears necessary to optimize the effectiveness of existing interventions. Women are also most likely to benefit from combination therapies that address some of the barriers noted above. They may benefit from adjunctive treatments for weight and depression, support from peers and professionals, and specific strategies to manage cues and situations unique to women smokers.

There is little evidence that specific cessation interventions are inappropriate or counterindicated for women, with the possible exception of some pharmacotherapies, particularly for pregnant women. Therefore, a completely separate tobacco control programme for women does not appear to be indicated. However, tailoring cessation to address the specific concerns of women may be needed to increase the effectiveness of intervention efforts for women smokers. In addition, some women smokers may prefer women-only groups, and these should be available as options.

This review suggests several specific ways to tailor cessation programming for women smokers. More extensive motivation and skills-based programming and the use of pharmacotherapy in conjunction with psychosocial treatments seem to be particularly beneficial for women smokers. Smoking cessation intervention specialists and counsellors should be trained in the needs and preferences of women smokers as part of their basic education and training. This is true for all counsellors, regardless of the type of contact they have with women smokers (e.g. whether they work through telephone or Internet contacts).

Medical settings, especially those in which a significant proportion of the patients are women, should have a state-of-the-art screening and brief-intervention component for smoking cessation, along with a network of referrals for more-intensive interventions. They should have the most current information, and their referral processes must be efficient and effective in connecting women smokers with the resources they need. The demand for creating an intervention component in medical settings is likely to be high throughout the world. In a survey pilot study, 87% to 99% of third-year health-profession students (e.g. dental, medical, nursing) in 10 countries reported that they had a responsibility to help patients quit smoking. However, only 5% to 37% received cessation training.[160]

Comprehensive approaches to smoking cessation, such as including family and partners in treatment, encouraging increases in healthy behaviours such as physical activity and healthy diets, and paying attention to the emotional and psychological needs of clients would be particularly helpful for female smokers. Self-help and mutual support groups may be particularly beneficial for women, providing both the material support (e.g. help with child care) and emotional support that have been identified as important for sustaining cessation.

The increase in women's smoking and the actual and potential disaster that certainly will follow for women's health increase the urgency of creating tobacco control programmes that can effectively address the unique and common challenges faced by smokers trying to break free of nicotine addiction. In addition to the policy and environmental interventions needed in a comprehensive tobacco control programme, tobacco control specialists are called to create the types of products and services for women consumers of tobacco cessation services that will effectively meet their needs and reduce mortality and morbidity worldwide.

References

1. *WHO report on the global tobacco epidemic: implementing smoke-free environments, 2009*. Geneva, World Health Organization, 2009,
2. Mayo Clinic Staff. *Women's health risks*. Rochester, MN, 2007 (http://www.mayoclinic.com/health/womens-health/WO00014#).
3. Thyrian JR et al. The relationship between smokers' motivation to quit and intensity of tobacco control at the population level: a comparison of five European countries. *BMC Public Health*, 2008, 8:2, published online 3 January 2008.
4. Centers for Disease Control and Prevention. Cigarette smoking among adults—United States, 2000. *Morbidity and Mortality Weekly Report*, 2002, 51:642–645.
5. Centers for Disease Control and Prevention, Cigarette smoking among adults—United States, 2004. *Morbidity and Mortality Weekly Report*, 2005, 54:1121–1124.
6. Fong GT et al. The near-universal experience of regret among smokers in four countries: findings from the International Tobacco Control Policy Evaluation Survey. *Nicotine and Tobacco Research*, 2004, 6 (Suppl. 3):341–351.
7. *WHO Framework Convention on Tobacco Control*. Geneva, World Health Organization, 2005.
8. *Women and smoking: a report of the Surgeon General*. Rockville, MD, US Department of Health and Human Services, 2001.
9. Global Youth Tobacco Survey Collaborating Group. Differences in worldwide tobacco use by gender: findings from the Global Youth Tobacco Survey. *Journal of School Health*, 2003; 207.
10. Samet J, Yoon S, eds., *Women and the tobacco epidemic: challenges for the 21st century*. Geneva, World Health Organization, 2001.
11. *Gender and tobacco control: a policy brief*. Geneva, World Health Organization, 2007 (http://www.idrc.ca/uploads/user-S/12097440371policy_brief.pdf).
12. Kessler DA et al. Nicotine addiction: a pediatric disease. *The Journal of Pediatrics*, 1997, 130:518–524.
13. Rock VJ et al. Cigarette smoking among adults—United States, 2006. *Morbidity and Mortality Weekly Report*, 2007, 56:1157–1161.
14. Federico B, Kunst AE, Costa G. Educational inequalities in initiation, cessation, and prevalence of smoking among 3 Italian birth cohorts. *American Journal of Public Health*, 2007, 97:838–845.
15. Schiaffino A et al. Gender and educational differences in smoking initiation rates in Spain from 1948 to 1992. *European Journal of Public Health*, 2003, 13:56.
16. Laaksonen M et al. Development of smoking by birth cohort in the adult population in eastern Finland 1972–97. *Tobacco Control*, 1999, 8:161–168.
17. Osler M et al. Socioeconomic position and smoking behaviour in Danish adults. *Scandinavian Journal of Public Health*, 2001, 29:32–39.
18. Barbeau EM, Leavy-Sperounis A, Balbach ED. Smoking, social class, and gender: what can public health learn from the tobacco industry about disparities in smoking? *Tobacco Control*, 2004, 13:115–120.
19. *Women and tobacco: global trends, Vol. 1–4*. Washington, DC, Campaign for Tobacco-Free Kids, 2007.
20. Centers for Disease Control and Prevention, Global youth tobacco surveillance, 2000–2007. *Morbidity and Mortality Weekly Report*, 2008, 57:1–21.
21. Mackay J, Eriksen M, Shafey O. *The tobacco atlas*, 2nd ed. Atlanta, GA, American Cancer Society, 2006.
22. Lando HA. et al. The landscape in global tobacco control research: a guide to gaining a foothold. *American Journal of Public Health*, 2005, 95:939–945.

23. Weber D et al. Smokers' attitudes and behaviors related to consumer demand for cessation counselling in the medical-care setting. *Nicotine & Tobacco Research*, 2007, 9:571–580.

24. Tauras J, Chaloupka F. The demand for nicotine replacement therapies. *Nicotine & Tobacco Research*, 2003, 5:237–243.

25. Ussher M, West R, Hibbs N. A survey of pregnant smokers' interest in different types of smoking cessation support. *Patient Education & Counselling*, 2004, 54:67–72.

26. Stead LF, Lancaster T. Interventions to reduce harm from continued tobacco use. *Cochrane Database of Systematic Reviews 2007.*

27. Hurt RD, Robertson CR. Prying open the door to the tobacco industry's secrets about nicotine: the Minnesota Tobacco Trial. *Journal of the American Medical Association*, 1998, 280:1173–1181.

28. US Department of Health and Human Services. Women and smoking: a report of the Surgeon General. *Morbidity and Mortality Weekly Report*, 2002, 51:1.

29. Orleans CT, Phillips T. *Innovations in building consumer demand for tobacco cessation products and services.* Washington, DC, Academy for Educational Development, 2007.

30. Perkins KA. Smoking cessation in women: special considerations. *CNS Drugs*, 2001, 15:391–411.

31. Bogart LM, Delahanty DL. Psychosocial models. In: Boll T et al., eds. *Handbook of clinical health psychology. Vol. 3. Models and perspectives in health psychology.* Washington, DC, American Psychological Association, 2004:201–248.

32. Glanz K, Rimer KB. *Theory at a glance: a guide for health promotion practice.* Bethesda, MD, US Department of Health and Human Services, Public Health Service, National Institutes of Health, National Cancer Institute, 1997.

33. Toll BA et al. Message framing for smoking cessation: the interaction of risk perceptions and gender. *Nicotine & Tobacco Research*, 2008, 10:195–200.

34. O'Hea EL, Wood KB, Brantley PJ. The transtheoretical model: gender differences across 3 health behaviors. *American Journal of Health Behavior*, 2003, 27:645–656.

35. Galvin KT. A critical review of the health belief model in relation to cigarette smoking behaviour. *Journal of Clinical Nursing*, 1992, 1:13–18.

36. Ajzen I. From intentions to actions: a theory of planned behavior. In: Beckman JKJ, ed. *Action-control: from cognition to behavior.* Heidelberg, Springer, 1985:11–39.

37. Ajzen I, Fishbein M. *Understanding attitudes and predicting social behavior.* Englewood Cliffs, NJ, Prentice-Hall, 1980.

38. Bandura A. *Social foundations of thought and action: a social cognitive theory.* Englewood Cliffs, NJ, Prentice-Hall, 1986 (Prentice-Hall Series in Social Learning Theory).

39. Hanson JS. An examination of ethnic differences in cigarette smoking intention among female teenagers. *Journal of the American Academy of Nurse Practitioners*, 2005, 17:149–155.

40. Norman P, Conner M, Bell R. The theory of planned behavior and smoking cessation. *Health Psychology*, 1999, 18:89–94.

41. DiClemente CC et al. The process of smoking cessation: an analysis of precontemplation, contemplation, and preparation stages of change. *Journal of Consulting and Clinical Psychology*, 1991, 59:295–304.

42. Prochaska JO. Diclemente CC. Norcross JC. In search of how people change: applications to addictive behaviors. *American Psychologist*, 1992, 47:1102–1114.

43. Prochaska JO, Diclemente CC. Stages and processes of self-change of smoking: toward an integrative model of change. *Journal of Consulting and Clinical Psychology*, 1983, 51:390–395.

44. Marlatt, GA, Donovan DM. *Relapse prevention: maintenance strategies in the treatment of addictive behaviors*, 2nd ed. New York, NY, Guilford Press, 2005.

45. Prochaska JO et al. Measuring processes of change: applications to the cessation of smoking. *Journal of Consulting and Clinical Psychology*, 1988, 56:520–528.

46. Diclemente CC. *Addiction and change: how addictions develop and addicted people recover.* New York, NY, Guilford Press, 2005 (Guilford Substance Abuse Series).

47. Etter J-FO. Prokhorov AV, Perneger TV. Gender differences in the psychological determinants of cigarette smoking. *Addiction*, 2002, 97:733.

48. Etter J-FO. The psychological determinants of low-rate daily smoking. *Addiction*, 2004, 99:1342–1350.

49. Clements-Thompson M et al. Relationships between stages of change in cigarette smokers and healthy lifestyle behaviors in a population of young military personnel during forced smoking abstinence. *Journal of Consulting and Clinical Psychology*, 1998, 66:1005–1011.

50. Perz CA, Diclemente CC, Carbonari JP. Doing the right thing at the right time? The interaction of stages and processes of change in successful smoking cessation. *Health Psychology*, 1996, 15:462–468.

51. Diclemente CC. Conceptual models and applied research: the ongoing contribution of the Transtheoretical Model. *Journal of Addictions Nursing*, 2005, 16:5–12.

52. O'Connor EA, Carbonari JP, Diclemente CC. Gender and smoking cessation: a factor structure comparison of processes of change. *Journal of Consulting and Clinical Psychology*, 1996, 64:130–138.

53. West R. Time for a change: putting the Transtheoretical (Stages of Change) Model to rest. *Addiction*, 2005, 100:1036–1039.

54. Etter, JF, Sutton S. Assessing "stage of change" in current and former smokers. *Addiction*, 2002, 97:1171.

55. *Reducing the health consequences of smoking: 25 years of progress. A report of the Surgeon General.* Rockville, MD, Centers for Disease Control, Center for Chronic Disease Prevention and Health Promotion, 1989.

56. Fiore M et al. Treating tobacco use and dependence: clinical practice guideline. In: *Clinical practice guideline.* Rockville, MD, United States Department of Health and Human Services, Public Health Service, Agency for Health Care Policy and Research, 2000.

57. Fiore M et al. Treating tobacco use and dependence: 2008 update. In: *Clinical practice guideline.* Rockville, MD, US Department of Health and Human Services, Public Health Service, 2008.

58. Maloni JA et al. Implementing evidence-based practice: reducing risk for low birth weight through pregnancy smoking cessation. *Journal of Obstetric, Gynecologic, & Neonatal Nursing*, 2003, 32:676.

59. Gill JM et al. Do physicians in Delaware follow national guidelines for tobacco counselling? *Delaware Medical Journal*, 2004, 76:297–308.

60. Stead L, Lancaster T. Group behaviour therapy programmes for smoking cessation. *Cochrane Database of Systematic Reviews,* 1998:CD001007.

61. Orleans CT, Alper J. Helping addicted smokers quit. In: Isaacs SL, Knickman JR, eds. *To improve health and health care.* San Francisco, CA, Jossey-Bass, 2003:125–148.

62. *Physician behavior and practice patterns related to smoking cessation.* Washington, DC, Association of American Medical Colleges, 2007.

63. Miller WR, Rollnick S. *Motivational interviewing: preparing people to change addictive behavior.* New York, NY, Guilford Press, 1991.

64. Miller W, Rollnick S. *Motivational interviewing: preparing people for change.* 2nd ed. New York, NY: Guilford Press, 2002.

65. Miller WR et al. *Motivational enhancement therapy manual: a clinical research guide for therapists treating individuals with alcohol abuse and dependence.* Rockville, MD, United States Department of Health, Public Health Service, 1992:121 (Project MATCH Monograph Series, Vol. 2).

66. Rollnick S, Miller WR, Butler CC. *Motivational interviewing in health care: helping patients change behavior (applications of motivational interviewing).* New York, NY, Guilford Press, 2008.

67. Haug NA, Svikis DS, DiClemente C. Motivational enhancement therapy for nicotine dependence in methadone-maintained pregnant women. *Psychology of Addictive Behaviors*, 2004, 18:289–292.

68. Stotts AL, DiClemente CC, Dolan-Mullen P. One-to-one: a motivational intervention for resistant pregnant smokers. *Addictive Behaviors*, 2002, 27:275–292.

69. Lancaster T, Stead L. Self-help interventions for smoking cessation. *Cochrane Database of Systematic Reviews*, 1998:CD001118. DOI.

70. Hughes JR, Keely J, Naud S. Shape of the relapse curve and long-term abstinence among untreated smokers. *Addiction*, 2004, 99:29–38.

71. Prochaska JO et al. Patterns of change: dynamic typology applied to smoking cessation. *Multivariate Behavioral Research*, 1991, 26:83.

72. Fiore MC. The new vital sign: assessing and documenting smoking status. *Journal of the American Medical Association*, 1991, 266:3183–3184.

73. Cobb N et al. Initial evaluation of a real-world Internet smoking cessation system. *Nicotine & Tobacco Research*, 2005, 7:207–216.

74. Strecher VJ, Shiffman S, West R. Randomized controlled trial of a web-based computer-tailored smoking cessation program as a supplement to nicotine patch therapy. *Addiction*, 2005, 100:682–688.

World Health Organization

75. Prochaska JO et al. Standardized, individualized, interactive, and personalized self-help programmes for smoking cessation. *Health Psychology*, 1993, 12:399–405.

76. Velicer WF, Prochaska JO. An expert system intervention for smoking cessation. *Patient Education and Counselling*, 1999, 36:119–129.

77. Prochaska JO et al. Stage-based expert systems to guide a population of primary care patients to quit smoking, eat healthier, prevent skin cancer, and receive regular mammograms. *Preventive Medicine*, 2005, 41:406–416.

78. Velicer WF, Prochaska JO, Redding CA. Tailored communications for smoking cessation: past successes and future directions. *Drug & Alcohol Review*, 2006, 25:49–57.

79. Velicer WF et al. An expert system intervention for smoking cessation. *Addictive Behaviors*, 1993, 18:269–290.

80. Meyer C et al. Proactive interventions for smoking cessation in general medical practice: a quasi-randomized controlled trial to examine the efficacy of computer-tailored letters and physician-delivered brief advice. *Addiction*, 2008, 103:294–304.

81. Schumann A. Computer-tailored smoking cessation intervention in a general population setting in Germany: outcome of a randomized controlled trial. *Nicotine & Tobacco Research*, 2008, 10:371.

82. Davis SW et al. The impact of tailored self-help smoking cessation guides on young mothers. *Health Education Quarterly*, 1992, 19:495–504.

83. Kessler RC, Brown RL, Broman CL. Sex differences in psychiatric help-seeking: evidence from four large-scale surveys. *Journal of Health and Social Behavior*, 1981, 22:49–64.

84. Pisinger C, Jorgensen T. Waist circumference and weight following smoking cessation in a general population: the Inter99 study. *Preventive Medicine*, 2007, 44:290–295.

85. Ortner R et al. Women addicted to nicotine. *Archives of Women's Mental Health*, 2002, 4:103–109.

86. Lancaster T, Stead LF. Individual behavioural counselling for smoking cessation. *Cochrane Database of Systematic Reviews* (online), 2005, :CD001292.

87. Wilhelm K et al. Prevalence and correlates of DSM-IV major depression in an Australian national survey. *Journal of Affective Disorders*, 2003, 75:155–162.

88. Lucksted A, Dixon L, Sembly J, A focus group pilot study of tobacco smoking among psychosocial rehabilitation clients. *Psychiatric Service*, 2000, 51:1544–1548.

89. Husky MM et al. Gender differences in the comorbidity of smoking behavior and major depression. *Drug & Alcohol Dependence*, 2008, 93:176–179.

90. Stead LF, Perera R, Lancaster T. A systematic review of interventions for smokers who contact quitlines. *Tobacco Control*, 2007, 16 (Suppl. 1):i3–i8.

91. Stead LF, Perera R, Lancaster T. Telephone counselling for smoking cessation. *Cochrane Database of Systematic Reviews* (online), 2006, 3:CD002850.

92. Rabius V et al. Effects of frequency and duration in telephone counselling for smoking cessation. *Tobacco Control*, 2007, 16 (Suppl. 1):i71–i74.

93. *Quitlines of North America and Europe*. Phoenix, AZ, North American Quitline Consortium, 2006.

94. Coffay AO. Smoking cessation: tactics that make a big difference. *Journal of Family Practice*, 2007, 56:817–824.

95. Rodgers A et al. Do u smoke after txt? results of a randomised trial of smoking cessation using mobile phone text messaging. *Tobacco Control*, 2005, 14:255–261.

96. Stead LF et al. Nicotine replacement therapy for smoking cessation. *Cochrane Database of Systematic Reviews* (online), 2008, 1:CD000146.

97. Evans SE et al. Transdermal nicotine-induced tobacco abstinence symptom suppression: nicotine dose and smokers' gender. *Experimental and Clinical Psychopharmacology*, 2006, 12:121–135.

98. Hughes JR, Stead LF, Lancaster T. Antidepressants for smoking cessation. *Cochrane Database of Systematic Reviews* (online), 2007, 1:CD000031.

99. Stack NM. Smoking cessation: an overview of treatment options with a focus on varenicline. *Pharmacotherapy*, 2007, 27:1550–1557.

100. Smith SS et al. Targeting smokers at increased risk for relapse: treating women and those with a history of depression. *Nicotine & Tobacco Research*, 2003, 5:99.

101. Levine MD, Marcus MD, Perkins KA. A history of depression and smoking cessation outcomes among women concerned about post-cessation weight gain. *Nicotine & Tobacco Research*, 2003, 5:69–76.

102. Jorenby DE et al. Efficacy of varenicline, an alpha4beta2 nicotinic acetylcholine receptor partial agonist, vs placebo or sustained-release bupropion for smoking cessation: a randomized controlled trial. *Journal of the American Medical Association*, 2006, 296:56–63.

103. Gonzales D et al. Effects of gender on relapse prevention in smokers treated with bupropion SR. *American Journal of Preventive Medicine*, 2002, 22:234.

104. Scharf D, Shiffman S. Are there gender differences in smoking cessation, with and without bupropion? Pooled- and meta-analyses of clinical trials of Bupropion SR. *Addiction*, 2004, 99:1462–1469.

105. Swan GE et al. Bupropion SR and counselling for smoking cessation in actual practice: predictors of outcome. *Nicotine & Tobacco Research*, 2003, 5:911–921.

106. Dale LC et al. Bupropion for smoking cessation: predictors of successful outcome. *Chest*, 2001, 119:1357–1364.

107. Tonstad S et al. Bupropion SR for smoking cessation in smokers with cardiovascular disease: a multicentre, randomized study. *European Heart Journal*, 2003, 24:946–955.

108. Gonzales D et al. Varenicline, an alpha4beta2 nicotinic acetylcholine receptor partial agonist, vs sustained-release bupropion and placebo for smoking cessation: a randomized controlled trial. *Journal of the American Medical Association*, 2006, 296:47–55.

109. Nides M et al. Maximizing smoking cessation in clinical practice: pharmacologic and behavioral interventions. *Preventive Cardiology*, 2007, 10, 2 (Suppl. 1):23–30.

110. Cahill K, Ussher M. Cannabinoid type 1 receptor antagonists (rimonabant) for smoking cessation. *Cochrane Database of Systematic Reviews* (online), 2007, 4:CD005353.

111. Cofta-Woerpel L, Wright KL, Wetter DW. Smoking cessation 3: multicomponent interventions. *Behavioral Medicine*, 2007, 32:135–149.

112. Chatkin JM et al. Abstinence rates and predictors of outcome for smoking cessation: do Brazilian smokers need special strategies? *Addiction*, 2004, 99: 778–784.

113. Cepeda-Benito A, Reynoso JT, Erath S. Meta-analysis of the efficacy of nicotine replacement therapy for smoking cessation: differences between men and women. *Journal of Consulting and Clinical Psychology*, 2004, 72:712–722.

114. Breslau N, Kilbey MM, Andreski P. Nicotine dependence, major depression, and anxiety in young adults. *Archives of General Psychiatry*, 1991, 48:1069–1074.

115. Kendler KS et al. Smoking and major depression: a causal analysis. *Archives of General Psychiatry*, 1993, 50:36–43.

116. Breslau N, Kilbey MM, Andreski P. Nicotine dependence and major depression: new evidence from a prospective investigation. *Archives of General Psychiatry*, 1993, 50:31–35.

117. Breslau N, Kilbey MM. DSM-III-R nicotine dependence in young adults: prevalence, correlates and associated psychiatric disorders. *Addiction*, 1994, 89:743–754.

118. Breslau N. Psychiatric comorbidity of smoking and nicotine dependence. *Behavior Genetics*, 1995, 25: 95–101.

119. Hurt RD et al. A comparison of sustained-release bupropion and placebo for smoking cessation. *New England Journal of Medicine*, 1997, 337:1195–1202.

120. Farrell M et al. Nicotine, alcohol and drug dependence and psychiatric comorbidity: results of a national household survey. *British Journal of Psychiatry*, 2001, 179:432–437.

121. Kandel DB, Davies M. Adult sequelae of adolescent depressive symptoms. *Archives of General Psychiatry*, 1986, 43:255–262.

122. *Diagnostic and statistical manual of mental disorders*. 4th ed. Washington, DC, American Psychiatric Association, 1994.

123. Blazer DG et al. The prevalence and distribution of major depression in a national community sample: the national comorbidity survey. *American Journal of Psychiatry*, 1994, 151:979–986.

124. Hemenway D, Solnick SJ, Colditz GA, Smoking and suicide among nurses. *American Journal of Public Health*, 1993, 83:249–251.

125. Niaura R et al. Symptoms of depression and survival experience among three samples of smokers trying to quit. *Psychology of Addictive Behaviors*, 2001, 15:13–17.

126. Breslau N, Kilbey M, Andreski P. Nicotine withdrawal symptoms and psychiatric disorders: findings from an epidemiologic study of young adults. *American Journal of Psychiatry*, 1992, 149:464–469.

World Health Organization

127. Ginsberg D et al. Mood and depression diagnosis in smoking cessation. *Experimental and Clinical Psychopharmacology*, 1995, 3:389–395.

128. Hall SM et al. Mood management and nicotine gum in smoking treatment: a therapeutic contact and placebo-controlled study. *Journal of Consulting and Clinical Psychology*, 1996, 64:1003–1009.

129. Gritz ER et al. Gender differences among smokers and quitters in the Working Well Trial. *Preventive Medicine*, 1998, 27: 553–561.

130. Covey LS, Glassman AH. Effect of history of alcoholism or major depression on smoking cessation. *American Journal of Psychiatry*, 1993, 150:1546.

131. Hall SM et al. Treatment for cigarette smoking among depressed mental health outpatients: a randomized clinical trial. *American Journal of Public Health*, 2006, 96:1808–1814.

132. *Gender, health and tobacco*. Geneva, World Health Organization, 2003 (http://www.who.int/gender/documents/Gender_Tobacco_2.pdf, accessed 7 March 2008).

133. Swan GE et al. Differential rates of relapse in subgroups of male and female smokers. *Journal of Clinical Epidemiology*, 1993, 46:1041–1053.

134. Meyers AW et al. Are weight concerns predictive of smoking cessation? A prospective analysis. *Journal of Consulting and Clinical Psychology*, 1997, 65:448–452.

135. Bowen DJ et al. Recruiting women into a smoking cessation program: who might quit? *Women & Health*, 2000, 31:41.

136. Strauss R, Mir H. Smoking and weight loss attempts in overweight and normal-weight adolescents. *International Journal of Obesity*, 2001, 25:1381–1385.

137. Tomeo CA, Field AE. Weight concerns, weight control behaviors, and smoking initiation. *Pediatrics*, 1999, 104:918.

138. French SA et al. Weight concerns, dieting behavior, and smoking initiation among adolescents: a prospective study. *American Journal of Public Health*, 1994, 84:1818–1818.

139. Perkins KA et al. Addressing women's concerns about weight gain due to smoking cessation. *Journal of Substance Abuse Treatment*, 1997, 14:173–182.

140. Borrelli B et al. Influences of gender and weight gain on short-term relapse to smoking in a cessation trial. *Journal of Consulting and Clinical Psychology*, 2001, 69:511–515.

141. Pisinger C, Jorgensen T. Weight concerns and smoking in a general population: the Inter99 study. *Preventive Medicine*, 2007, 44:283–289.

142. Pleis J, Lethbridge-Cejku M. Summary health statistics for US adults: National Health Interview Survey, 2005. In: *Vital Health Statistics*. Washington, DC, Centers for Disease Control and Prevention, National Center for Health Statistics, 2006.

143. Sanchez-Johnsen LAP. Smoking cessation, obesity and weight concerns in black women: a call to action for culturally competent interventions. *Journal of the National Medical Association*, 2005, 97:1630–1638.

144. Carpenter MJ et al. Menstrual cycle phase effects on nicotine withdrawal and cigarette craving: a review. *Nicotine & Tobacco Research*, 2006, 8:627–638.

145. Allen SS et al. Symptomatology and energy intake during the menstrual cycle in smoking women. *Journal of Substance Abuse*, 1996, 8:303–319.

146. Franklin TR et al. Retrospective study: influence of menstrual cycle on cue-induced cigarette craving. *Nicotine & Tobacco Research*, 2004, 6:171–175.

147. Fiore,MC. A clinical practice guideline for treating tobacco use and dependence: a US Public Health Service report. *Journal of the American Medical Association*, 2000, 283: 3244–3254.

148. Schwartz R., Leppin A. Social support and health: a meta-analysis. *Psychological Health*, 1989, 9:1–15.

149. Stockton MC, Mcmahon SD, Jason LA. Gender and smoking behavior in a worksite smoking cessation program. *Addictive Behaviors*, 2000, 25:347–360.

150. Reynoso J, Susabda A, Cepeda-Benito A. Gender differences in smoking cessation. *Journal of Psychopathology & Behavioral Assessment*, 2005, 27:227–234.

151. Thompson KA. Women's perceptions of support from partners, family members and close friends for smoking cessation during pregnancy—combining quantitative and qualitative findings. *Health Education Research*, 2004, 19:29.

152. Mullen PD, Quinn VP, Ershoff DH. Maintenance of nonsmoking postpartum by women who stopped smoking during pregnancy. *American Journal of Public Health*, 1990, 80:992–994.

153. Turner LR et al. Social support as a moderator of the relationship between recent history of depression and smoking cessation among lower-educated women. *Nicotine & Tobacco Research*, 2008, 10:201–212.

154. Murray RP et al. Social support for smoking cessation and abstinence: the Lung Health Study. Lung Health Study Research Group. *Addictive Behaviors*, 1995, 20:159–170.

155. Cummings KM et al. Reports of smoking withdrawal symptoms over a 21 day period of abstinence. *Addictive Behaviors*, 1985, 10:373–381.

156. Nides MM. Update on pharmacologic options for smoking cessation treatment. *American Journal of Medicine*, 2008, 121:S20.

157. Hitsman B et al. History of depression and smoking cessation outcome: a meta-analysis. *Journal of Consulting and Clinical Psychology*, 2003, 71:657–663.

158. Perkins KA et al. Sex differences in nicotine effects and self-administration: review of human and animal evidence. *Nicotine & Tobacco Research*, 1999, 1:301–315.

159. Benowitz NL et al. Gender differences in the pharmacology of nicotine addiction. *Addiction Biology*, 1998, 3:383.

160. Costa da Silva V et al. Tobacco use and cessation counselling—Global Health Professionals Survey Pilot Study, 10 countries, 2005. *Morbidity and Mortality Weekly Report*, 2005, 54:505–509.

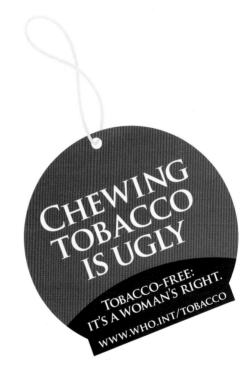

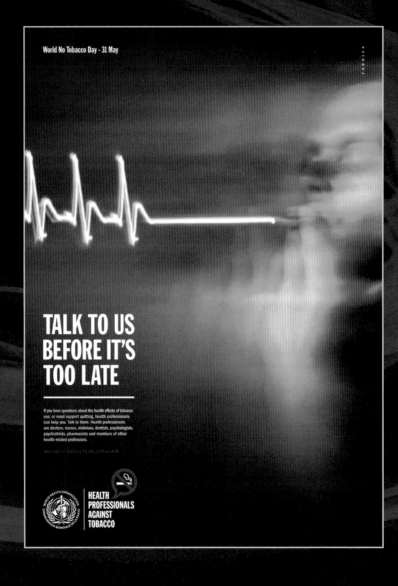

9. Pregnancy and Postpartum Smoking Cessation

Introduction

For female smokers and their partners, pregnancy represents an opportunity to re-evaluate lifestyles and a variety of health behaviours, including smoking. Most women smokers in industrialized countries are aware of health warnings about the serious consequences of cigarette smoking during pregnancy for the health and well-being of the newborn child.[1–3] Smoking and smoke exposure during pregnancy have important deleterious effects on the fetus and on the baby at birth and throughout his or her early development, including miscarriage, stillbirth, placental abruption, placenta previa, low birth weight, cognitive impairment, and risk of death from certain conditions such as sudden infant death syndrome (SIDS).[4,5] Children living in homes where the mother and/or father continues to smoke during the postnatal and early childhood period are at greater risk for respiratory illnesses, middle-ear infections, and reduced lung growth.[6–9] A 2001 study[10] estimated that 27% of children in the United States 6 years of age and younger lived with smokers. Additional risks are death and injury resulting from fires caused by cigarettes, exacerbation of asthma, and accidental poisonings from ingestion of cigarettes or other tobacco products.[11,12]

Birth asphyxia caused 23% of neonatal deaths world-wide in 2004, while low birth weight (primarily due to prematurity) caused 31% of neonatal deaths.[13] Clearly, these two causes of death reflect not only maternal ciga-rette smoking but also the many other factors contributing to premature birth and asphyxia. However, studies on risks of smoking during pregnancy indicate that a signifi-cant percentage of these deaths is attributable to smoking by the mother and others in the family environment.[14,15] Studies from laboratories around the world are exploring the physiological mechanisms linking smoking exposure during pregnancy to adverse neurodevelopmental effects that occur well into adulthood.[9] Detrimental effects are caused by exposure to carbon monoxide (CO), tar, benzene, and heavy metals, as well as by nicotine, the addictive substance in tobacco products that affects ges-tation and can cross the placenta to directly affect fetal tissue. In their review of the animal and human research

on smoking during pregnancy and fetal outcomes, Shea and Steiner[9] concluded that these negative consequences "involve a cascade of events causing not only dysregulation of the nicotinic and muscarinic, but also the catecho-laminergic and serotonergic neurotransmitter systems". A deeper understanding is needed of how smoke exposure in utero affects long-term regulation of behaviour, emotions, and attention.[9,15]

Because smoking during pregnancy and in the postpartum period has serious consequences for children, smoking cessation by women and their partners during the prenatal, perinatal, and postnatal periods offers multiple, significant benefits. Those benefits have been demonstrated in numerous studies showing that smoking cessation interventions significantly reduce the frequency of low birth weight, increase mean birth weight, and reduce the frequency of pre-term births.[16] There is also evidence of a dose-response relationship between numbers of cigarettes smoked during pregnancy and low birth weight.[17–19] Thus, a significant reduction (usually more than 50%) in smoking and the resulting decrease in exposure during pregnancy can significantly increase birth weight.[20]

Over the past 20 years, numerous clinical trials and observational studies in the United States, the United Kingdom, Europe, Australia, Sweden, and other countries have demonstrated the effectiveness of smoking cessation interventions early in pregnancy.[16,17,19,21–29] Other studies have highlighted the cost-effectiveness of such prenatal and perinatal interventions in terms of birth outcomes.[30,31] Moreover, interventions in paediatric settings that target new mothers who continue to smoke or relapse to smoking during the postpartum period have begun to demonstrate modest success,[32,33] although efficacy is not well established. Finally, intervention studies are beginning to target partners who smoke and to include fathers in family interventions.[34–37] Studies of smoking cessation in the context of pregnancy and the birth of a child have yielded important information about the course and process of smoking cessation during pregnancy and the postpartum period.[38,39]

This chapter outlines conceptual and practical considerations for smoking cessation with regard to pregnancy and infancy. It reviews recent literature and highlights the multiple opportunities to intervene during the entire period prior to, during, and after pregnancy. It also describes what is known about smoking cessation

 World Health Organization

and pregnancy and discusses ways to promote effective, evidence-based strategies throughout and after pregnancy to create smoke-free families.

Smoking During Pregnancy

Pregnant smokers constitute a subset of a larger population of female smokers of childbearing age. Demographic characteristics of this group vary from country to country. Epidemiological data provide insights into characteristics of pregnant women who smoke and into the subpopulations at risk for the consequences of smoking during pregnancy and in the postpartum period. Age-standardized estimates from the *WHO Report on the Global Tobacco Epidemic, 2009*[40] indicate that the current prevalence of tobacco smoking among female adults ranges from less than 1% in countries such as Algeria and Morocco and less than 5% in Armenia, Bahrain, Chad, China, the Congo, Guatemala, Thailand, and Uganda to over 20% in Belgium, Germany, Iceland, Ireland, Israel, Latvia, Spain, and Uruguay and over 30% in Bosnia and Herzegovina and Chile. The prevalence rate in the United States is 19.0%. The wide range of prevalence indicates a need for targeting by national and international smoking control agencies to maximize the impact and cost-effectiveness of their efforts.

In some subpopulations, smoking rates may be higher among younger women of childbearing years than in the general population; thus, total population rates may underestimate the true prevalence of women at risk for smoking during pregnancy in countries where subpopulations may also smoke at higher or lower rates because of their particular determinants of smoking. For example, in the United States, the prevalence of smoking during pregnancy is particularly high among Caucasian women in the lower socioeconomic strata of society.[41–43] Among Afro-American, Hispanic, and Asian populations of women, cigarette smoking is generally less prevalent across all age ranges, with few exceptions.[42] Knowledge of smoking rates and prevalence among subpopulations of women of childbearing age can inform strategies for creating targeted anti-smoking advertising and other programmes.[44]

For effective intervention, we need to understand why rates of initiation are highest and rates of cessation lowest among certain subgroups of women smokers.[41,43,45,46] First, younger smokers tend to be less worried about the long-

term health effects of smoking and are more vulnerable to the advertising of the tobacco industry, which focuses on different themes depending on the age of the target population. Brands for younger women stress freedom, camaraderie, independence, and self-confidence and feature young women as smokers; brands for older women stress weight reduction, relaxation, and needs for pleasure.[47] This is elaborated in the chapter in this monograph on global perspectives on the marketing of tobacco to women. Second, women appear to seek some unique consequences of smoking (e.g. weight and affect management) that make smoking part of their way of coping with life and increase their dependence on nicotine.[48] Some of these factors are particularly salient for pregnant women. Third, younger women in many cultures have multiple demands and stressors related to performing the competing roles of mother, homemaker, and employee.[46] For some women of childbearing age, smoking becomes a stress-coping strategy that can assist them in asserting independence, managing negative emotions, and providing weight management, as well as creating a particular image. Fourth, many women who smoke are influenced by support systems that encourage nicotine use, and they are often surrounded by smokers in their social networks.[49]

Younger women who decide to smoke in the context of the current anti-smoking climate and social norms constitute a subgroup of the population that may not be affected by simple educational interventions and is therefore probably resistant to quitting. This group's motivations for smoking need to be better understood,[50] particularly in countries where smoking is increasing among youth and specifically among young women. Interventions are needed that are based on a better understanding of the needs and perspectives of young women to interfere with the initiation of tobacco dependence and to be effective in promoting cessation. Interventions to reach these at-risk women even before they become pregnant represent the most effective strategy to prevent smoking during pregnancy. However, the interventions will have to be potent and multifaceted and will have to include comprehensive approaches that range from protective and restrictive policy interventions to prevention and cessation efforts as outlined in the WHO Framework Convention on Tobacco Control (WHO FCTC).[51]

There are multiple points of entry and targets of intervention for control of smoking during pregnancy. Ruggiero et al.[52] screened a group of low-income pregnant women (n = 1105) who were ever-smokers. Of this group, 22% quit before they became pregnant, 27% quit after becoming pregnant, and 52% were smoking on entry into prenatal care. Table 9.1 offers a view of smoking during pre-pregnancy, pregnancy, and postpartum periods and interventions to be considered. In addition to reducing risks for babies, interventions should focus on the health and well-being of the mother, the father or partner, and the extended family. It is critical to search for teachable moments throughout the lives of smokers and to use them to promote cessation.[53]

Pre-Pregnancy Quitters

Women smokers of childbearing years follow a number of different paths in managing their smoking as they anticipate becoming pregnant. Some women con-

sider the option of stopping smoking and modifying other behaviours that increase risks to becoming and staying pregnant. This group usually consists of women who anticipate pregnancy or who have already created plans and expectations that when they become pregnant, they will stop smoking either permanently or, at the very least, for the duration of the pregnancy.[41] This level of concern, planning, and forethought is a positive indicator for successful cessation of smoking during pregnancy but does not ensure sustained cessation.[20,54] Although the actual number of women who quit smoking prior to becoming pregnant is not known, anecdotal and observational data indicate that many women stop smoking prior to becoming pregnant or while trying to become pregnant. Self-reported rates of smoking on entry to obstetric care are generally lower than overall population rates. In the early 1990s, when the smoking rate of the female population in the United States was

Table 9.1. Opportunities and Targets of Intervention for Young Women Smokers

Smoking Status	Interventions
Smokers (age 15–45)	Use policy and interventions to promote pre-pregnancy quitting.
Early-pregnancy smokers	Promote early first-trimester cessation. Offer cessation help (5 As) in obstetric care.
Early-pregnancy quitters	Provide support to sustain cessation during pregnancy and postpartum. Promote spouse and family quitting and exposure reduction. Shift motivation to include mother, not just baby.
Late-pregnancy smokers	Provide intensive interventions to promote cessation. Support reduction even late in the pregnancy. Involve the family in protecting the fetus and preparing for the baby.
Pregnancy quitters	Engage family and spouse smokers to quit. Offer relapse prevention immediately postpartum.
Continuing smokers	Prevent return to pre-pregnancy levels. Provide interventions during paediatric visits. Promote smoke-free home policies.
Postpartum relapsers	Support recycling and cessation. Highlight protection and smoke-free policies.

 World Health Organization

over 20%, the rate for women in obstetric care was estimated to be 13.6%.[55]

There are two challenges for designing interventions that target women who stop smoking immediately prior to becoming pregnant: promoting pre-pregnancy quitting, and supporting cessation throughout pregnancy and preventing relapse during the difficult postpartum period.[56] Strategies to promote pre-pregnancy smoking cessation among women of childbearing age include creating and displaying media messages that highlight the links between smoking during pregnancy and fetal health; demonstrating how smoking can adversely affect fertility and how cessation can prevent loss of the fetus; and emphasizing the long-term neurodevelopmental effects of smoking on the child. Another important strategy would be to engage medical and other professionals who have regular contact with pre-pregnancy smokers to promote smoking cessation. The smoking cessation guidelines calling for 5 As (Ask, Advise, Assess, Assist, and Arrange for follow-up) should be used in office practice. Emphasis should be given to the benefits of cessation before women become pregnant.[57] This type of message could have a particularly strong impact in more-industrialized countries where women often have careers outside the home and delay pregnancy until they are older and consequently have concerns about fertility. In countries where access to obstetric and gynaecological medical care may be limited and where childbirth may be less medicalized, other providers, such as midwives, elders, and indigenous health-care providers, should be trained to promote quitting smoking before pregnancy.[58,59]

The challenge of preventing relapse must be addressed by the health-care providers who look after women during pregnancy.[1,60] When women who have quit smoking prior to their pregnancy come to the first prenatal visit, they are likely to report that they do not smoke. Unless a full smoking history is obtained, these women are likely to be considered as either never-smokers or former smokers and therefore are not counselled about the need to avoid re-starting smoking, although they are highly vulnerable to doing so. This group has not been well studied, as the women are usually not identified and included in pregnancy smoking cessation studies and are not followed by researchers. However, they seem more conscious of health risks of smoking both for themselves and for their babies and are often committed to becoming smoke-free not only for the pregnancy but for their entire life.[41] Pre-pregnancy

quitters typically sustain cessation throughout the pregnancy and postpartum period. Nevertheless, depending on the strength of the smoking habit and the depth of their motivation to quit, these women are vulnerable to a return to smoking, particularly if they experience a stressful event or a shift in environmental support during or after the pregnancy.[61] Although interventions and services for women who quit before pregnancy are clearly a lower priority than interventions and services for those who continue to smoke during pregnancy, a comprehensive approach to smoking cessation in pregnancy should recognize that these women have greater risks from smoking than never-smokers have, and they may need support to prevent postpartum relapse.

Newly Pregnant Spontaneous Quitters

Another group of women smokers quit smoking upon learning that they are pregnant or soon after, usually during the first trimester of pregnancy. They have been called "spontaneous quitters", and most are highly motivated to protect their babies from tobacco smoke.[62] They quit primarily for the health and welfare of the baby and often only secondarily for themselves.[63] These women who stop smoking "spontaneously" or without a formal intervention generally have higher socioeconomic status (SES) and educational attainment than those who do not stop.[55] In fact, there are often dramatic differences between the spontaneous quitters and the pregnant women who continue to smoke. Race, educational level, income, and employment status are primary characteristics on which the spontaneous quitters differ from those who continue to smoke.[54,64] For example, in the United States, less-educated, lower-SES, Caucasian, unemployed women who are more dependent on nicotine have the greatest risk of continued smoking during pregnancy.[41] In addition, the strength of nicotine addiction, measured by years of smoking and level of cotinine (a specific nicotine metabolite) in the body, is a predictor of whether a woman will continue smoking or will quit.[65] Finally, partner smoking is another important factor that influences whether a woman will quit spontaneously.[62,66] Spontaneous quitting or stopping smoking for the welfare of the baby usually happens early in the pregnancy and thus offers significant protection for the fetus. Therefore, women of childbearing age who become pregnant need to be reached with warnings and messages about the risks of smoking and the benefits of cessation. Depending on the methods for confirming pregnancy in various societies, messages could be delivered during pregnancy testing or during any contact or conversations with extended family or other pregnancy support systems, such as midwives.

In each country, detailed information should be gathered about spontaneous quitters and the motivations that enable them to stop smoking for extended periods of time, in order to understand the cultural forces and values that will promote early-pregnancy quitting. It should be noted that pregnant women in family-oriented cultures with involvement of extended families in the pregnancy often have lower smoking rates.[67,68] Cultural factors may include values and pressures that promote spontaneous quitting. Cultural sensitivity is critical in accessing the decisional factors that have the personal relevance and cultural support to tip decision-making towards change of an addictive behaviour.[69]

Most spontaneous quitters (80% to 85%) are able to maintain cessation of smoking throughout the pregnancy.[20,54,64,70] However, the majority of these women return to smoking during the postpartum period at rates that are high, considering the extended period of abstinence from cigarettes they have experienced.[61,71,72] Their rates of return to smoking by 6 months after the birth of the baby exceed 50% and can be as high as 80%; the relapse rate may be higher among the lower-SES mothers who were able to stop smoking during the pregnancy.[61,73]

In a 1996 study of return to smoking, researchers examined process-of-change variables (decisional balance, self-efficacy, and processes of change) among a group of women in Texas who quit smoking early in their pregnancies and compared them with those of women who were not pregnant but were in the process of quitting smoking. They found that many of the pregnant women were not actually quitting smoking but appeared to be simply stopping or suspending their smoking for the duration of the pregnancy.[39] When compared with non-pregnant women who were in various stages of change in the process of quitting smoking, the pregnant women who stopped smoking in early pregnancy looked like non-pregnant women smokers who were in earlier contemplation or preparation stages of change and were not similar to the non-pregnant women in the action stage of smoking cessation.[39,74] Many women who stop smoking while

pregnant suspend their smoking to provide protection for the fetus and are not engaged in intentionally quitting smoking for the rest of their lives. The lack of action-oriented cessation coping activities during the period of pregnancy may explain the very high relapse rate in the first 6 months of the postpartum period.[21,61,70]

The challenge for tobacco control is to prevent the postpartum return to smoking of these spontaneous quitters by shifting motivational considerations from an almost exclusive focus on protecting the baby to greater consideration of cessation for the health and well-being of the mother. This shift from more extrinsic to intrinsic considerations might increase specific cognitive and behavioural process activity during the last trimester of pregnancy and, most important, in the transition between pregnancy and the postpartum period. Stotts et al. found that by asking spontaneous quitters during their pregnancy about their postpartum goal related to cigarette smoking (to never smoke again, to smoke occasionally, or to return to smoking after breastfeeding) and about their self-efficacy to remain abstinent postpartum, they were able to predict the rate of return to smoking after the birth of the baby.[75] Most smoking cessation programmes and efforts to stop smoking during pregnancy, however, do not address the needs of spontaneous quitters. The smoking status of spontaneous quitters, like that of women who are pre-pregnancy quitters, is often ignored after the initial obstetric visit. These women receive few or no services to support cessation or to prevent relapse in the postpartum period. At the very least, relapse prevention services should be offered to these women at the beginning of the postpartum period.[76,77] A significant number of them resume smoking within 2 to 3 months (~ 45%) or 6 months (60 to 70%) postpartum or after they have stopped breastfeeding.[41,78-80]

Women Who Continue To Smoke During Pregnancy

Women who continue to smoke during pregnancy pose a challenge different from that of women who quit spontaneously either while preparing for pregnancy or upon learning that they are pregnant. The pregnant women who continue to smoke may differ substantially in socioeconomic characteristics from both those who stop and those of childbearing age generally.[41] The largest numbers of pregnant women who continue to smoke come from the subgroup of addicted smokers that includes lower-SES women smokers with fewer resources and more psychosocial problems, although this profile may vary by country. These continuing smokers may have multiple and complex problems, in addition to nicotine addiction.[43,46,73] They tend to have more psychological and emotional problems, less social support and financial resources, more family problems, and less residential stability than those who stop smoking.[64,65] Pregnancy is an additional stress producer because of the multiple problems these women already have, and smoking, for them, is a perceived stress reducer. Women who continue to smoke throughout a pregnancy also typically live in more smoke-filled home environments. Reaching pregnant women who continue to smoke with sustained, effective interventions that address the complicated context of their real-life problems has been a significant challenge.

Although difficult, it is not impossible to persuade women who continue to smoke even after they discover that they are pregnant to quit.[21,29] In fact, there is ample evidence that a significant number of women can be helped to quit smoking early in pregnancy with effective, low-intensity interventions. The literature strongly supports the efficacy of 5- to 15-minute cessation counselling sessions delivered by trained providers and accompanied by pregnancy-specific self-help materials. These brief interventions are significantly more effective than simple advice in increasing cessation rates of pregnant smokers.[81] A meta-analysis showed a summary risk ratio (weighted by the precision of each study's risk ratio) of 1.7 (95% CI = 1.3, 2.2) for successful cessation during pregnancy, an average improvement in cessation of 70% over standard practice; the confidence interval suggests that the outcome (cessation) was at least 30% higher in the treated groups than in the untreated groups. Studies included in this meta-analysis came from the United States, the United Kingdom, Sweden, Australia, and Canada. Moreover, there was a dose-response relationship, with contact time ranging from a half hour to an hour and a half. However, more-intensive periods of contact provided no additional benefit. A brief intervention strategy was least successful with more-dependent or addicted smokers.

Similar results have been highlighted in other reviews.[19,82] Lumley et al.,[16] in their Cochrane Collaboration review of interventions that promote smoking cessation in pregnancy, examined 64 trials that included 51 randomized control trials and six cluster-randomized trials with more than 28 000 participants. The smoking cessation intervention trials with cessation validated biochemically showed a significant reduction in smoking, with a relative risk (RR) of 0.94 (95% CI = 0.92, 0.95). Two trials that used reward plus social support achieved a greater smoking reduction than the others, resulting in a relative risk of 0.77 (95% CI = 0.72, 0.82).

Brief interventions early in pregnancy (less than 20 to 24 weeks) have helped women to quit smoking and thus have increased the pool of early-pregnancy quitters. Some interventions are based on the clinical practice guidelines promulgated by the Agency for Health Care Policy and Research.[83] These guidelines include a 5-step process that should be used in all health-care settings to the extent possible (see Table 9.2). The steps can be completed in five to 10 minutes in the health-care provider's office prior to or during pregnancy. *Ask*, the first step, includes checking on smoking status to determine if the pregnant woman is a never-smoker, quit before finding out she was pregnant, stopped after learning about the pregnancy, reduced her smoking during the pregnancy, or smoked about the same before the pregnancy as she does now. *Assessment* of readiness and motivation to quit follows firm but empathetically delivered *Advice* that emphasizes the fact that it would be in the best interest of the woman and the developing child for her to quit smoking. The *Assist* step usually connects the smoker with resources to choose from, including self-help materials specifically tailored for pregnant women and their families, nicotine replacement or other pharmacological aids (when medically appropriate), and referral to groups of other types of cessation programmes, quit lines, or other specific intervention, depending on the needs and requests of the smoker. *Arranging* for some type of follow-up and checking on progress over time is the critical last step in this intervention. These components have been determined to be helpful and to increase cessation among both the general population of smokers and pregnant women smokers.[81]

These interventions are also cost effective. Windsor et al.[30,84] have demonstrated the effectiveness of brief, well-executed interventions that use medical advice, videos, and self-help materials. They estimated that the cost of delivering a brief intervention on a large scale would be approximately US$ 6.00 per pregnant smoker in year 2000 dollars. According to their estimates, the cost–benefit ratio for an intervention that achieved a 15% smoking cessation rate, compared with the 5% cessation rate of usual practice, would be US$ 11 in savings for each US$ 1 of investment[19] although the costs of the programme and the savings from preventing the expenses for care of low-birth-weight babies would vary by country. The evidence shows that a brief, empirically supported intervention can have low delivery costs and can yield significant benefits, not only for the child and his or her family but for the entire health-care system.[3]

A number of countries have implemented national programmes that are based on the demonstrated efficacy of brief interventions and that combine pregnancy interventions with policy initiatives and other types of incentives and programmes for pregnant smokers. A 2005 conference highlighted these efforts in the United Kingdom,[85] New Zealand,[86] and Sweden.[87] In some programmes, midwives deliver cessation messages, often during home visits, while in others, the messages are delivered by the physician or nurse in the health-care setting. Most programmes include a variety of resources for women smokers, such as free or low-cost pharmacotherapy, access to telephone counselling through quit lines, self-help materials specifically tailored to women or more specifically to pregnant women, and, at times, more-intensive smoking cessation group or individual treatment.[16,88,89] Comprehensive programming offers the potential for synergy of effects. However, if resources are limited, introduction of a brief health-care-provider-based intervention that can reach the majority of women smokers should be the first priority for a community or nation to reduce the risks of tobacco exposure during pregnancy.

Later-Pregnancy Continuing Smokers

Cessation is very difficult for pregnant women who continue to smoke up to the third trimester, and they are not responsive to minimal interventions. Promoting cessation is even more difficult with women who have already had a child and smoked during the first pregnancy. These multiparous smokers typically believe that the harm of smoking is exaggerated because of their personal experiences of "successful" pregnancies while smoking, even if the previous children had low birth weight. In the Birmingham Trial II study, none of the women recruited between 24 and 32 weeks of gestation quit or significantly reduced their smoking.[30] More-dependent, heavier smokers have a greater probability of continuing to smoke, while light or moderate smokers are better able to stop earlier in a pregnancy.[65] The type and intensity of interventions needed to assist women who continue to smoke during the last trimester of pregnancy to quit have not been established. Several studies have focused on second- and third-trimester continuing smokers and examined different types of interventions. One study evaluated an intervention consisting of motivational interviewing strategies delivered over the telephone and enhanced with personalized feedback for continuing, resistant smokers.[90] Findings of lower cotinine levels at the end of pregnancy for the women who received the full programme of two telephone calls and a personalized feedback letter were promising. However, it was difficult to deliver the full intervention to these smokers, particularly in the last trimester. Women who continue to smoke late

---

Table 9.2. Agency for Health Care Policy and Research Guidelines: the 5 As

Step 1:	**Ask** about the smoking history and current smoking pattern of women in health-care settings. Record that information so that it is accessible throughout the pregnancy.
Step 2:	**Advise** each and every woman who smokes of the value of stopping and the risks of continuing in an empathetic, sensitive, clear, and personalized manner.
Step 3:	**Assess** the woman's motivation and thoughts related to smoking cessation or reduction.
Step 4:	**Assist** the smoker in any attempts to quit, with office-based, mailed, or other materials and the offer of referral to specific services to assist her in her efforts, from quit lines to more-intensive individual or group-focused programmes.
Step 5:	**Arrange** for a follow-up contact and continued contact throughout the pregnancy and postpartum period, through telephone calls, office or home visits, or the Internet.

World Health Organization

in pregnancy may need more-intensive interventions, but they are not motivated to stop smoking and are difficult to reach and engage, and they tend to believe that they are protecting the fetus in other ways.

Many pregnant women who continue to smoke throughout a pregnancy reduce the number of cigarettes smoked during that time.[91,92] The data indicate that they can reduce nicotine levels significantly (50% or more) and can sustain the reductions throughout the pregnancy. Reduction of smoking during pregnancy offers some measure of protection for the child.[91] Although reducing is less desirable than complete cessation and never provides as much protection, decreased exposure to the effects of smoking in utero is better for the developing fetus, especially in the later weeks of the pregnancy when significant fetal growth and development takes place. It may even be possible to gain some benefit for the fetus if the mother stops smoking right before the birthing, when needs for oxygen are high and smoking presents a greater threat. Whether it would be possible to influence continuing smokers to stop completely during the final days of pregnancy so that the actual delivery would be uncomplicated by the ingestion of smoke, nicotine, carbon monoxide, and smoking-related chemicals has not been tested. However, if cessation cannot be achieved, harm-reduction strategies such as stopping smoking for brief periods of time either during the pregnancy or at the delivery, significantly reducing the number of cigarettes smoked, and engaging in other health-protection behaviours, including taking vitamins and exercise,[93] should be considered as interventions.[29]

Postpartum Relapse and Cessation

The most problematic change in smoking status during the first 12 months of the postpartum period is a return to smoking by women who stopped during pregnancy. Equally troubling is an increase in the number of cigarettes smoked by those who reduced their amount of smoking significantly during pregnancy. Although increasing numbers of pregnant women are stopping or reducing smoking to protect their babies, the overall yield in terms of permanent reduction in smoking prevalence among women as a result of pregnancy leaves much to be desired, because of postpartum relapse.

During the postpartum period, many, if not most, spontaneous quitters and intervention-assisted quitters resume smoking. This return is delayed if women breastfeed, but estimates are that 50% to 70% of the women who stop smoking during pregnancy return to smoking regularly 6 to 12 months postpartum.[61,71–73]

In the general population, relapse prevention has not been very successful for smokers who quit for short periods of time or who stop smoking for a particular event such as pregnancy. The Cochrane Collaboration review of relapse prevention interventions concluded, "We detected no benefit of brief and 'skills-based' relapse prevention interventions for women who have quit smoking due to pregnancy or for smokers undergoing a period of enforced abstinence".[94] These authors also concluded that at present there is insufficient evidence to support the use of relapse prevention strategies for those who quit on their own or through cessation programmes.

The return to smoking postpartum is a significant problem, since the child of the smoker will be exposed to second-hand smoke (SHS). Preventing relapse simply by focusing on skills-based or cue-management strategies delivered to women is problematic. Although the evidence is not conclusive on the effectiveness of interventions, a variety have been designed to address this problem, including approaches that target the transition period between late pregnancy and immediately postpartum; are delivered in the paediatric-care system to reach parents of newborns and young children; include innovative efforts focusing on the environment and the partner who smokes; and attempt to incorporate pharmacotherapy for smoking cessation either during the pregnancy or immediately after the birth of the child.

Few interventions recognize and utilize the critical transition from pregnancy to the postpartum period marked by the birth of the baby as the opportunity for intervening to prevent a return to smoking. However, some interventions use nurses who deliver messages in the hospital after delivery, midwives who visit homes and assist during the immediate postpartum period, and messages that are delivered during well-baby visits.[37,77,95,96] Trials using these approaches have had mixed results, and even intensive, state-of-the-art motivational interventions delivered in women's homes by midwives have not always been successful.[97] One randomized, controlled trial, Project PANDA, developed an intervention in which videos and newsletters were mailed to the women and their partners, timed to arrive at intervals during the final weeks of pregnancy and the first six weeks postpartum.[63] The goal of this intervention was to prevent women who quit smoking for the pregnancy from returning to smoking at the time they were most vulnerable. Results from Project PANDA indicated significantly greater abstinence over the entire follow-up period and at the 12-month follow-up by the participants in the intervention group (55% vs 45%), supporting the idea that it is possible to decrease the return to smoking among these women. Women in the experimental condition were significantly more likely to be abstinent at almost every follow-up point than women in a standard-care control group. However, the total number of women who benefited from the intervention was small, and almost half returned to smoking. The period immediately after the birth of the child is a particularly difficult one for a new mother. The return to smoking appears to be facilitated by stress, lack of sleep, concerns about weight, and the ability to protect the baby from SHS. Interestingly, mothers who breastfeed seem to postpone the return to smoking until the baby is weaned.[77] Although the early postpartum period is a difficult time, some women who stop smoking during pregnancy might be motivated to stop permanently.[23,61,98,99]

The shift to new-baby and paediatric care offers another opportunity to intervene with women smokers who are now new mothers. Some women who continued to smoke during pregnancy may be able to quit during the postpartum period,[32] although few do so. Postpartum cessation is best related to increasing awareness of the effects of SHS on small babies or some problematic birth outcome that might be related to smoking. The 2006 US Surgeon General's report on involuntary exposure to tobacco smoke offers a strong rationale for preventing passive smoking exposure and offers strategies to address such exposure.[5] Unfortunately, however, the number of women who relapse during the postpartum period exceeds by far the number of women who smoked during pregnancy and quit postpartum.[71] Much needs to be done to decrease the SHS exposure of children living in households in which family members smoke. Increasing emphasis on partners and families can be helpful in addressing the exposure issue, as well as in promoting women's cessation of smoking.

Partner Smoking

Having a partner who smokes is probably the most important facilitator of a woman's continued smoking during pregnancy and her return to smoking during the postpartum period.[35,61,66,73] Most interventions for smoking during pregnancy concentrate on the woman and seldom offer messages about smoking in the home, and few address partner smoking. However, some interventions are beginning to use a partner's pregnancy as an opportunity to promote quitting by men. At a minimum, these interventions encourage male partners who are smoking to support and not undermine their partner's cessation during pregnancy and the postpartum period. One example of such an approach is Project PANDA. A secondary goal of that project was to provide an intervention to address partner smoking. Partners identified by the pregnant women were sent a set of video and print materials, similar to those sent to the pregnant smoker but tailored to the male perspective on pregnancy and child care, which tends to be more instrumental and focused on child-rearing. Materials were designed to promote cessation in light of impending fatherhood and to evoke support for the women during pregnancy; some emphasis on SHS exposure was also included. An initial evaluation of these materials indicated greater cessation among the men reported by the women in the intervention group than among those reported by the control-group women. Men appeared to read and use the materials sent to them, and the intervention appeared to make a small but significant difference in smoking; 28% of these men were not smoking at 3 months postpartum, compared with 14% of the control-group men. However, no differences were reported by the women at the 6- and 12-month follow-up visits.[34] Cessation of smoking by partners or spouses is critical for protecting newborns from exposure to tobacco smoke and offers another opportunity for the development and evaluation of innovative interventions.[34,35,62,99]

Using Nicotine Replacement or Pharmocotherapy During Pregnancy

There is growing evidence of the effectiveness of pharmacotherapy for quitting smoking in the general population of smokers. The findings point to equivalent

World Health Organization

efficacy for women and men.[3] Since the advent of these medications, tobacco control advocates have been interested in the feasibility of using nicotine replacement therapy (NRT) or cessation medications to help pregnant women stop smoking and sustain cessation.[81] To date, only a limited number of trials have examined the use of different forms of NRT or either bupropion or varenicline among pregnant women, and therefore definitive recommendations cannot be made. However, we review some of the current information about these pharmacological options below.

Both animal and human studies have demonstrated that nicotine has adverse neurodevelopmental effects on the fetus. These effects vary by dose and are found for exposure to both smoking and smokeless tobacco.[14,15,100] In a review of nicotine's effects during pregnancy, Wickstrom[15] concluded that even though nicotine obtained from NRT is safer than nicotine obtained from smoking, it is the total dose of nicotine received by the fetus that determines the effect on brain development. There is a concern, moreover, that higher doses of NRT and longer-acting replacement products may lead to higher doses of nicotine than those delivered by smoking. If NRT is viewed as a less risky alternative to smoking, it might encourage use of smokeless products and the promotion of new, "reduced exposure" products by tobacco companies. The use of NRT should always be envisaged only as a harm-reduction strategy for women who continue to smoke during pregnancy, in that it reduces exposure to other chemicals and, in particular, the CO generated by smoking cigarettes. There is no safe level of exposure to nicotine for the fetus. However, in cases where it is not possible to eliminate exposure to nicotine from cigarette smoking, verified reduced exposure would be a somewhat salutary goal for pregnant tobacco users.

Some studies have examined the effectiveness of adding NRT to behavioural treatments for smoking cessation. An open-label randomized trial called Baby Steps examined the addition of NRT to cognitive behavioural therapy (CBT) for 181 pregnant smokers who could choose between patch, gum, or lozenge.[101] Investigators found that women in the CBT + NRT group were significantly more likely to have biochemically validated cessation at two pregnancy time points (24% vs 8% after 7 weeks and 18% vs 7% at 38 weeks). However, differences were not significant at the 3-month postpartum follow-up

(20% vs 14%). This trial was suspended early because of some indication of a higher rate of negative birth outcomes in the NRT cohort, although this was found not to be significant when the rates were adjusted for prior history of pre-term births. Several other studies, reviewed by Schnoll et al.,[3] found that the nicotine patch had limited efficacy for pregnant women.

Nicotine gum is currently classified by the Food and Drug Administration (FDA) as a pregnancy category C drug (i.e. risks cannot be ruled out, but there are no adequate human studies to confirm this, and potential benefits may outweigh potential risks). Other formulations are category D (evidence of risk from human studies, but potential benefits may still outweigh potential risks).[3] Some important differences between the sexes also affect NRT efficacy. Women report more severe withdrawal from NRT than men, and pregnant women metabolize nicotine much faster than men and may require higher-dose patches. This need for more nicotine and larger doses of NRT raises concern about the risk to the fetus from nicotine exposure. There are no clear guidelines for the use of NRT by pregnant women,[102] and more research is needed to understand whether and how NRT should be used by them.

In addition to the nicotine-based medications, two medications currently on the market have shown sufficient efficacy for modifying smoking behaviour to be evaluated by the FDA, and bupropion was approved for the treatment of tobacco dependence in 1997.[3] The few studies that examined use of this drug for smoking cessation during pregnancy had inconclusive results.[103] Bupropion is currently rated as FDA pregnancy category C. Varenicline has also been approved for treating tobacco dependence and has an FDA pregnancy category C rating. No data are available on the safety of its use during pregnancy, but studies indicate that there are no differences in its efficacy between men and women.[3]

If medications or NRT can be used safely during pregnancy, they could offer some hope of increased cessation and possible assistance to prevent postpartum relapse. Additional studies are needed to evaluate these pharmacotherapy options. At present, we can recommend only that these medications and NRT be considered and studied to evaluate whether they can safely lessen the risk of smoke exposure for some women who are heavy smokers.

Conclusions and Actions

Most of the benefits of smoking cessation during pregnancy have focused on the fetus and the child. However, cessation programmes also help to improve the health and long-term well-being of mothers and fathers by reducing the incidence of cancer and other chronic illnesses caused by smoking. Pregnancy provides an opportunity for change. The challenges lie in finding the best methods to create a complete and comprehensive set of community and health-care programmes to eliminate smoking during pregnancy and fetal exposure, to protect newborn and developing children, to preserve the health and well-being of parents, and to create truly smoke-free families.

Reducing the personal and financial costs of smoking, particularly during pregnancy and following the birth of a child, are also important societal and economic goals. What are the critical approaches to interventions needed to meet these challenges? First, it is important to promote smoking cessation among women and men who are considering having a child by emphasizing cessation of tobacco use either prior to or as close to the beginning of pregnancy as possible. Potential parents can be reached in a variety of medical settings (especially gynaecological and obstetric settings), as well as through programmes and other health-care providers such as midwives, nurse practitioners, and genetic counsellors. Women of childbearing age and young families can also be targeted through media messaging about the benefits of smoking cessation. Such messages can even be incorporated into wedding preparations. These efforts would emphasize quitting smoking before becoming pregnant. This suggestion is consistent with recommendations for preconception counselling made a decade ago by an expert panel on the content of prenatal care.[60]

Cessation of smoking prior to pregnancy offers the best protection for infants and maximizes the possibility that women and men will integrate intrinsic motives about quitting for their own health with the motivation of quitting for their babies' health.[39,104] Including smoking cessation interventions in family planning programmes, in the distribution of various methods of birth control, and in pregnancy testing done at home or in clinic offices would provide opportunities to reach women smokers and their partners prior to pregnancy. In addition, with tobacco control messages that incorporate a focus on the health of both mother and baby, it may be possible to motivate quitting that will be more durable postpartum.

Second, tobacco control programmes should reach a pregnant smoker as early as possible in the pregnancy and follow her throughout the pregnancy to promote and support sustained smoking cessation. Women who have the most difficulty stopping smoking often are burdened by multiple life problems and a lack of adequate resources. Providing access to obstetric care as early as possible and embedding smoking cessation interventions in a comprehensive approach to these women's problems would appear to have the greatest chance of success. However, more intervention is not necessarily more efficacious.[105]

Three critical issues need to be addressed when creating pregnancy smoking cessation programmes. First, the identification of pregnant women at risk must incorporate a broad definition of smoking risk that includes women who quit before becoming pregnant. If women are concerned that labelling will bring harassment, they may be reluctant to self-identify as former smokers, and interventions will not reach and influence those most in need of them.[74,106,107] Sensitivity and tact are needed when addressing the issue of smoking with these women. Second, although many spontaneous quitters sustain cessation on their own throughout pregnancy, some need additional assistance. Sensitive probes and offers of support throughout the pregnancy rather than only at the first prenatal visit could be helpful to these women. Lastly, it is essential to create and sustain systems that ensure reliable, early, recurrent, and effective delivery of interventions throughout the pregnancy to all pregnant smokers. The system should include training of doctors, nurses, and staff in ob-gyn clinics, as well as midwives, nurse practitioners, and other alternative providers, in effective methods for counselling pregnant women about smoking. Educating them about the process of change and the windows of opportunity for intervention should be considered minimal preparation. They should also learn motivational and behavioural strategies to address each woman's concerns. Creating office, clinic, and home-care systems that institutionalize identification and intervention protocols is critical. While this is an ambitious agenda, the payoff would be significant in terms of both quality of life and health-care costs.[108] Research and clinical programmes that have already demonstrated efficacy can be used as models for creating intervention programmes for pregnant women in both public and private settings.[107]

Third, it is necessary to create interventions that shift the focus for women who stop smoking for the duration of their pregnancy to maintenance of cessation immediately after the birth and throughout the postpartum period. These interventions should be initiated near the end of the pregnancy, continue into the early postpartum period, and extend to at least one year postpartum, since many women return to smoking during this period. The interventions should shift motivational considerations from only protecting the fetus to protecting the health of the mother. Women who stop smoking only to protect the baby during the pre-pregnancy and pregnancy periods are the most vulnerable to relapse. Motivation and coping activities should shift to protecting the woman's health and longevity and should include creating a smoke-free family.[39, 73, 107]

Fourth, tobacco control programmes need to create a specific strategy and set of interventions for women who continue to smoke during the later stages of pregnancy. Intervention efforts should promote behaviours such as smoking reduction and abstinence during critical periods immediately prior to the birthing process. They should also encourage other health-protection behaviours, such as taking vitamins and exercising, and should emphasize the opportunity to stop smoking during the postpartum period. Many women who continue to smoke during pregnancy are concerned about the health of the baby but find it very difficult to stop. Some have had prior births with few serious or obvious consequences from smoking. Others are overwhelmed by emotional, financial, and family problems. Working with these women to achieve possible rather than optimal outcomes can contribute to the overall goals of protecting the baby and promoting cessation. Harm-reduction strategies are appropriate here and can facilitate movement towards optimal goals.[29,45,46] Newer cessation tools, such as medications and NRT, need to be explored for their potential utility with the difficult population of women who continue smoking during pregnancy.

Finally, and most important, tobacco control programmes must focus more on one of the most ignored targets of intervention: the spouse or partner of the woman smoker. Regardless of his or her smoking status, the spouse or partner of the pregnant woman is, in almost all cases, an important part of the pregnancy. Despite the fact that partners who smoke have been identified as a risk factor for women's smoking during pregnancy and

for postpartum relapse,[66] few interventions include them. Cessation efforts during pregnancy should include spouses or partners as important targets and allies in the effort to create a smoke-free family. Pregnancy may be a very opportune time to intervene in smoking and other health habits of the partner. Parenthood brings a re-evaluation of lifestyle and family needs that offers an ideal opportunity to engage other members of the family in a discussion of values and health behaviours.

In sum, pregnancy offers multiple windows of opportunity for smoking cessation intervention. The course of pregnancy and the reality of the postpartum period create a prime target for cessation efforts. The goal of creating smoke-free families, however, must be achieved through a comprehensive tobacco control programme based on early prevention, as well as gender-specific service delivery. Understanding the process of change for smoking during pregnancy and using empirically supported treatments can provide guidance about how to promote healthy lifestyles for the entire family.

References

1. *The health consequences of smoking for women. a report of the Surgeon General.* Rockville, MD, US Public Health Service, Office on Smoking and Health, 1980.
2. Floyd RL et al. A review of smoking in pregnancy: effects on pregnancy outcomes and cessation efforts. *Annual Review of Public Health*, 1993. 14:379–411.
3. Schnoll R, Patterson F, Lerman C. Treating tobacco dependence in women. *Journal of Women's Health*, 2007, 16:1211–1218.
4. US Department of Health and Human Services. *2004 Surgeon General's report—the health consequences of smoking.* Atlanta, GA, Centers for Disease Control and Prevention, 2004 (http://www.cdc.gov/tobacco/data_statistics/sgr/sgr_2004/chapters.htm).
5. *The health consequences of involuntary exposure to tobacco smoke: a report of the Surgeon General.* Rockville, MD, US Department of Health and Human Services, Centers for Disease Control and Prevention, 2006.
6. Tager IB, Ngo L, Hanrahan JP. Maternal smoking during pregnancy. Effects on lung function during the first 18 months of life. *American Journal of Respiratory and Critical Care Medicine*, 1995, 152:977–983.
7. Hu FB et al. Prevalence of asthma and wheezing in public schoolchildren: association with maternal smoking during pregnancy. *Annals of Allergy, Asthma & Immunology*, 1997, 79:80–84.
8. Moshammer H et al. Parental smoking and lung function in children: an international study. *American Journal of Respiratory and Critical Care Medicine*, 2006, 173:1255–1263.
9. Shea A, Steiner M. Cigarette smoking during pregnancy. *Nicotine & Tobacco Research*, 2008, 10:267–278.
10. Aligne CA, Stoddard JJ. Deaths and injuries from house fires. *New England Journal of Medicine*, 2001, 345:14; reply 1065.
11. Farber HJ et al. Second hand tobacco smoke in children with asthma: sources of and parental perceptions about children's exposure, and parental readiness to change. *Chest*, 2008, 133:1367–1374.
12. Campaign for Tobacco-Free Kids. *Women and tobacco: global trends*, 2007 (http://tobaccofreecenter.org/sites/default/files/WomenandTobacco.pdf).
13. *The global burden of disease: 2004 update.* Geneva, World Health Organization, 2008.

World Health Organization

14. Slotkin, TA. If nicotine is a developmental neurotoxicant in animal studies, dare we recommend nicotine replacement therapy in pregnant women and adolescents? *Neurotoxicology and Teratology*, 2008, 30:1–19.

15. Wickstrom R. Effects of nicotine during pregnancy: human and experimental evidence. *Current Neuropharmacology*, 2007, 5:213–222.

16. Lumley J et al. Interventions for promoting smoking cessation during pregnancy. *The Cochrane Database of Systematic Reviews*, 2004, 3.

17. Sexton M, Hebel R. A clinical trial of change in maternal smoking and its effect on birth weight. *Journal of the American Medical Association*, 1984, 251:911–915.

18. Kramer MS. Determinants of low birth weight: methodological assessment and meta-analysis. *Bulletin of the World Health Organization*, 1987, 65:663–737.

19. Windsor RA. Smoking, cessation and pregnancy, in women and the tobacco epidemic: challenges for the 21st century. In: Samet JM, Yoon SY, eds. *Women and the tobacco epidemic: challenges for the 21st century*. Geneva, World Health Organization, 2001.

20. Li CQ et al. The impact on infant birth weight and gestational age of cotinine-validated smoking reduction during pregnancy. *Journal of the American Medical Association*, 1993, 269:1519–1524.

21. Dolan-Mullen P, Ramirez G, Groff J. A meta-analysis of randomized trials of prenatal smoking cessation interventions. *American Journal of Obstetrics & Gynecology*, 1994, 171:1328–1334.

22. Ershoff D, Mullen P, Quinn V. A randomized trial of a serialized self-help smoking cessation program for pregnant women in an HMO. *American Journal of Public Health*, 1989, 79:182–187.

23. Secker-Walker RH et al. Reducing smoking during pregnancy and postpartum: physician's advice supported by individual counselling. *Preventive Medicine*, 1998, 27:422.

24. Kendrick J et al. Integrating smoking cessation into routine public prenatal care: the Smoking Cessation in Pregnancy Project. *American Journal of Public Health*, 1995, 85:217–222.

25. Lowe JB, Balanda K, Clare G. Evaluation of antenatal smoking cessation programmes for pregnant women. *Australian and New Zealand Journal of Public Health*, 1998, 22:55–59.

26. Valbo A, Nylander G. Smoking cessation in pregnancy: intervention among heavy smokers. *Acta Obstetricia et Gynecologica Scandinavica*, 1994, 73:215–219.

27. Walsh RA et al. A smoking cessation program at a public antenatal clinic. *American Journal of Public Health*, 1997, 87:1201.

28. Windsor RA et al. The effectiveness of smoking cessation methods for smokers in public health maternity clinics: a randomized trial. *American Journal of Public Health*, 1985, 75:1389–1392.

29. Windsor RA, Boyd NR, Orleans CT. A meta-evaluation of smoking cessation intervention research among pregnant women: improving the science and art. *Health Education Research*, 1998, 13:419–438.

30. Windsor RA et al. Health education for pregnant smokers: its behavioural impact and cost–benefit. *American Journal of Public Health*, 1993, 83:201–206.

31. Windsor RA, Warner KE, Cutter GR. A cost-effectiveness analysis of self-help smoking cessation methods for pregnant women. *Public Health Reports*, 1988, 103:83–87.

32. Severson HH et al. Reducing maternal smoking and relapse: long-term evaluation of a paediatric intervention. *Preventive Medicine*, 1997, 26:120–130.

33. Stephenson KR, Allen PJ. The role of paediatric primary care providers in parental smoking cessation: assessing and motivating parents to quit. *Paediatric Nursing*, 2007, 33:434–441.

34. DiClemente CC et al. Intervention effects on pregnant quitters' partners' smoking. *Proceedings of the Annual Meeting of the Society of Behavioural Medicine, New Orleans, 9–12 March 1998*.

35. Wakefield M, Jones W. Effects of a smoking cessation program for pregnant women and their partners attending a public hospital antenatal clinic. *Australian and New Zealand Journal of Public Health*, 1998, 22:313–320.

36. Depue JD et al. Assessment of parents' smoking behaviours at a paediatric emergency department. *Nicotine & Tobacco Research*, 2007, 9:33–41.

37. Hannover W, Roske K, Thyrian JR, eds. *Smoking cessation and relapse prevention in women post partum: minutes from the International Workshop in Greifswald, September 2005*. Lengerich, Pabst Science Publishers, 2007.

38. DiClemente CC, Dolan-Mullen P, Windsor, RA. The process of pregnancy smoking cessation: implications for interventions. *Tobacco Control*, 2000, 9 (Suppl. 3):III16–21.

39. Stotts A et al. Pregnancy smoking cessation: a case of mistaken identity. *Addictive Behaviours*, 1996, 21:459–471.

40. *WHO report on the global tobacco epidemic, 2009: implementing smoke-free environments*. Geneva, World Health Organization, 2009.

41. Kahn RS, Certain L, Whitaker RC. A reexamination of smoking before, during, and after pregnancy. *American Journal of Public Health*, 2002, 92:1801–1808.

42. Bergen AW, Caporaso N. Cigarette smoking. *Journal of the National Cancer Institute*, 1999, 91:1365–1375.

43. Mullen PD et al. Relations among psychosocial variables, addiction, and self-efficacy in lower and higher income pregnant smokers. *Proceedings of the Annual Meeting of the Society for Research on Nicotine and Tobacco*, 1999:5–7.

44. Manfredi C et al. A path model of smoking cessation in women smokers of low socio-economic status. *Health Education Research*, 2007, 22:747–756.

45. Walsh R et al. Predictors of smoking in pregnancy and attitudes and knowledge of risks of pregnant smokers. *Drug & Alcohol Review*, 1997, 61:41–67.

46. Paarlberg K et al. Smoking status in pregnancy is associated with daily stressors and low well-being. *Psychology & Health*, 1999, 14:87–96.

47. Anderson SJ, Glantz SA, Ling PM. Emotions for sale: cigarette advertising and women's psychosocial needs. *Tobacco Control*, 2005, 14:127–135.

48. Levine MD et al. Weight concerns affect motivation to remain abstinent from smoking postpartum. *Annals of Behavioural Medicine*, 2006, 32:147–153.

49. Berman B, Gritz E. Women and smoking: current trends and issues for the 1990's. *Journal of Substance Abuse*, 1991, 3:221–238.

50. Nichter M et al. Smoking among low-income pregnant women: an ethnographic analysis. *Health Education & Behaviour*, 2007, 34:748–764.

51. *WHO report on the global tobacco epidemic, 2008: the MPOWER package*. Geneva, World Health Organization, 2008.

52. Ruggiero L et al. Identification and recruitment of low-income pregnant smokers: who are we missing? *Addictive Behaviours*, 2003, 28:1497–1505.

53. Mcbride CM, Emmons KM, Lipkus IM. Understanding the potential of teachable moments: the case of smoking cessation. *Health Education Research*, 2003, 18:156–170.

54. Quinn VP, Mullen PD, Ershoff DH. Women who stop smoking spontaneously prior to prenatal care and predictors of relapse before delivery. *Addictive Behaviours*, 1991, 6:153–160.

55. National Center for Health Statistics/Center for Disease Control, Smoking during pregnancy, 1990–96. *National Vital Statistics Reports*, 1998, 47:1–12.

56. Hymowitz N et al. Postpartum relapse to cigarette smoking in inner city women. *Journal of the National Medical Association*, 2003, 95:461–474.

57. Schnoll RA, Patterson F, Lerman C. Treating tobacco dependence in women. *Journal of Women's Health (2002)*, 2007, 16:1211–1218.

58. Cookson T. Partnerships in general practice - the MATPRO experience. *New Zealand Family Physicians*, 1998, 25:33–34.

59. Mcleod D et al. Can support and education for smoking cessation and reduction be provided effectively by midwives within primary maternity care? *Midwifery*, 2004, 20:37–50.

60. *Caring for our future: the content of prenatal care*. Washington, DC, US Department of Health and Human Services, 1989.

61. Mullen P et al. Postpartum return to smoking: who is at risk and when. *American Journal of Health Promotion*, 1997, 11:323–330.

62. Appleton P, Pharoah P. Partner smoking behaviour change is associated with women's smoking reduction and cessation during pregnancy. *British Journal of Health Psychology*, 1998, 3:361–374.

63. Dolan-Mullen PD, DiClemente CC, Bartholomew LK. Theory and context in project PANDA: a program to help postpartum women stay off cigarettes. In: *Intervention mapping: designing theory- and evidence-based health promotion programmes*. Mountain View, CA, Mayfield, 2001:453–476.

64. Panjari M et al. Women who spontaneously quit smoking in early pregnancy. *Australian and New Zealand Journal of Obstetrics and Gynecology*, 1997, 37:271–278.

World Health Organization

65. Woodby LL et al. Predictors of smoking cessation during pregnancy. *Addiction*, 1999, 94:283–292.

66. McBride C et al. Partner smoking and pregnant smoker's perceptions of support for and likelihood of smoking cessation. *Health Psychology*, 1998, 17:63–69.

67. McLeod D, Pullon S, Cookson T. Factors that influence changes in smoking behaviour during pregnancy. *The New Zealand Medical Journal*, 2003, 116:U418–U418.

68. Walsh RA, Lowe JB, Hopkins PJ. Quitting smoking in pregnancy. *The Medical Journal of Australia*, 2001, 175:320–323.

69. DiClemente CC. *Addiction and change: how addictions develop and addicted people recover.* New York, NY, The Guildford Press, 2003.

70. Fingerhut L, Kleinman J, Kendrick J. Smoking before, during and after pregnancy. *American Journal of Public Health*, 1990, 80:541–544.

71. McBride CM, Pirie PL. Postpartum smoking relapse. *Addictive Behaviours*, 1990, 15:165–168.

72. Polanska K, Hanke W, Sobala W. Smoking relapse one year after delivery among women who quit smoking during pregnancy. *International Journal of Occupational Medicine and Environmental Health*, 2005, 18:159–165.

73. Ko, M, Schulken, ED. Factors related to smoking cessation and relapse among pregnant smokers. *American Journal of Health Behaviours*, 1998, 22:83–89.

74. DiClemente CC et al. Toward a comprehensive, transtheoretical model of change: stages of change and addictive behaviours. In: Miller W, Heather N, eds. *Treating Addictive Behaviours*, 2nd ed. New York, NY: Plenum Press, 1998, 3–24.

75. Stotts AL et al. Postpartum return to smoking: staging a "suspended" behaviour. *Health Psychology*, 2000, 19:324.

76. Mullen PD. How can more smoking suspension during pregnancy become lifelong abstinence? Lessons learned about predictors, interventions, and gaps in our accumulated knowledge. *Nicotine & Tobacco Research*, 2004, 6 (Suppl. 2):217–S238.

77. Ratner PA et al. Twelve-month follow-up of a smoking relapse prevention intervention for postpartum women. *Addictive Behaviours*, 2000, 25:81–92.

78. Mullen PD, Quinn VP, Ershoff DH. Maintenance of nonsmoking postpartum by women who stopped smoking during pregnancy. *American Journal of Public Health*, 1990, 80:992–994.

79. Letourneau A et al. Timing and predictors of postpartum return to smoking in a group of inner-city women: an exploratory pilot study. *Birth*, 2007, 34:245–252.

80. Colman GJ, Joyce T. Trends in smoking before, during, and after pregnancy in ten states. *American Journal of Preventive Medicine*, 2003, 24:29–35.

81. Melvin C et al. Recommended cessation counselling for pregnant women who smoke: a review of the evidence. *Tobacco Control*, 2000, 9:80–84.

82. Melvin C, Gaffney C. Treating nicotine use and dependence of pregnant and parenting smokers: an update. *Nicotine & Tobacco Research*, 2004, 6 (Suppl. 2):S107–S124.

83. Fiore MC (Chair, Guideline Panel). *AHCPR supported clinical practice guidelines. 18. Treating tobacco use and dependence: 2008 update.* Rockville, MD, Agency for Healthcare Research and Quality, US Department of Health and Human Services, 2008.

84. Windsor R et al. The effectiveness of smoking cessation methods for smokers in public health maternity clinics: a randomized trial. *American Journal of Public Health*, 1985, 75:1389–1392.

85. Percival J. Smoking: tackling the silent epidemic. *Journal of Family Health Care*, 2007, 17:109–110.

86. McLeod D. Putting theory into practice. In: Hannover W, Roske K, Thyrian JR, eds. *Smoking cessation and relapse prevention in women post partum: minutes from the international workshop in Greifswald, September 2005.* Lengerich, Pabst, 2007.

87. Lennartsson U. Smoke-free children: a report from the successful 10-year project in Sweden. In: Hannover W, Roske K, Thyrian JR, eds. *Smoking cessation and relapse prevention in women post partum: minutes from the international workshop in Greifswald, September 2005.* Lengerich, Pabst, 2007.

88. Hegaard HK et al. Multimodal intervention raises smoking cessation rate during pregnancy. *Acta Obstetricia et Gynecologica Scandinavica*, 2003, 82:813–819.

89. Pullon S et al. Smoking cessation in New Zealand: education and resources for use by midwives for women who smoke during pregnancy. *Health Promotion International*, 2003, 18:315–325.

90. DiClemente CC, Mullen PD, Stotts AL. One-to-one: a motivational intervention for resistant pregnant smokers. *Addictive Behaviours*, 2002, 27:275.

91. Li C et al. The impact on birthweight and gestational age of cotinine validated smoking reduction during pregnancy. *Journal of the American Medical Association*, 1993, 269:1519–1524.

92. Windsor R et al. The use of significant reduction rates to evaluate health education methods for pregnant smokers: a new harm reduction behavioural indicator? *Health Education & Behaviour*, 1999, 26:648–662.

93. Hanna E, Faden V, Dufour M. The effects of substance use during gestation on birth outcome, infant and maternal health. *Journal of Substance Abuse*, 1997, 9:111–126.

94. Hajek P et al. Relapse prevention interventions for smoking cessation. *Cochrane Database of Systematic Reviews*, 2005, 1.

95. Johnson JL et al. Preventing smoking relapse in postpartum women. *Nursing Research*, 2000, 49:44–52.

96. French GM et al. Staying smoke free: an intervention to prevent postpartum relapse. *Nicotine & Tobacco Research*, 2007, 9:663–670.

97. Tappin DM et al. Randomised controlled trial of home based motivational interviewing by midwives to help pregnant smokers quit or cut down. *British Medical Journal*, 2005, 331:373–377.

98. Mullen PD et al. *Project PANDA: Maintenance of prenatal smoking abstinence 12 months postpartum.* 1999 (unpublished manuscript).

99. McBride CM et al. Prevention of relapse in women who quit smoking during pregnancy. *American Journal of Public Health*, 1999, 89:706.

100. Dempsey DA, Benowitz NL. Risks and benefits of nicotine and other medications to aid smoking cessation in pregnancy. *Drug Safety*, 2001, 24:277–322.

101. Pollack KI et al. Nicotine replacement and behavioural therapy for smoking cessation in pregnancy. *American Journal of Preventive Medicine*, 2007, 33:297–305.

102. Coleman T, Britton J, Thornton J. Nicotine replacement therapy in pregnancy is probably safer than smoking. *British Medical Journal*, 2004, 328:965–966.

103. Chan B, Einarson A, Koren G. Effectiveness of bupropion for smoking cessation during pregnancy. *Journal of Addictive Diseases*, 2005, 24:19–23.

104. DiClemente C. Motivation for change: implications for substance abuse treatment. *Psychological Science*, 1999, 10:209–213.

105. Ershoff D et al. The Kaiser Permanente prenatal smoking cessation trial: when more isn't better, what is enough? *American Journal of Preventive Medicine*, 1999, 17:161–168.

106. Solomon LJ et al. Stages of change in smoking during pregnancy in low-income women. *Journal of Behavioural Medicine*, 1996, 19:333–344.

107. Mullen PD, Maternal smoking during pregnancy and evidence-based intervention to promote cessation. *Primary Care*, 1999, 26:577–589.

108. Institute of Medicine. *Ending the tobacco problem: a blueprint for the nation.* Washington, DC, National Academies Press, 2007.

World Health Organization

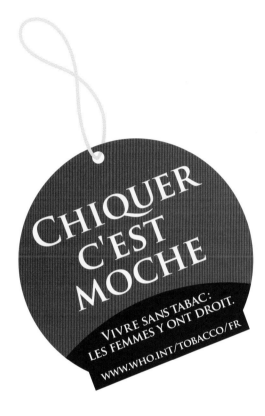

CHIQUER C'EST MOCHE

VIVRE SANS TABAC :
LES FEMMES Y ONT DROIT.
WWW.WHO.INT/TOBACCO/FR

SMOKING
IS UGLY

WWW.WHO.INT/TOBACCO

Style? No, gangrene.

Protect women from
tobacco marketing
and smoke.

31MAY: WORLDNOTOBACCODAY

World Health
Organization

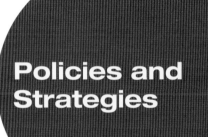

Policies and Strategies

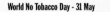

10. How to Make Policies More Gender-Sensitive

Introduction

Although tobacco control policies have been on record since the late 1800s, most of the early tobacco control legislation focused on policies banning sales of tobacco to youth. For example, an 1890 District of Columbia ordinance prohibited the sale of cigarettes to minors in the United States,[1] and in 1900, smoking by persons under 20 years of age was prohibited in Japan, where the sale of cigarettes to minors was also banned.[2] Once the epidemiological evidence on the relationship between smoking and lung cancer and other diseases emerged,[3–6] tobacco control initiatives began to focus more broadly on prevention and cessation of smoking for the public's health.

Until recently, tobacco control initiatives did not reflect the population's diversity and did not specifically address women's concerns. Diversity was lacking in policy largely because it was missing in the early epidemiological research that fuelled such policy. Because the smoking epidemic started primarily among upper-class men in industrialized countries, men were hit first by its devastating health consequences, making them prime targets for research. At the time, women were considered a minority of the smoking population and were not of great interest to clinicians. As a result, a significant opportunity was lost in early research to study ways in which smoking might affect women's health. Because of this missing research demographic, most policies were crafted without concern for the rates of smoking or tobacco-related disease among women. Fortunately, this male-centred approach has since been challenged, and new directions are being sought.

This chapter examines a policy model for understanding the relationship between gender and tobacco control with a focus on women. In addition, it highlights the tobacco control policies of four countries—China, South Africa, Sweden, and the United Kingdom—to provide four distinct case-studies that depict the incorporation (or non-incorporation) of gender into health policy. These countries were selected because they exemplify industrialized and developing countries at differing stages of tobacco control

programme development with varying rates of smoking prevalence among women.

South Africa and China represent expanding markets for the tobacco industry, and women are being specifically targeted by marketing efforts. Sweden provides an interesting case-study, as it is one of the few countries in which the smoking prevalence of women is higher than that of men.[7] Finally, the United Kingdom, though similar to other industrialized countries in terms of smoking prevalence rates, provides some contrast to those countries because of its relatively late adoption of stringent tobacco control policies.

While the four countries selected as case-studies in no way represent the full diversity of political, economic, and social contexts or the diversity of tobacco control policies, they do offer insights into ways in which the content of tobacco policies can address both gender inequality and women as a group. While there are considerable gaps in national data concerning the effects of tobacco control policies on women, current evidence points to interesting trends and advocacy issues for the future. Table 10.1 presents age-standardized smoking prevalence among adult (15 years and older) males and females in the four countries.

A Framework for Gender-Sensitive Policy

Gender has long been established as a major factor in women's health, affecting the occurrence, etiology, treatment, and eventual outcome of illness. The concept of gender refers specifically to men's and women's socially determined roles and responsibilities.[8,9] It is distinct from men's and women's biological and reproductive characteristics, because it is shaped by historical, cultural, economic, and political constructs. By definition, then, gender constructs can be changed and may permeate institutions as well as influence individual actions. It is important to note that the sex-based (or biology-based) differences between men and women also impact men's and women's morbidity and mortality.[9]

As described by Greaves and Jategaonkar[10] and in the chapter on a gender equality framework in this monograph, gender has become an important factor in smoking

World Health Organization

behaviour. Historically, men have had higher rates of smoking prevalence than women. However, data from the Global Youth Tobacco Survey (GYTS) suggest that smoking rates of adolescent females are higher than those of adolescent males in the United States, as well as in some countries in Europe and South America. The survey also indicates women's differential exposure to second-hand smoke (SHS) in households and workplaces. In some settings, women may be unable to avoid environmental tobacco smoke because of power imbalances between men and women. There is also an interaction between socio-economic status (SES) and gender, which influences the motivations for smoking initiation and smoking cessation. This interaction underlies much of the current policy debate surrounding gender-sensitive policies.[10–14]

The tobacco control policies of the four countries examined in this chapter can be classified according to their gender sensitivity. According to Kabeer,[15] whose work has shaped much of the research and action on gender equality in the development field, the first step in analysis is to look at the different ways that gender is present or absent in policies.

Gender-blindness is the ignoring of the socially determined gender roles, responsibilities, and capabilities of men and women. Gender-blind policies, though they may appear to be unbiased, are often, in fact, based on information derived from men's activities and/or the assumption that women affected by the policies have the

---

Table 10.1. **Age-Standardized Current Tobacco Smoking Prevalence of Men and Women in China, South Africa, Sweden, and the United Kingdom**

Smoking prevalence (%)

Country	Men	Women
China	59	4
South Africa	29	9
Sweden	17	23
United Kingdom	26	24

Source: Ref. 22.

---

same needs and interests as men.[16] For example, policies that target a particular population of smokers (e.g. all smokers or young smokers) may be based exclusively on men's experiences and needs.

> *Gender-blind policies, though they may appear to be unbiased, are often, in fact, based on information derived from men's activities and/or the assumption that all persons affected by the policies have the same needs and interests as males.*

In contrast to gender-blind policies, *gender-sensitive policies* take gender relations into account. Kabeer's framework describes three types of gender-sensitive policies: gender-neutral, gender-specific, and gender-redistributive. Gender-sensitive policies take into account the different social roles of men and women that lead to women and men having different needs. The three types of policies are described below.

Gender-neutral policies are not aimed specifically at either men or women and are assumed to affect both sexes equally. A gender-neutral policy allocates resources to meet specific goals, such as reducing the number of young people who initiate smoking. Gender-neutral legislation could include the banning of tobacco advertising and control of SHS through regulation of smoking in public places and workplaces. Taxation of tobacco and restrictions on places where smoking is permitted may be viewed as gender-neutral policies. While these types of policies are gender-neutral by design, their impact may, in fact, be gendered.

Gender-specific policies acknowledge that women's gender-related needs have been neglected in the past and advocate on behalf of gender equality. Such policies identify specific strategies that are appropriate for women. Gender-specific tobacco control policies acknowledge the different socioeconomic and cultural factors that contribute to tobacco use among women, as compared with men. Under these policies, specific programmes are implemented that address the needs and interests of women, while continuing to address the needs of men. For example, since health-worker interventions have proven effective in influencing clients to stop smoking, some tobacco control policies train health workers to use smoking cessation methods and messages that are specific to pregnant women. These programmes improve the health of both the women and their fetuses. Programmes that target pregnant women are by their nature gender-specific (owing to women's biological capacity for reproduction).[12]

Gender-redistributive policies recognize that because of political and economic inequality, women are often excluded or disadvantaged in terms of access to social and

economic resources and involvement in decision-making. The goal of gender-redistributive policies is to rebalance the power structure to create a more balanced relationship between men and women. The policies therefore target both sexes, either simultaneously or separately. Implicit in gender-redistributive policies is the notion that they have the potential to "create supportive conditions for women to empower themselves".[17] For example, granting microcredit loans to women is a redistributive policy, as it changes the balance of financial resources between men and women in the household. Greaves and Tungohan[11] suggest that combining tobacco control with housing or child-care programmes has the potential to "transform gender relations", which is the ultimate goal of redistributive policies.

Figure 10.1. Kabeer's Framework for Gender-Sensitive Policies

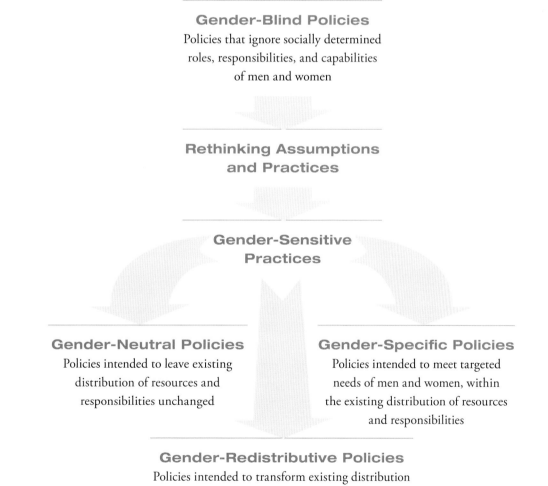

Gender-Blind Policies
Policies that ignore socially determined
roles, responsibilities, and capabilities
of men and women

**Rethinking Assumptions
and Practices**

**Gender-Sensitive
Practices**

Gender-Neutral Policies
Policies intended to leave existing
distribution of resources and
responsibilities unchanged

Gender-Specific Policies
Policies intended to meet targeted
needs of men and women, within
the existing distribution of resources
and responsibilities

Gender-Redistributive Policies
Policies intended to transform existing distribution
of resources to create balanced gender relationships

Source: Adapted from March, Smyth, and Mukhopadhyay.[17]

World Health Organization

It should be noted that in circumstances where the norm has been gender-blind policies, gender-neutral policies could represent a step forward. It is also possible that gender-redistributive policies may not be the best solution in all circumstances.[17]

Figure 10.1 presents a framework for Kabeer's gender-sensitive policies.

Ideally, tobacco control policy could lead to the transformation of gender relations in other domains. More often than not, however, tobacco policy tends to exploit existing gender relations or accommodate and reinforce them.[11] For example, tobacco control policies that specifically target women for "protection" can be viewed as paternalistic. Likewise, marketing that focuses on women's independence or liberation exploits existing gender inequalities. Programmes that target pregnant women or smoking at home in the presence of children can be viewed as accommodating and reinforcing women's traditional gender roles without doing anything to change them. Tobacco control has the potential to go beyond simply reducing women's vulnerabilities to tobacco and to move towards the achievement of greater gender equity.[11]

> *Gender-redistributive policies recognize that because of political and economic inequality, women are often excluded or disadvantaged in terms of access to social and economic resources and involvement in decision-making.*

The WHO Framework Convention on Tobacco Control (WHO FCTC)[18,19] specifically calls for women's participation in policy-making and policy implementation. Articles 6–17 of the WHO FCTC[18] detail policy measures that should be enacted to reduce both the supply and demand of tobacco. The following discussion highlights the supply- and demand-side measures that provide the greatest opportunity for gender-sensitive policy development.

Measures Favouring Gender-Sensitive Policy Development

Price and Tax Measures

The effect of imposing taxes is indicated by price elasticity, a measure of change in consumption in response to a specified change in price. Depending on the population of smokers surveyed, the price elasticity of tobacco ranges from –0.4 to –0.8, meaning that a 10% increase in cigarette price will yield a 4% to 8% decrease in the number of cigarettes smoked.[20] Studies have shown that one of the clearest and most immediate influences on tobacco use is the price of tobacco products. Tobacco control policies that include taxation of tobacco products therefore reduce tobacco consumption.[21] This is elaborated in the chapter in this monograph on taxation and the economics of tobacco control.

Article 6 of the WHO FCTC[18] encourages Parties to adopt price and tax measures as an "effective and important means of reducing tobacco consumption by various segments of the population". The treaty is very direct in saying that this measure is intended to curtail smoking among young people who are most sensitive to price changes. Studies from the United States confirm the consistent price sensitivity of young people. The fact that young female smokers outnumber young male smokers in many industrialized countries indicates that young women are substantially affected by increases in tobacco prices.[22]

Adults are also affected by increasing cigarette prices. Although evidence is mixed as to whether adult women are more sensitive than men to changes in price, it is clear that individuals from lower socioeconomic backgrounds are more price-sensitive than their wealthier counterparts. In the United States, adolescent males are more sensitive to price than adolescent females are, while in the United Kingdom, females are more sensitive to price. In the lowest socioeconomic groups, smoking prevalence among both males and females is correlated with the price of tobacco products.[23]

Although measures to increase tobacco prices are applied equally to men and women (i.e. are gender-neutral), it is important to recognize that the consequences of such measures are gender-specific—more women than men are affected by increasing prices, because a greater proportion of the poor are women.[24] Greaves and Tungohan[11] suggest that in addition to assistance in implementing taxes or raising prices, assistance with cessation or social support to ensure that addicted women are not doubly disadvantaged by gender and income inequalities should be included as countries implement the provisions of the WHO FCTC.

All four of the countries examined in this chapter have some form of consumer-incurred tobacco tax, but the degree to which taxation is used as a tobacco control measure varies greatly. Sweden increased taxes on tobacco in 1996 and 1997, and consumption decreased with each increase in price. Taxation was reduced in 1998, however, because of a perceived increase in smuggling (and a lack of public support for the tax increases).[25] Interestingly and somewhat unexpectedly, the overall prevalence of smoking remained similar in the years before and after the tax repeal (19.1% in 1998 and 19.3% in 1999) and continued to decrease through 2005.[26]

Limiting cigarette consumption by increasing taxation was the primary focus of South Africa's first tobacco control strategy in the 1990s.[27] In South Africa and the United Kingdom, consumption decreased with an increase in taxation that raised the real price of cigarettes.[28] However, changes in consumption were not compared across sex and age. An oversight in the taxation policy in South Africa is the exclusion of snuff, which is used primarily by rural women.

China, the largest grower of tobacco leaf in the world, has been reluctant to increase tobacco taxes for fear of damaging its own economy. At present, China has some of the world's lowest taxes on tobacco products.[22] The Chinese government has acknowledged the health risks of smoking and has discussed a variety of tobacco control options (e.g. bans on advertising) but has failed to increase tobacco taxes to reduce consumption.[29] Upon ratifying the WHO FCTC, the Chinese government issued a statement indicating that non-price measures would be its first tobacco control priority.

Protection from Exposure to Tobacco Smoke

In countries where smoking rates are high among men and low among women, such as some countries in Asia and Africa, women are more likely than men to be exposed involuntarily to tobacco smoke and to be at increased risk for a number of smoking-related diseases. This issue is described in the chapter on SHS in this monograph.

Article 8 of the WHO FCTC[18] calls upon Parties to provide protection from SHS in public transport, indoor workplaces, indoor public places, and other public areas. Some advocates question the effectiveness of restrictions on smoking in public places and workplaces in countries where women traditionally do not work outside the home. While regulations affecting public places may not appear to affect women's exposure to smoke in the home, such restrictions can create a social climate in which it is not acceptable to smoke indoors.[30,31] This can empower non-smoking women to limit smoking in their homes. Education aimed at male smokers is still needed to increase awareness of the health risks to their families from SHS.

While regulations affecting public places may not appear to affect women's exposure to smoke in the home, such restrictions can create a social climate in which it is not acceptable to smoke indoors.

In 1993, the Swedish Tobacco Act called for smoke-free workplaces, although special smoking rooms were permitted in most cases.[32] In 2004, an amendment to this act was passed whereby restaurants and bars were required to be smoke-free by 2005, with the option of building separately ventilated smoking rooms. By 2005, smoking bans were in place in health-care facilities, educational facilities, government facilities, restaurants, pubs and bars, indoor workplaces and offices, theatres, and cinemas.[32]

China's 1991 Tobacco Monopoly Act requires smoking to be banned or restricted on public transport and in transport-related public places. The 1991 Act for Protection of Minors also bans smoking in the classrooms and dormitories of middle schools, elementary schools, and kindergartens.[33] Federal legislation in China is generally very weak, by international standards, and

World Health Organization

is not strongly enforced. Therefore, many municipalities have taken it upon themselves to introduce and monitor their own smoking bans. By 1996, more than 70 cities in China had introduced piecemeal legislation to ban smoking in places such as theatres, video halls, music venues, indoor sports stadia, reading rooms, exhibition halls, shopping malls, waiting rooms, public transport, schools, and nurseries.[34] By October 2006, 46% of Chinese cities had bans on public smoking that were more stringent than the national law.[33] Unfortunately, the rationale behind these efforts may not be reaching the general population. A 2007 study of low-income workers found that only 25% were aware of the dangers of passive smoking, despite the fact that most of the workers surveyed were subject to workplace smoking restrictions.[35] Workplace smoking has not been addressed by the Chinese government, either federally or locally, although some groups (e.g. health-care institutions) have adopted voluntary smoke-free policies. There were plans for a "smoke-free Olympics" in Beijing in 2008,[36] but reports leading up to the games indicated that legislators had created sizeable exemptions (e.g. for bars and restaurants).[37]

The United Kingdom's *Smoking Kills: A White Paper on Tobacco*[38] revealed that smoking restrictions in public places were weak in the 1990s. At the time, the United Kingdom's tobacco control policy placed greater emphasis on the individual's right to smoke than on health. However, some underground trains, buses, aboveground trains, workplaces, shops, banks, and post offices went smoke-free (despite the lack of national regulation) in response to customer demands.[31] Bans on smoking in public places changed dramatically when the Republic of Ireland went smoke-free in 2004.[39] Scientific studies quickly assuaged fears that smoking was being driven "inside the home" by demonstrating that in-home smoking rates were no different between Ireland and the United Kingdom.[40] Scotland, Wales, Northern Ireland, and England became smoke-free soon afterwards, each having a comprehensive ban in effect by 2007.[41]

South Africa's 1993 Tobacco Products Control Act (implemented in 1995) banned smoking on public transport.[42] A 1999 amendment included bans on smoking in workplaces; currently, South Africa bans smoking in all public places except bars and restaurants.[22]

Packaging and Labelling of Tobacco Products

Mandatory health warnings on cigarette packages are used to alert the public to the dangers of tobacco use. Article 11 of the WHO FCTC describes the treaty's requirements for the packaging and labelling of tobacco products.[18] Within three years of signing the WHO FCTC, Parties are required to provide health warnings that cover a minimum of 30% of tobacco-product packaging and to remove misleading package labels that imply "healthier" products (e.g. "low tar" or "light"). So-called "health-conscious" tobacco products are more likely to be adopted by women, suggesting that removal of these misleading labels will have a greater impact on women.[43] Additionally, because the majority of the world's illiterate population is female,[44] the policies created regarding tobacco packaging and labelling should include pictorial or other non-written messaging in order to be gender-sensitive.

Iceland and Canada led the world in the incorporation of pictograms into tobacco package warnings.[31] The European Union has given each of its 25 countries the option to include pictorial warnings on cigarette packages. Accordingly, the United Kingdom developed its own pictograms that went into effect in October 2008.[45] Seventeen countries have adopted pictograms, including some developing nations, such as India, Brazil, and Jordan.[45] This has great implications for women's access to health messages in these countries.

South Africa also requires health warnings on packages of cigarettes.[46] Examples include "Smoking causes lung cancer" and "Smoking is addictive". These warnings attempt to reach broad audiences.

China's first anti-tobacco law, which went into effect in January 1992, mandated the printing of tar levels and health warnings on domestic and imported cigarettes. Even the most ardent Chinese tobacco control advocates are reluctant to see graphic warning labels on cigarette packages, however, for fear that "ugly pictures would mar the packs traditionally given as presents to wedding guests".[36] Nevertheless, by signing the WHO FCTC, China agreed that by 2008, clear health warnings would occupy more than 30% of the surface of every cigarette pack sold.

World Health Organization

Education, Communication, Training, and Public Awareness

Article 12 of the WHO FCTC[18] promotes public information, training, and education campaigns. Specifically, it imposes a legal obligation on Parties to promote access to information about the dangers of tobacco consumption and the benefits of cessation. Public awareness efforts can target specific groups, including children, young adults, and pregnant women. Because men and women cite different motivations for smoking initiation and because adolescent males and females have different predictors for initiation,[47] there is good reason to believe that prevention messages should be gender-specific. This is not to say that entire programmes must be gender-specific, but health professionals (i.e. instructors and clinicians) should understand the gender differences in smoking initiation, so that prevention efforts can be maximized. Hoving et al.[47] point to the need for continuing to teach girls skills that will build self-efficacy and allow them to resist social pressure; boys may need more messages regarding the negative consequences of smoking and may need programmes that simultaneously target other risk-taking behaviours such as alcohol consumption.

In addition to different initiation rates and rationales, other gender differences must be addressed by national education and health-worker training programmes. As Greaves and Tungohan suggest,[11] the substantially higher illiteracy rates among women in developing nations may prevent women from accessing messages about the risks of using tobacco products. They suggest that tobacco control programmes should work with organizations that promote female literacy to ensure that appropriate messages are developed and transmitted via multiple types of media.[11]

Policies in all four of our case-study countries include health promotion. Unlike anti-tobacco laws and regulations, which require small amounts of money for monitoring and evaluation, health education programmes can be very costly. The state of prevention programmes, educational efforts, and health-worker training in the four countries varies greatly, largely as a result of the financial resources available (or made available) for tobacco control.

Sweden's strong tobacco health education activities include school-based programmes about the health hazards of tobacco use and public awareness campaigns revolving around the annual World No Tobacco Day and the national non-smoking day.[7]

Before the publication of its white paper on tobacco in 1998, the UK government allocated resources to various health education agencies for anti-tobacco campaigns.[48] The white paper outlined extensive health-promotion activities, including mass media and education campaigns. The latter included the training of health workers and teachers through initiatives such as the Healthy Schools Campaign. The United Kingdom also has a highly successful national public awareness campaign to help people quit smoking—the annual UK No Smoking Day, which is now in its twenty-fifth year.[31]

In South Africa, a number of health education efforts have been undertaken to prevent smoking. In 2002, the National Council Against Smoking sponsored a "Quit & Win" campaign that awarded substantial prizes to a pool of eligible former smokers, all of whom had successfully quit smoking for at least four weeks.[49] The National Council Against Smoking also runs a tobacco/health information hotline and provides online advice regarding smoking cessation.

In 2005, cigarette sales in China generated US$ 32.5 billion in taxes and profits, yet the national government spent less than US$ 31 000 on tobacco control measures, including national public awareness campaigns.[36] Although China did participate in the 21st annual World No Tobacco Day in 2008 by asking taxi drivers to post no-smoking signs in their windows,[50] it is difficult to identify other nationally guided smoking prevention programmes.

Health promotion is a key area for the implementation of gender-sensitive policy. Unlike laws and regulations that must be gender-neutral in design and application, health promotion has the distinction of being able to purposefully target gender differences in smoking initiation rationales in order to maximize prevention efforts. For example, women are the focus of gender-specific programmes such as Scotland's Women, Low Income, and Smoking project.[38] Given the higher rates of smoking among women in Sweden, several health education programmes there also specifically target women. Sweden has published self-help manuals for different target audiences, including pregnant women, parents, young girls, and older women, which touch upon topics such as how to give up smoking

World Health Organization

199

without gaining weight.[51] Since 1996, all candidates for the title of Miss Sweden have had to be non-smokers.[52] The finalists for the competition receive training from the Swedish National Institute of Public Health about how to convey anti-smoking messages to children on their tours of local schools.[53]

> *Some women's groups have raised objections to focusing women's anti-smoking programmes solely on pregnant women, noting that too often the motivation for such targeting has not been the reduction of smoking among women, but rather the protection of the fetus.*

Tobacco Advertising, Promotion, and Sponsorship

Article 13 of the WHO FCTC mandates that Parties undertake a comprehensive ban or, in cases of constitutional limitations, a restriction of all tobacco advertising, promotion, and sponsorship.[18] Evidence suggests that in both industrialized and developing countries, advertising bans have a negative effect on tobacco consumption: decreases of approximately 6% have occurred when comprehensive advertising restrictions are in place.[54] Partial advertising restrictions have little to no effect on overall smoking consumption, because the tobacco industry quickly shifts marketing efforts to non-restricted media.[54,55] Advertising restrictions are gender-neutral in their design, but because of the specific targeting of women by the tobacco industry, the restrictions may in fact be gender-sensitive in their effect.

Tobacco advertising on Chinese television and radio and in magazines was banned in 1992, but the restriction only encouraged tobacco companies to shift marketing

funds into non-restricted areas, such as sponsorship of sports, art, and music.[56] The 1996 Prevalence Survey of Smoking in China specifically highlighted the need to maintain low smoking rates among women through aggressive campaigns to counter the targeting of women by the tobacco industry.[34] However, it is not clear that any campaigns have been successful. China still permits a variety of advertising avenues that are considered highly female-targeted, including the free distribution of tobacco products by mail, promotional discounts on tobacco products, and the branding of non-tobacco products with tobacco brand names.[22] All forms of tobacco advertising will be banned in China by 2010.[36]

South Africa has never permitted the direct advertising of cigarettes on television, and it also bans tobacco advertising in local and international magazines and newspapers.[22] Industry-sponsored sports and music events, such as Rothman's soccer, circumvented the television advertising bans until 1999, when South Africa's Tobacco Control Act of 1993 was amended to include bans on all tobacco advertisements, including indirect advertising and promotional events.[42] The proposed 2008 amendment to the Tobacco Control Act further restricts advertising and increases the fines for those failing to meet the requirements of the Act.[57]

Sweden's first restrictions on tobacco advertising were introduced in the 1960s. These included the restriction of advertising in theatres, cinemas, sports arenas, and sporting events and on sports pages in magazines and newspapers. In the 1970s, tobacco companies were forbidden to use human models in their advertisements. By the end of that decade, health warnings became mandatory on advertisements for tobacco products, and the advertising of tobacco products on national television and radio was banned. Sweden, like the rest of Europe, still has not banned advertising on international television and radio. Although Sweden does not allow the free distribution of tobacco products or the branding of non-tobacco products with tobacco brand names, it does allow for promotional discounts on tobacco products.[22]

The United Kingdom originally banned the advertisement of cigarettes on television in 1964, and it banned such advertising on the radio in 1973. Successive governments wanted to follow a voluntary approach, but more recently, between 2002 and 2005, the United

Kingdom phased in an advertising and sponsorship ban. This new ban forbids billboard and press advertising and extends to the sponsorship of sports. Unlike Sweden, the United Kingdom bans promotional discounts on tobacco products.[22]

A total ban on the advertising of and sponsorship by tobacco products reduces smoking in most groups, making it a gender-neutral policy. But since it is clear from tobacco industry documents that women are being specifically targeted, enforcement of a complete ban on advertising and promotion across all tobacco products and in all media is recommended as an integral part of a comprehensive, gender-sensitive tobacco control policy.

Tobacco Dependence and Cessation Measures

Article 14 of the WHO FCTC encourages Parties to design and implement effective programmes aimed at promoting the cessation of tobacco use. While the treaty does not specifically mention the need for gender sensitivity in such programmes, current research indicates that gender-specific cessation messages, counselling services, and health-worker training may be as important as prevention activities. Although nicotine dependency is equally strong in men and women, the difficulty of smoking cessation does appear to differ by gender. Women report using cigarettes more frequently with other women, meaning that group dynamics and a desire for socialization may hinder the quitting process for women. Additionally, studies show that women report greater fears of weight gain associated with quitting and have higher rates of depression, which may create additional barriers to cessation.[58] These differences demonstrate the need for gender-specific cessation programmes that target the quitting "hurdles" unique to women.

Some women's groups have raised objections to focusing women's anti-smoking programmes solely on pregnant women, noting that too often the motivation for such targeting has not been the reduction of smoking among women, but rather the protection of the fetus. Women are thus considered only in their procreative role. As a result, programmes that aim to reduce smoking by pregnant women have sometimes been labelled as "victim

blaming", and their designers have been accused of using guilt to encourage women to stop smoking. Nevertheless, programmes that seek to integrate pregnant women into larger cessation efforts are highly effective in reducing the number of women who smoke during pregnancy. In 2003, fewer than 10% of Swedish women reported smoking daily during pregnancy, a reduction of more than 50% from the level in the 1990s.[59]

The 1998 UK white paper recognized the need to provide support to prevent relapse into smoking by mothers after a baby's birth.[38] The UK policy increasingly seeks to encourage women to quit smoking during pregnancy as a way of breaking the cycle of health inequalities, since the vast majority of these women smokers are poor, young, and undereducated. The government tries to reach them through the National Health Service's Stop Smoking Services, as well as through social programmes that target infant and child health and development, such as Sure Start. Stop Smoking Services were launched countrywide in 2000 and 2001; they include a national help line, a dedicated web site, the provision of cessation prescriptions, and one-on-one counselling and support groups in local centres.[60] The annual 2004–2005 expenditure on this programme was £46.8 million, excluding the cost of prescriptions. Despite such a strong government stance on smoking cessation, the Service has been called to task for its failure to provide adequate services to underage smokers, of whom females constitute the majority. A 2003 survey found that fewer than 7% of all service providers in England accepted referrals from underage smokers,[61] indicating that beliefs about "propriety" may be overshadowing public health needs.

State funding for cessation programmes is nonexistent in China. The US$ 31 000 the Chinese government spent on tobacco control in 2005 was intended for prevention and cessation programming[36] for the country's 1.3 billion residents. The overwhelming majority of the poor are uninsured and rely on out-of-pocket payments for health care,[35] making cessation programmes somewhat of a luxury. One study of smoking cessation among lower-income Chinese workers found that of 333 former smokers, none had used nicotine replacement therapy.[35] Additionally, a study of female microelectronics workers found that the "smoking culture" of the workplace applies to women in much the same way that it applies to men, with rates of smoking increasing among blue-collar working women.[62]

Both studies indicate that much more needs to be done in China to increase support for smokers who want to quit, and there is a very specific niche for workplace cessation programmes, which have the potential to impact vulnerable women.

Currently, 55% of all tobacco leaf is grown by only three countries—China, Brazil, and India. The effects of this shift are gendered in nature, with women being most vulnerable to the health and economic harms of tobacco production.

Reducing the number of women who smoke during pregnancy is an important public health intervention, and policies targeting pregnant women are gender-sensitive. Pregnancy is a good entry point for reaching women and their partners who smoke, but support in maintaining cessation after birth should be an integral part of cessation programmes. Women need gender-sensitive programmes that focus on their entire lifespan, not solely on their reproductive lifespan. Moreover, additional strategies that target young women and non-pregnant women must be developed.

Sales of Tobacco To and By Minors

Article 16 of the WHO FCTC includes a variety of policy recommendations intended to limit youth access to tobacco. The policies include the restriction of direct sales to minors, requiring identification when making sales, and prohibition of tobacco vending machines. This Article also includes policies that are not minor-specific but do seek to limit the ease of access and appeal of cigarettes to youth. These policies restrict the sale of individual cigarettes, prohibit the distribution of free tobacco products, and ban the manufacturing of sweets and toys in the form of tobacco products (e.g. candy cigarettes). Although the policies are gender-neutral in design, their successful implementation can produce gendered results. Studies show that underage females are less likely to attempt to purchase cigarettes than their male peers are, but these same studies also show that females are more likely to be successful in such purchases if they are attempted.[10] In this example, the strong enforcement of identification laws would be gender-neutral in application but gender-sensitive in result.

South Africa's first tobacco control act, implemented in 1995, included the banning of cigarette sales to youth.[42] The 2008 amendment further elaborates on the restriction of cigarette sales to persons under 16 years of age.[57]

A UK law has restricted the supply of tobacco to young people since 1908. Under current legislation in the Children and Young Persons (Protection from Tobacco) Act of 1991, it is against the law to sell tobacco to anyone under 16 years of age.[60]

A minimum-age law was passed in Sweden in 1997, restricting tobacco purchases to persons 18 years of age and older.[63] A study comparing students before and after the law was enacted found that after enactment, all adolescents reported greater difficulty in buying tobacco near their homes, but only adolescent females reported a statistically significant decrease in tobacco purchases. Unfortunately, the proportion of adolescents who bought tobacco from friends increased during the same time period.

As of 2006, no federal law prohibited the sale of tobacco products to minors in China, although many local municipalities have addressed the issue with their own regulations.[64] The existence of local restrictions, however, does not imply widespread knowledge of them. In Wuhan province, a survey found that only 23% of parents of high-school students were aware that Wuhan had a law prohibiting the sale of cigarettes to adolescents.[65] Cigarette use by young people is considered normal in China, since children are often asked to buy cigarettes for their parents, and they are often given cigarettes as gifts on special occasions.

Support for Economically Viable Alternatives to Tobacco Production

Tobacco production has shifted primarily to lower- and middle-income countries and affects the millions of

 World Health Organization

poor women working in tobacco production. Currently, 55% of all tobacco leaf is grown by only three countries—China, Brazil, and India.[66] The effects of this shift are gendered in nature, with women being most vulnerable to the health and economic harms of tobacco production.[11,67] It is noteworthy that Article 17 of the WHO FCTC calls upon Parties to "promote, as appropriate, economically viable alternatives for tobacco workers, growers and, as the case may be, sellers".[18]

Surveys that analyse the revenue-to-cost ratio of various crops show that tobacco farming is far from the most lucrative option for Chinese farmers. Fruit, mulberries, silkworms, rice, wheat, vegetable oil, and beans all have higher revenue-to-cost ratios than tobacco, indicating that tobacco may not always produce the best economic returns for China. According to Hu et al.,[29] "this is a prime time for the Chinese government to encourage less profitable tobacco farmers to produce other crops".

As members of the European Union, Sweden and the United Kingdom operate under the jurisdiction of the Common Agriculture Policy of 2003. This policy eliminated a system of product-specific farm subsidies (e.g. subsidies provided to farmers based on the quantity of tobacco they produced) and now provides single-farm subsidies that are product-blind. The overall goal is to allow producers to adjust to a situation in which product support will be phased out. The transition from tobacco-specific subsidies to "decoupled" subsidies is gradual, and it is hoped that farmers will adjust their crop selection accordingly for maximum profit.[66]

According to a Campaign for Tobacco-Free Kids report, the world's excess tobacco production is driving many families into deep poverty.[67] Family farms that contract with tobacco companies for advance purchases of seed and fertilizer are then bound to sell their crops to those same companies for very low "market" prices—barely enough to pay off the debts they accrued prior to planting. The tobacco industry works throughout developing countries to convince farmers to grow tobacco exclusively. As a result, rates of malnutrition among children have increased in tobacco-growing regions of Kenya, for example, because families are planting tobacco instead of traditional food crops in the hope of escaping poverty.

Additionally, tobacco-leaf companies in Brazil have specifically requested that school systems shorten their

terms to permit children to help their families in the field.[67] In countries where disparities in schooling and nutrition already exist between boys and girls, tobacco farms will only exaggerate the problem. In all these tobacco-producing countries, alternatives to growing tobacco have great potential for changing the educational, economic, and health prospects of women.

Given that the WHO FCTC entered into force in February 2005, the question remains as to whether countries have successfully incorporated its call for gender sensitivity into their national programmes and policies.

Conclusion

Given that the WHO FCTC entered into force in February 2005, the question remains as to whether countries have successfully incorporated its call for gender sensitivity into their national programmes and policies. Monitoring and evaluation will be the key to making such a determination. Specifically, monitoring and evaluation efforts *must* include collection of sex-disaggregated data on the initiation, maintenance, and cessation of tobacco use at the national level. Findings that reveal gender differences must then be used to inform research and to strengthen or modify existing policies and programmes.

The WHO FCTC has been a major accomplishment for international tobacco control. In the four countries examined here, ratification of the treaty has clearly brought a new commitment to tobacco control policy and programme creation and implementation. Even before these countries became Parties to the treaty, all four made progress in strengthening national legislation in many areas of tobacco control, including advertising and promotion, exposure to SHS, and information, education and communication.

World Health Organization

The four countries offer insights into how the content of tobacco policies can ignore or address both gender inequality and women as a group. These countries have achieved varying degrees of gender sensitivity in their policies: all have a variety of gender-neutral policies (e.g. advertising bans), and all have at least some gender-specific policies. Sweden appears to have the most gender-specific policies and programmes, e.g. programmes targeting pregnant women for smoking cessation. The challenge for China will be to address smoking among vulnerable groups. In addition, the four case-studies highlight the fact that the design of policies may often be gender-neutral, while the impact of those policies may be highly gendered, affecting women more than men. Advertising bans are an excellent example of this. Although advertising restrictions are applied equally to both men and women, some measures will have a greater likelihood of decreasing smoking prevalence among women, based on gender norms, roles, and relations.

In some realms, it may be appropriate to expect gender-redistributive policies, but movement from gender-blind to gender-neutral policies and from gender-neutral to gender-specific policies may be more readily attainable and should be considered progress in the area of tobacco control.[10]

While it is not the focus of this chapter, there is clear evidence that tobacco control policies and programmes should be developed that include strong consideration of SES, in addition to gender.[68,69] Graham et al.[69] suggest that women's smoking status in developing countries is influenced by "biographies of disadvantage". Women's initiation of smoking, persistence, and cessation are influenced by childhood disadvantage, educational trajectories, and reproductive careers. Graham et al. suggest that policies regarding tobacco control need to focus on these social conditions that affect smoking status. Greaves, Vallone, and Velicer[12] suggest the use of gender-redistributive policies that link "housing, welfare, child-care, training and economic policies and programmes" to address the needs of low-SES women and girls.

Finally, in the implementation of Article 20 of the WHO FCTC related to research, surveillance, and exchange of information, there is a need for research on the development and implementation of tobacco control policies that are gender-specific with a focus on women. More case-studies related to how gender policies are financed, monitored, and evaluated will help guide policy-makers as the WHO FCTC is implemented. The active participation of gender experts in policy-related research will also enrich the knowledge concerning how tobacco control can benefit women as well as men of all ages.

References

1. *Legislative action to combat smoking around the world: a survey of existing legislation.* Geneva, World Health Organization, 1976.
2. Roemer R. *Legislative action to combat the world tobacco epidemic.* Geneva, World Health Organization, 1995.
3. Royal College of Physicians of London. *Summary of a report of the Royal College of Physicians of London on smoking in relation to cancer of the lung and other diseases.* London, Pitman Medical Publishing Co. Ltd., 1962.
4. US Department of Health, Education and Welfare. *Smoking and health: report of the Advisory Committee to the Surgeon General.* Washington, DC, US Government Printing Office, 1964, (DHEW Publication (PHS) 1103).
5. US Department of Health and Human Services. *The health benefits of smoking cessation: a report of the Surgeon General.* Washington, DC: US Government Printing Office, 1990.
6. Doll R, Hill AB. Mortality in relation to smoking: ten years' observations of British Doctors. *British Medical Journal,* 1964, 1:1399-1410.
7. *The European tobacco control report 2007.* Copenhagen, World Health Organization Regional Office for Europe, 2007.
8. *Gender, health and tobacco.* Geneva, World Health Organization, (Fact sheet November 2003; http://www.who.int/gender/documents/Gender_Tobacco_2.pdf).
9. Bird CE, Rieker PP. *Gender and health: the effects of constrained choices and social policies.* New York, NY, Cambridge University Press, 2008.
10. Greaves L, Jategaonkar N. Tobacco policies and vulnerable girls and women: toward a framework for gender sensitive policy development. *Journal of Epidemiology and Community Health,* 2006, 60 (Suppl. 2):ii57–ii65.
11. Greaves L, Tungohan E. Engendering tobacco control: using an international public health treaty to reduce smoking and empower women. *Tobacco Control,* 2007, 16:148–150.
12. Greaves L, Vallone D, Velicer W. Special effects: tobacco policies and low socioeconomic status girls and women. *Journal of Epidemiology and Community Health,* 2006, 60 (Suppl. 2):ii1–ii2.
13. Pampel F. National income, inequality and global patterns of cigarette use. *Social Forces,* 2007, 86:445–466.
14. Pampel FC. Global patterns and determinants of sex differences in smoking. *International Journal of Comparative Sociology,* 2006, 47:466–487.
15. Kabeer N. Gender-aware policy and planning: a social relations perspective. In: Macdonald M, ed. *Gender planning in development agencies: meeting the challenge.* Oxford, Oxfam, 1994.
16. Kabeer N. *Gender mainstreaming in poverty eradication and the millennium development goals: a handbook for policy-makers and other stakeholders.* Ottawa, The Commonwealth Secretariat, 2003 (New Gender Mainstreaming Series on Development Issues).
17. March C, Smyth I, Mukhopadhyay M. *A guide to gender-analysis frameworks.* Oxford, Oxfam, 1999.
18. *WHO Framework Convention on Tobacco Control.* Geneva, World Health Organization, 2003.
19. *Full list of Signatories and Parties to the WHO Framework Convention on Tobacco Control.* Geneva, World Health Organization (http://www.who.int/fctc/signatories_parties/en/index.html, accessed 7 July 2008).
20. Jha P, Chaloupka FJ. The economics of global tobacco control. *British Medical Journal,* 2000, 321:358-361.
21. Saloojee Y. South Africa National Council Against Smoking: annual report, 1995 (unpublished).
22. *WHO report on the global tobacco epidemic, 2009: implementing smoke-free environments.* Geneva, World Health Organization, 2009.
23. Main C et al. Population tobacco control interventions and their effects on social inequalities in smoking: placing an equity lens on existing systematic reviews. *BMC Public Health,* 2008, 8:178.

24. *State of the world population—people, poverty and possibilities: making development work for the poor.* Geneva, United Nations Population Fund, 2002.

25. Joossens L, Raw M. How can cigarette smuggling be reduced? *British Medical Journal*, 2000, 321:947–950.

26. *European health for all database (HFA-DB).* World Health Organization Regional Office for Europe (http://www.euro.who.int/hfadb, accessed 2 June 2009).

27. van Walbeek C, Blecher E, van Graan M. Effects of the Tobacco Products Control Amendment Act of 1999 on restaurant revenues in South Africa—a survey approach. *South African Medical Journal*, 2007, 97:211.

28. Townsend J. The role of taxation policy in tobacco control. In: Abedian I, van der Merwe R, Wilkins N, eds. *The economics of tobacco control: towards an optimal policy mix.* Cape Town, Applied Fiscal Research Centre, University of Cape Town, 1998.

29. Hu TW et al. China at the crossroads: the economics of tobacco and health. *Tobacco Control*, 2006, 15 (Suppl. 1):i37–i41.

30. Borland R et al. Determinants and consequences of smoke-free homes: findings from the International Tobacco Control (ITC) Four Country Survey. *Tobacco Control*, 2006, 15 (Suppl. 3):iii42–iii50.

31. Sandford A. Government action to reduce smoking. *Respirology,* 2003, 8:7–16.

32. *The Tobacco Act. 581.* Stockholm, Swedish Ministry of Health and Social Welfare, 1993.

33. Gan Q et al. Effectiveness of a smoke-free policy in lowering secondhand smoke concentrations in offices in china. *Journal of Occupational and Environmental Medicine*, 2008, 50:570–575.

34. Chinese Academy of Preventive Medicine (CAPM), Chinese Association of Smoking and Health (CASH). *Smoking and health in China: 1996 National Prevalence Survey of Smoking Patterns.* Yunnan, China Science and Technology Press, 1997.

35. Hesketh T et al. Smoking, cessation and expenditure in low income Chinese: cross sectional survey. *BMC Public Health*, 2007, 7:29.

36. Wright AA, Katz IT. Tobacco tightrope—balancing disease prevention and economic development in China. *New England Journal of Medicine*, 2007, 356:1493–1496.

37. Xiaohuo C. Restaurants exempt from smoking ban. *China Daily,* 14 April 2008 (http://www.chinadaily.com.cn/olympics/2008-04/14/content_6613463.htm, accessed 7 July 2008).

38. *Smoking kills: a white paper on tobacco.* London, UK Department of Health, 1998.

39. *Smokefree England* (http://www.smokefreeengland.co.uk/smokefreeworld/ireland.html, accessed 7 July 2008).

40. Hyland A et al. Does smoke-free Ireland have more smoking inside the home and less in pubs than the United Kingdom? Findings from the international tobacco control policy evaluation project. *European Journal of Public Health*, 2008, 18:63–65.

41. United Kingdom, Department of Health. *The Smoke-free (Premises and Enforcement) Regulations 2006. No. 3368. 1 July 2008* (http://www.opsi.gov.uk/si/si2006/20063368.htm).

42. *The surveillance and monitoring of tobacco control in South Africa.* Geneva, World Health Organization, 2003 (Paper SAFR2003).

43. Carpenter CM, Wayne GF, Connolly GN. Designing cigarettes for women: new findings from the tobacco industry documents. *Addiction*, 2005, 100:837–851.

44. UNESCO Literacy Portal (http://portal.unesco.org, accessed 7 July 2008).

45. Physicians for a Smoke-Free Canada. *Cigarette warnings in the United Kingdom* (http://www.smoke-free.ca/warnings/United%20Kingdom%20-%20health%20warnings.htm, accessed 7 July 2008).

46. *The tobacco atlas.* Geneva, World Health Organization, 2002.

47. Hoving C, Reubsaet A, de Vries H. Predictors of smoking stage transitions for adolescent boys and girls. *Preventive Medicine*, 2007, 44:485–489.

48. Calnan M. The politics of health: the case of smoking control. *Journal of Social Policy*, 1984, 13:279–296.

49. *Fabulous prizes to quit smoking* (http://www.againstsmoking.org/press%20releases/NCASprizes%20for%20quitting.html, accessed 7 July 2008).

50. *China Marks World Tobacco Day* (http://english.cri.cn/4026/2008/06/01/1721@364117.htm, accessed 7 July 2008).

51. United Nations Commission for Europe. *Gender statistics web site for Europe and North America* (http://www.unece.org/stats/gender/genpols/keyinds/health/tobacco.htm, accessed 1 July 2008).

52. *Progress and challenge in tobacco control (Swedish Style): disarming a deadly weapon.* Stockholm, Health Professionals Against Tobacco, 2003.

53. Steimle S. New EU report: more women are smoking. *Journal of the National Cancer Institute*, 1999, 91:212–213.

54. Jha P, Chaloupka FJ. *Curbing the epidemic: governments and the economics of tobacco control.* Washington, DC, The World Bank, 1999.

55. Lewis MJ, Delnevo CD, Slade J. Tobacco industry direct mail marketing and participation by New Jersey adults. *American Journal of Public Health*, 2004, 94:257–259.

56. Mackay J, Amos A. Women and tobacco. *Respirology*, 2003, 8:123–130.

57. *Tobacco Products Control Amendment Act, 2007. No. 247.* Cape Town, Parliament of the Republic of South Africa, 2008.

58. Hunter S. Quitting. In: Samet J, Yoon SY, eds. *Women and the tobacco epidemic: challenges for the 21st century.* Geneva, World Health Organization, 2001:121–146.

59. Post A et al. Maternal smoking during pregnancy: a comparison between concurrent and retrospective self-reports. *Pediatric and Perinatal Epidemiology*, 2008, 22:155–161.

60. Denscombe M. UK health policy and "underage" smokers: the case for smoking cessation services. *Health Policy*, 2007, 80:69–76.

61. Coleman T et al. Implementing a national treatment service for dependent smokers: initial challenges and solutions. *Addiction*, 2005, 100 (Suppl. 2):12–18.

62. Lin YP et al. Emerging epidemic in a growing industry: cigarette smoking among female micro-electronics workers in Taiwan. *Public Health*, 2005, 119:184–188.

63. Sundh M, Hagquist C. Effects of a minimum-age tobacco law—Swedish experience. *Drugs: education, prevention and policy*, 2005, 12:501–510.

64. Embassy of the People's Republic of China in Australia. *China planning ban on tobacco, alcohol sales to children* (http://au.china-embassy.org/eng/xw/t268608.htm, accessed 7 July 2008).

65. Unger JB et al. Peer influences and access to cigarettes as correlates of adolescent smoking: a cross-cultural comparison of Wuhan, China, and California. *Preventive Medicine*, 2002, 34:476–484.

66. Commission of the European Communities. *Accomplishing a sustainable agricultural model for Europe through the reformed CAP—the tobacco, olive oil, cotton and sugar sectors.* Brussels, European Commission, 2003:554.

67. *Golden leaf, barren harvests: the costs of tobacco farming.* Washington, DC: Campaign for Tobacco-Free Kids, 2001.

68. Harrell JS et al. Smoking initiation in youth: the roles of gender, race, socioeconomics, and developmental status. *Journal of Adolescent Health*, 1998, 23:271–279.

69. Graham H et al. Pathways of disadvantage and smoking careers: evidence and policy implications. *Journal of Epidemiology and Community Health*, 2006, 60 (Suppl. 2):ii7–12.

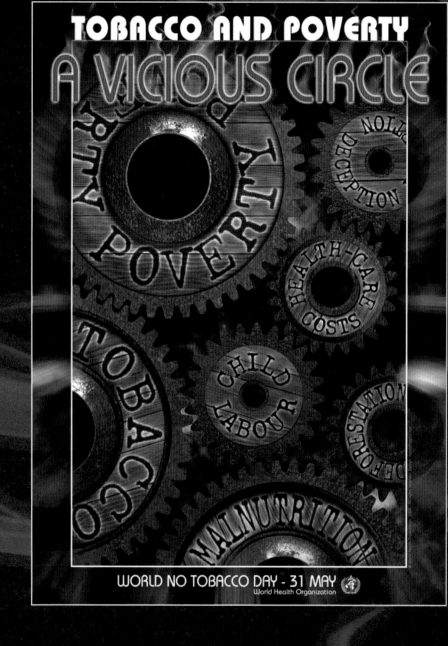

11. Taxation and the Economics of Tobacco Control

Introduction

The relevance of economic research and analysis to tobacco control, whether directed at the general population or specifically at women, is becoming increasingly understood. The World Health Organization (WHO) 2009 report on the global tobacco epidemic noted, "While more data and analysis are needed on tobacco's costs and economic burden, it is clear that its economic impact on productivity and health care—already disproportionately felt by the poor—will worsen as tobacco use increases".[1] This chapter highlights findings and presents a gender analysis with a focus on women where data are available. Specifically, it reviews costs of tobacco use and the global evidence of the effects of taxation on the consumption of tobacco, in particular the effects of taxes on smoking. Little research on the economic aspects of tobacco has focused specifically on gender and women or the wide range of tobacco products used, including chewing tobacco, snuff, and bidis. Indeed, in some areas of the world, women and men use other tobacco products more than they use cigarettes. For example, in India, 12% of women chew tobacco, whereas only 2.4% of women smoke manufactured cigarettes.[2] Because many economic concepts, policies, and practices are relevant to a gender analysis, they are presented here to identify gaps needing to be addressed in further research.

Regardless of which subgroup is targeted, tobacco control programmes need to address the economic forces influencing tobacco production and consumption, including the role that tobacco production and sales play in employment, tax revenues, and trade balances in some countries. Tobacco control policies also need to acknowledge the health effects and other costs of tobacco use and to incorporate measures to reduce demand through higher prices. Debate continues about several aspects of the economics related to the consumption of tobacco, including concerns about the equity and efficiency of cigarette taxation.

The first section of this chapter discusses the costs of tobacco consumption. This topic is relevant to millions of women, particularly in developing countries, because tobacco use exacerbates poverty conditions and negatively affects women's roles as family providers. The costs of treating tobacco-related illnesses and the resulting loss of productivity are leading economic arguments for tobacco control policies. This is especially true for the costs related to illnesses caused by exposure to second-hand smoke (SHS)—costs that are borne by both those exposed to SHS and society in general.

The costs of treating tobacco-related illnesses and the resulting loss of productivity are leading economic arguments for tobacco control policies.

The second section covers various issues concerning taxation and price. Although taxation is a "blunt" instrument that may not have a gender-specific goal, it influences women's consumer behaviour and is an important source of revenue for governments and public health programmes.

Costs of Tobacco

Costs of Tobacco Consumption

From a policy perspective, it is important to understand how to maintain women's relatively low smoking rates in the face of greater female autonomy, higher incomes, increased female labour force participation, and increased marketing efforts by tobacco companies in low- and middle-income countries. Moreover, it is imperative to understand how to decrease women's tobacco use and the costs imposed by tobacco use in countries that have higher prevalence of female tobacco use.

As noted in the chapter on a gender equality framework, tobacco use undermines progress made in social and economic development and creates hardship for the millions of people in the world who live in poverty, the majority of whom are women. Women worldwide are

World Health Organization

the main producers of food, while also being home-care providers and caregivers of children. Tobacco-related diseases impose serious burdens on their care responsibilities, and the costs of care compete for scarce resources needed to feed families. When mothers of young children die from tobacco-related diseases, the loss is social as well as economic. Within the household, expenditures for tobacco may reduce the resources available for necessities, including food and clothing. Tobacco use, in short, is a development issue with economic costs.

At the household level, in Indonesia, where smoking is most common among the poor, 15% of the total expenditure of the lowest income group is for tobacco, while the poorest 20% of households in Mexico spend nearly 11%.

The health costs of tobacco use fall into two broad categories: the financial consequences of tobacco use for health care, life insurance, pensions, and other collective programmes; and the health costs associated with exposure to SHS, which is also referred to as environmental tobacco smoke (ETS).[3] The indirect and intangible psychological costs of pain and suffering arising from smoking-caused disease are particularly difficult to quantify.

Estimates of the treatment costs and productivity losses associated with diseases caused by smoking provide potentially powerful evidence for implementing tobacco control. These costs are borne by individuals and society, generally consequent to the sale of an addicting product for profit. A societal perspective—including individuals, households, employers, government, and society in general—is the most comprehensive perspective. However, data limitations restrict many costing studies to specific perspectives, such as the health-care system, government, or households.

Cost estimates vary by the categories of costs included. One key distinction is between *direct* costs—including payment for tobacco products and medical care—and *indirect* costs, which include forgone earnings due to inability to work and productivity losses at the societal level. How deaths that are causally related to smoking are treated is a sensitive methodological point. If smokers die prematurely, there can be a "death benefit" in terms of saved pension costs. However, moral objections aside, these savings are counterbalanced by forgone productivity and increased costs of medical treatment while smokers are alive.

Productivity losses, including lost wages due to time off work for smokers and their caregivers and lower quality of life due to smoking-related illnesses, represent a substantial category of costs. For example, a study using household survey data from the 2005 Albania Living Standards Monitoring Survey found that after controlling for other observable factors, smokers' wages were 20% lower than those of similar non-smokers.[4]

Data from other countries also provide a basis for concern. The WHO report on the global tobacco epidemic notes that in the United States in 2008, the economic costs related to tobacco use approximated US$ 193 billion per year.[1] In China, the economic costs of smoking were estimated to be US$ 5.0 billion in 2000, equivalent to US$ 25.43 per smoker over the age of 35. Direct costs accounted for US$ 1.7 billion (34% of the total), equivalent to 3.1% of total national health spending in China. Productivity losses related to illness amounted to US$ 0.4 billion (8%), and productivity losses caused by death were US$ 2.9 billion (58%). The direct costs of smoking accounted for an estimated 3.1% of China's national health expenditures in 2000.[5]

A study conducted in the United States found that smoking-attributable neonatal costs were almost US$ 367 million (in 1996 dollars).[6] This estimate implies that a mother who smokes incurs additional neonatal costs of more than US$ 700 (in 1996 dollars). As discussed in the chapter on the impact of tobacco use on women's health, women who smoke during pregnancy are at increased risk of premature rupture of membranes, abruptio placentae, placenta previa, and pre-term delivery. Moreover, infants of mothers who smoke during pregnancy are more likely to have lower average birth weight, are more likely to be small for gestational age, and are at increased risk of stillbirth and perinatal mortality than are the infants of non-smoking women.

As the chapter on a gender equality framework for tobacco control notes, tobacco production causes diseases among agricultural workers, many of whom are women. The diseases include acute nicotine poisoning, known as green tobacco sickness. These health ailments tend to be more common in developing countries, where regulation of tobacco companies for the protection of farmers may be weak or poorly enforced. Tobacco-related diseases in conjunction with injuries incurred while farming impose significant costs on agricultural workers. While the evidence on disease and injury costs is scant, one study conducted in Kentucky between 1992 and 1999 found that hospital costs for tobacco workers averaged US$ 403.[7] Physician fees, rehabilitation charges, and other fees related to injuries were not included in the assessment, so this estimate of the health-care cost of treating tobacco workers should be considered conservative. Much more attention needs to be paid to the costs of health care for tobacco-related diseases among women tobacco workers in developing countries.

Costs of Exposure to Second-Hand Smoke

In the chapter on SHS, the authors state that the majority of victims of SHS, particularly in developing countries, are women and children. The costs of SHS exposure are thus very relevant to a gender perspective on tobacco control. While the costs of medical treatment for smoking-related illnesses are well documented, the economic impact of SHS on health-care costs is less well understood. The 2006 US Surgeon General's report documents in detail the evidence causally linking specific medical conditions to exposure to SHS.[8] In Minnesota, the cost of direct medical treatment for conditions for which the Surgeon General's Office found sufficient evidence to conclude that there was a causal link with exposure to SHS, including lung cancer and coronary heart disease, was estimated to be US$ 228.7 million (in 2008 dollars), equivalent to US$ 44.58 per Minnesota resident.[9]

A study in China, Hong Kong Special Administrative Region, found that the total costs associated with SHS—including direct medical costs, long-term care, and productivity losses—were US$ 156 million in 1998, for a population of 6.5 million. A study in Marion County,

Indiana, found that costs related to health care and premature loss of life totalled US$ 53.9 million, equivalent to US$ 62.68 per capita annually.[10]

A report from the American Society of Actuaries calculated that US$ 2.6 billion was spent on non-smokers in the United States for medical care for lung cancer and heart disease (including heart attacks) caused by exposure to SHS.

A report from the American Society of Actuaries calculated that in 2004, billions of dollars were spent on non-smokers in the United States for medical care for lung cancer and heart disease (including heart attacks) caused by exposure to SHS. The report calculated that exposure to SHS resulted in an additional US$ 3.2 billion of economic losses—including lost wages, benefits, and household services—to individuals and governments. On a per capita basis, this is equivalent to US$ 9.02 for medical care and US$ 11.10 for additional economic losses.[11,12] More research is needed on such costs related to women and men in developing countries.

As discussed in the section below on smoking and pregnancy, many studies have found that exposure of non-smoking pregnant women to SHS is associated with negative consequences,[13] including decreased average mean birth weight, which has been associated with increased costs.[14] A study in New York City calculated annual costs of US$ 99 million related to infants' developmental delays caused by prenatal exposure to SHS.[15]

Why Tax Tobacco Products?

Given the economic burden that tobacco use places on societies, policy-makers have increasingly looked to

World Health Organization

209

economists to provide input into public health policies. While the taxation of tobacco products around the world is a nearly universal practice, it is not always effectively implemented.

From the public health perspective, tobacco taxation has been clearly shown to prevent non-smokers from starting, to prevent former users from re-starting, and to lead current users to try to quit.

Taxes serve different objectives and have different effects on consumption, depending on the prevalence of smoking, the behavioural impact of the tax, and pricing effects. In most countries, for a given tax increase, the price of tobacco products will rise by an amount equal to or greater than the tax increase. This pricing pattern has been attributed to the addictive nature of the product and the coordinated oligopolistic nature of the tobacco industry in many countries.[16]

One of the fundamental principles of economics is that of the downward-sloping demand curve. A demand curve that slopes downwards implies that an inverse relationship exists between the real price of a good and the amount of the good that is consumed. Some researchers once believed that because of the addictive properties of nicotine, tobacco products might be an exception to this fundamental principle. However, many econometric studies conducted over the past four decades, including several that have explicitly modelled the addictive nature of cigarettes, have shown that cigarettes are not an exception to the economic law of demand. The inverse relationship between price and consumption has important policy implications. That is, by increasing the real price of cigarettes, a cigarette tax increase has tremendous potential to be an effective policy lever for decreasing cigarette consumption.

There are several justifications for taxation of tobacco products, from the economic and public health points of view. From the public health perspective, tobacco

taxation has been clearly shown to prevent non-smokers from starting, to prevent former users from re-starting, and to lead current users to try to quit. Higher taxes also reduce consumption among those who do continue to smoke. In addition, taxation generates revenues for governments, given the relatively inelastic demand for smoking (see below), which can be used to offset both the society-level costs of treating illnesses related to smoking and exposure to SHS and the loss of productivity associated with these illnesses.

Because of the inelasticity of demand, tobacco is an ideal product to tax. The taxes provide a relatively stable, predictable, and sustained source of revenue, and in general, cigarette excise taxes are inexpensive to implement and are administratively relatively easy to apply. Given the price sensitivity of demand for cigarettes, significant taxes can produce substantial public health benefits by discouraging smoking, particularly among children and the poor. Taxation can also blunt one of the most potent weapons the tobacco industry employs—differential pricing to divide and attract segments of the market that have different levels of price sensitivity.[17] However, as documented in the WHO report on the global tobacco epidemic,[1] taxes in most countries are well below the levels of those in countries that have used them as part of a comprehensive strategy for reducing tobacco use. Indeed, at least some countries adopt tax structures that tax low-price cigarettes at relatively low rates in order to keep prices low, making the cigarettes more accessible by the poor.

While the strongest rationale for using taxation as a tobacco control measure is that smoking imposes net costs on society, taxation also provides a mechanism to partially recoup these costs from smokers. In addition, the strong negative externalities associated with tobacco use, including illnesses and related medical care for conditions caused by exposure to SHS, provide a strong justification for taxation.

The Economic Perspective

Tobacco taxation is a complex topic, partly because of the variety of taxes that are possible. The most common are excise taxes, value-added or ad valorem sales taxes, import duties, and, in the case of state-owned industries, monopoly profits.

The impact of excise taxes on cigarette demand depends on the extent to which changes in the taxes are reflected in cigarette prices and the responsiveness of cigarette demand to price (the price elasticity of demand, discussed below). Excise tax increases will discourage smoking to the extent that the increases are passed on to smokers in the form of higher prices; there is substantial evidence that a tax increase often leads to a more than proportional increase in retail price.[18]

Ad valorem and specific taxes are the most common excise taxes levied by countries. Ad valorem is levied as a percentage of retail or wholesale price, whereas a specific tax is an absolute value (e.g. US$ 2, or £0.75) levied on packs (e.g. 10, 20, 25 pieces) or number of cigarettes (e.g. per 1000 pieces). In 2008, 33% of countries (60 out of 182) relied on ad valorem taxes, while 30% (55 out of 182) relied on specific excises. Some countries relied on both excises by imposing a mixture of specific and ad valorem excises (48 out of 182). There is still a significant number of countries that do not levy excise on tobacco products (19 out of 182) (WHO database, 2008).

A number of countries impose differential taxes on cigarettes and other tobacco products, based on characteristics of the cigarettes or tobacco products (e.g. price, length, packaging, type of tobacco content, content of cigarettes). In previous years, the United Kingdom imposed differential taxes on cigarettes with high tar and nicotine content.[3] A differential tax system, however, may be prone to tax avoidance: the industry may alter an aspect of a brand, such as retail price, that subsequently reclassifies the brand into a lower tax bracket. Just such a phenomenon was recently observed in Egypt, where an international brand lowered its price just enough to be reclassified into a lower tax bracket.

Excise taxes are relatively easy to collect and therefore have low administrative costs. However, specific excise taxes are susceptible to losing value; they must keep up with inflation in order for their real value not to be eroded. Thus, specific excise taxes must be regularly updated to ensure that their real value is maintained over time. In recent years, a number of countries have shifted to specific excise taxes on tobacco products. However, among 55 countries that rely solely on specific excise taxes, only two (Australia and New Zealand) have automatic inflation adjustment mechanisms in place. A failure to adjust the excise taxes led to a problem in South Africa, as discussed below. Excise taxes there did not keep pace with inflation, leading to a fall in the real price of cigarettes and a concomitant rise in consumption prior to 1991.

In contrast, the real value of an ad valorem tax is maintained when the prices of tobacco products rise in conjunction with those of other goods and services. Thus, the real value of revenues generated by ad valorem taxes stays relatively stable over time, and they are favoured by the tobacco industry, which can maintain the base price, and therefore the tax, at a relatively low level. Similar to a differential tax system, ad valorem taxes are also prone to tax avoidance, since they rely on retail or wholesale price.

Tobacco tax rates differ widely across industrialized and developing countries. The tax rates of most countries that have used taxation as part of a comprehensive approach to reducing tobacco consumption have been around 65% to 75% of the retail price of cigarettes. However, many lower-income countries still have tax rates that fall well below 50% of the price of cigarettes, and many middle-income countries have rates that fall below 25% of the price.

Smokers may engage in compensating behaviours to sustain nicotine intake as a result of tax and price increases. They may smoke longer cigarettes or cigarettes with higher tar and nicotine content; or, because cigarettes and other tobacco products may substitute for one another as a source of nicotine, they may switch to hand-rolled cigarettes, pipes, snuff, chewing tobacco, or other forms of smokeless tobacco. Thus, tax increases need to be applied symmetrically across all types of tobacco products in a manner that equalizes their retail prices, so that consumers will not turn away from relatively high-priced products towards those with relatively lower prices.

Price Elasticity

To fully understand how taxation policies work, it is necessary to understand the concept of elasticity. Economists use the price elasticity of demand to measure the responsiveness of cigarette consumption to changes in the inflation-adjusted price of cigarettes. The price elasticity of demand is defined as the percentage change in the number of cigarettes consumed that results from a 1% increase in the inflation-adjusted price of cigarettes.

The reductions in cigarette use in response to price increases reflect not only increased smoking cessation and decreased smoking initiation, but also reduced relapse among former smokers and decreased average consumption by individuals who continue to smoke despite the higher prices.

Elastic demand is defined as an elasticity that is less than –1.0, or, alternatively, whose absolute value is greater than 1.0. In other words, the change in consumption is greater, in percentage terms, than the change in price. *Inelastic demand*, on the other hand, refers to situations in which consumption does go down when the price increases, but by a relatively smaller amount—the percentage change in consumption is less than the percentage change in the price. Inelastic demand is therefore defined as having an elasticity between 0.0 and –1.0.

There is a difference between short-term elasticities and long-term elasticities. In the long term, individuals are more elastic, meaning they will reduce consumption proportionately more than in the short term.[3] Most studies, however, measure demand in the short term only. While a majority of econometric studies of the effect of price on cigarette consumption use aggregate data, a growing number of such studies, particularly in high-income countries, are using individual-level data, which enables assessment of the impact of cigarette prices on smoking in subgroups of the population, such as by age, income, and gender.

Price Elasticity Estimates

Most of the econometric studies conducted in high-income industrialized countries, such as the United States, the United Kingdom, and Canada, conclude that the overall price elasticity of demand ranges from –0.5 to –0.25, implying that a 10% increase in the price of cigarettes will decrease overall cigarette consumption in these countries by between 5.0% and 2.5%.[3] Many of these studies used individual-level data to examine the determinants of cigarette demand. Several recent studies that employed individual-level data concluded that approximately one half of the overall impact of price on demand results from decreases in smoking prevalence, and the remainder results from reductions in average cigarette consumption by smokers.

Price Elasticity and Youth

The use of individual-level data allows researchers to examine differences in the price elasticity of demand by socioeconomic and demographic characteristics. Numerous studies in the United States have used individual-level data to explore differences in the price elasticity of demand by age. As noted in the chapter on the prevalence of tobacco use and factors influencing its initiation and maintenance, tobacco use among youth is rising, and in some countries, rates are the same for boys and girls. Measuring the impact of economic policies on youth smoking is thus an important global priority. Given that most regular smokers start smoking in their youth, it is important to try to understand the influence of price on this age group. There is a growing body of evidence indicating that adolescents and young adults are substantially more price-elastic than older adults.

Although some studies, such as those of Chaloupka,[19] Wasserman et al.,[20] and Townsend et al.,[21] found either that younger people were less price-sensitive than adults or that there was no statistically significant difference between youth and adult price-responsiveness, most other studies have found youth to be much more price-sensitive than adults. Young people in industrialized countries generally have relatively low incomes, of which a high proportion is available for discretionary expenditure, so changes in relative price are likely to affect their smoking patterns. Ross and Chaloupka found, in fact, that young people's demand for smoking in the United States, with an elasticity between –0.67 and –1.02, is more elastic than adult demand and that the perceived price of cigarettes is the largest single factor affecting teen smoking.[22]

Most researchers assume that price effects on youth reflect the impact of price on smoking initiation, while the estimate for adults reflects the effects of price on smoking cessation. Although some studies examining smoking initiation found that prices had an insignificant effect on initiation by young people,[23–25] some of these studies suffered from econometric problems associated with the use of retrospective data. Studies in which missing data are imputed[26] and which use larger samples that include a number of determinants of cigarette demand (such as restrictions on smoking)[27,28] have found relatively conclusive evidence that price increases will

World Health Organization

reduce not only the number of cigarettes smoked but also the overall prevalence of smoking among young people.

In fact, a majority of the studies that examine the economic determinants of cigarette consumption among youth and young adults have concluded that this age group is more price-responsive than adults, suggesting that excise tax increases leading to price increases would be a very effective means of reducing and discouraging cigarette smoking among adolescents. This would lead to permanent reductions in smoking in all age groups. The aforementioned studies are from the United States and the United Kingdom, high-income countries. However, a small but growing number of studies about the response to price and tax increases among youth in low- and middle-income countries have found evidence consistent with that from high-income countries on an inverse relationship between age and price-responsiveness. For example, Krasovsky et al. estimated differences in the price elasticity of cigarette demand by age and income in Ukraine[29] and found younger smokers to be more responsive to price changes than older smokers at each income level. Ross also estimated cigarette demand equations for students in Ukraine[30] and concluded that their price elasticities for smoking prevalence ranged from −0.29 to −0.51, while the estimated price elasticities for average smoking were considerably higher, from −1.42 to −1.83. Karki et al. estimated the joint demand for cigarettes and bidis by age in Nepal[31] and found that young people (15 through 24 years of age) were more than twice as responsive to price as the overall population and that price-responsiveness generally fell with age. Kyaing estimated price elasticities of smoked tobacco products in Myanmar[32] and found the price elasticity for youth and young adults to be approximately 50% greater than that for the overall population. Ross[33] estimated the price elasticity of demand for students in Moscow to be −1.15, well above the estimates provided in the limited studies of the impact of price on adult smoking in the Russian Federation.

Economic theory predicts that youth will respond more to price and tax increases than adults, and the evidence from the United States and the United Kingdom is very relevant to low- and middle-income countries, to which the tobacco epidemic is steadily shifting. In recent years, tobacco manufacturers have turned their attention to young women and girls in these countries— their largest untapped market. Given the documented effects of price increases on youth, increases in cigarette taxes can be a powerful tool for protecting young women and girls in low- and middle-income countries from the hazards of smoking.

Economic theory predicts that youth will respond more to price and tax increases than adults, and the evidence from the United States and the United Kingdom is very relevant to low- and middle-income countries, to which the tobacco epidemic is steadily shifting.

Lewit et al. suggest that young people are likely to be more price-sensitive than adults because they have been smoking for a shorter time and so can adjust more quickly to price changes than long-time smokers who are strongly addicted can.[34] Moreover, the fraction of disposable income spent on cigarettes by the young smoker is likely to be greater than that of an adult smoker. These are all important reasons for young smokers to be more affected by price increases than adults. These reasons create an important opportunity to discourage young people from taking up smoking. Because youth have higher discount rates than adults, they do not internalize risks and give less weight to future consequences from their current tobacco consumption.

Youth may also be influenced more easily than adults by bandwagon or peer-group effects.[34] That is, they are more likely to smoke if their parents, siblings, or peers smoke. Higher prices could discourage young people from smoking by the price mechanism's working through the same peer or bandwagon channel; that is, a price increase will not only reduce a youth's smoking but will also reduce peer smoking. Given evidence that individuals are far less likely to start smoking after they reach their mid-twenties, young smokers who never begin to smoke because of a price increase may well never become regular smokers. As a result, over a longer period of time, aggregate smoking and the detrimental health effects it imposes would be dramatically reduced.

Price Elasticity and Income

Some studies have used individual-level data to examine differences in the price elasticity of demand by income, socioeconomic status (SES), and education. These studies generally find that individuals who have lower income, have less education, or are of lower SES respond more to price changes than do individuals who have higher income, have more education, or are of higher SES, respectively.[19,21,35]

An inverse relationship between income and response to cigarette prices has also been found when comparing price-elasticity estimates of low- and high-income countries. A recent review of the literature suggests that the price-elasticty estimates for low- and middle-income countries are approximately double those for high-income countries.[3] That is, for low- and middle-income countries, demand is generally found to be more elastic, and estimates of the average price elasticity centre around –0.8.

> *Researchers found a positive relationship between income and cigarette consumption in all income groups in Turkey. Their results show that income elasticity declines with household income level.*

Income Effect on Demand

When factors that increase demand (such as rising per capita income) are taken into consideration, the full expected effect of higher prices on cigarette consumption may not be achieved. Evidence from many countries (e.g. Indonesia, Malaysia, Turkey, Viet Nam, and China) shows that changing per capita income significantly affects smoking prevalence, as well as cigarette demand.[36] Onder and Yurekli found a positive and significant relationship between income and frequency of cigarette smoking in all income groups in Turkey except for the richest group.[37] Their results suggest that as income increases, the prevalence of smoking increases more for the poorest group (0.11) than for the better-off groups (fourth quartile) (0.06), but the richest households decrease their smoking as their income increases (–0.02). Similarly, Adioetomo et al.[38] and Djutahara et al.[39] estimated that a rise in incomes in Indonesia would increase the number of smokers by causing more potential smokers to decide to take up smoking. They estimated that a 10% increase in daily income would raise the current number of smoking households* from 60.2% to 60.8% and would increase the quantity of cigarettes smoked by current smokers by 6.5%.**

Onder and Yurekli found a positive relationship between income and cigarette consumption in all income groups in Turkey.[37] Their results show that income elasticity declines with household income level. Adioetomo et al. also found a significant and positive relationship between income and the demand for cigarettes in Indonesia.[38] The income elasticity (e) was 0.65 in Adioetomo et al., and it varied between 0.46 and 0.21 in Djutahara et al.[39] As expected, Adioetomo et al. estimated that Indonesian smokers in low-income households were more sensitive to income increases (e= 0.9) than were smokers in high-income households (e= 0.3). Adioetomo et al. estimated that a 10% increase in income would increase the quantity of cigarettes smoked by 9% in low-income households, 3% in middle-income households, and less than 1% in high-income households.

The inverse relationship between price and demand and the positive relationship between income and demand will cause a simultaneous per capita income increase and cigarette price increase to have opposing effects on cigarette demand. In order to reduce consumption by a desired amount, the percentage increase in price will need to be higher if income is increasing. If cigarette prices remain unchanged while income increases, the demand for cigarettes will rise.

---

* The unit of measurement was households; the data indicate whether there are smokers in the household but do not indicate who smokes. So instead of using the criterion "smokers, non-smokers", the study refers to "smoking households" (where there are smokers) and "non-smoking households" (where there are no smokers). The results show that as daily income increases by 10%, the ratio between smoking and non-smoking households increases 63%, meaning at least one member of a non-smoking household will smoke, and the household will become a smoking household.

** A 10% increase in daily income will increase the log odd ratio by 2.64% for overall household level and 7.25% for low-income households. When evaluated at the mean values of all the variables, the 10% increase in income would increase the proportion of current households' smokers from 60.2% to 60.8%, and for low-income households, from 61.1% to 62.8%.

World Health Organization

Figure 11.1. Consumption and Price of Cigarettes in China, 1990–2005[50,51]

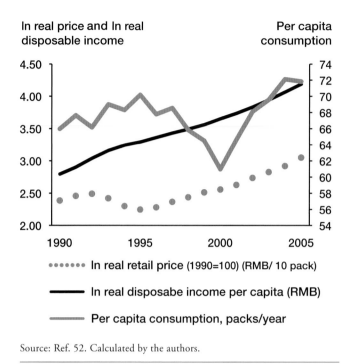

In real price and In real
disposable income

Per capita
consumption

•••••••• In real retail price (1990=100) (RMB/ 10 pack)

——— In real disposabe income per capita (RMB)

——— Per capita consumption, packs/year

Source: Ref. 52. Calculated by the authors.

One of the first studies of the impact of tobacco taxes on the demand for cigarettes and other tobacco products was conducted by Chapman and Richardson in 1990.[40] Using annual data from 1973 to 1986 for Papua New Guinea, they estimated tax elasticities of demand for cigarettes and other tobacco products to be –0.71 and –0.50, respectively. These estimates are lower than the true price elasticity of demand because the tobacco taxes are less than 100% of the price of the products. If half of the price is accounted for by the tax, the estimated price elasticity of demand for cigarettes and other tobacco products would be –1.42 and –1.0, respectively, significantly higher than the consensus estimate for high-income countries.

Since the publication of Chapman and Richardson's paper, interest in tobacco tax and price effects in low- and middle-income countries has been growing. A number of studies have examined the effects of tobacco taxes and prices on the demand for tobacco in these countries, and most, but not all, have shown that the demand for tobacco products is more responsive to price and tax changes there than it is in high-income countries. Studies from China,[41-43] Viet Nam,[44] South Africa,[45,46] Zimbabwe,[47] Morocco,[48] Myanmar,[32] Bulgaria,[49] and other low- and middle-income countries have estimated tax or price effects in excess of the consensus estimate for high-income countries. Several studies have examined the differential price response by income level. For example, Sayginsoy et al. estimated cigarette demand elasticities of –1.33, –1.00, and –0.52 for low-, middle-, and high-income individuals, respectively, in Bulgaria.[49] Van Walbeek estimated price

Figure 11.2. Relationship Between Cigarette Consumption and Excise Tax Rate in South Africa, 1980–2006[1,53]

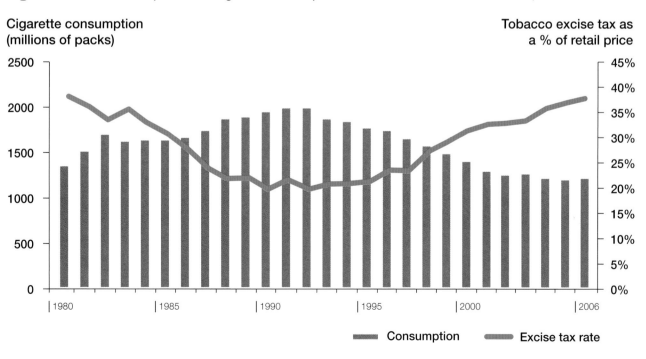

Cigarette consumption
(millions of packs)

Tobacco excise tax as
a % of retail price

▬▬ Consumption   ▬▬ Excise tax rate

Figure 11.3. Consumption and Price of Cigarettes in the United States, 1970–2006[54]

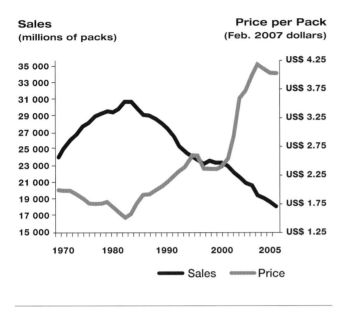

Sales (millions of packs)   **Price per Pack** (Feb. 2007 dollars)

relationship can also be seen graphically with bivariate scatter plots. For example, Figures 11.1, 11.2, and 11.3 plot cigarette price and cigarette consumption in China, South Africa, and the United States, respectively, and show a very strong inverse relationship between consumption and price.

Price Elasticty and Gender

Of particular importance in this chapter is the relationship between cigarette prices and smoking and patterns of tobacco use among women and men. The relationship between smoking and gender is a complex one that tends to change with changes in the labour force. Demand for cigarettes may increase as more women and girls in developing countries enter the wage labour force and have more disposable income. When the increases in retail prices of cigarettes fall behind the increases in inflation and increases in income, cigarettes become more affordable, and demand increases. This is the case in many countries where the smoking epidemic is highest among men and increasing among women (see Figure 11.4).

elasticities of demand by income quartile in South Africa and found that the lowest quartile was more elastic (–1.39) than the highest quartile (–0.81).[51]

While the aforementioned studies found inverse relationships between consumption and price by using multivariate analyses that control for a host of other factors thought likely to affect cigarette demand, the inverse

It is clear that the epidemiological pattern needs to be analysed in relation to the differential effects of economic development and consumer patterns on women and men. As noted in the chapter on prevalence of tobacco use and factors influencing initiation and maintenance among women, there is now a significant opportunity to prevent a

Figure 11.4. Cigarette Affordability in Selected Countries

Affordability, GDP per capita/retail price per pack, 1990=1

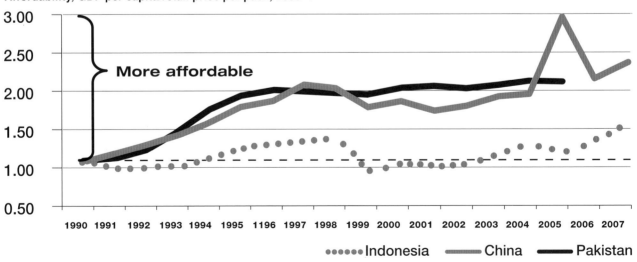
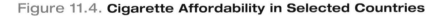

Source: WHO calculations using data from papers prepared as part of the Bloomberg Initiative to Reduce Tobacco Use (http://www.worldlungfoundation.org/publications.php).

World Health Organization

Table 11.1. Findings of Selected Studies of the Elasticity of Demand for Smoking by Sex

Date	Study	Country	Elasticity Estimate for Females	Elasticity Estimate for Males	Comment
Studies of Prevalence and Average Smoking					
1973	Atkinson and Skegg	UK	−0.34	No significant response	Aggregate-level annual data on cigarette sales in UK for years 1951–1970
1982	Lewit and Coate	USA	No significant response	Aged 20–25, -1.4; aged 35+, -0.45	1976 Health Interview Survey
1990	Chaloupka	USA	No significant response	−0.60 long-run price elasticity	Second National Health and Nutrition Examination Survey
1994	Townsend, Roderick, and Cooper	UK	−0.61	−0.47	General Household Survey 1972–1990
1997	Lewit et al.	USA	No significant response	−1.51	Ninth-grade students from 21 North American communities, 1990–1992
1998	Farrelly and Bray	USA	−0.19	−0.26	National Health Interview Surveys 1976–1993
1999	Chaloupka and Pacula	USA	−0.595	−0.928	8th-, 10th-, and 12th- grade students, Monitoring the Future Surveys 1992–1994
2000	Hersch	USA	−0.38	−0.54	Tobacco Use Supplement to the Current Population Survey 1992–1993
2001	Farrelly and Bray	USA	−0.32	−0.18	National Health Interview Surveys 1976–1993
2001	Stephens et al.	Canada	−0.3	−0.5	National Population Health Survey
2007	Stehr	USA	−0.51	−0.26	Behavioural Risk Factor Surveillance System 1985–2000
Studies of Smoking Transitions					
2001	Tauras and Chaloupka	USA	0.34 to 0.71 price elasticity of cessation	0.27 to 0.92 price elasticity of cessation	Longitudinal component of the Monitoring the Future Surveys 1976–1995
2004	Cawley, Markowitz, and Tauras	USA	No significant response	−0.86 to −1.49 price elasticity of initiation	National Longitudinal Survey of Youth 1997 Cohort (1997–2000)
2004	Cawley, Markowitz, and Tauras	USA	No significant response	−1.20 price elasticity of initiation	Children of the National Longitudinal Survey of Youth 1979 Cohort (1988–2000)
Studies of Smoking During Pregnancy					
1999	Evans and Ringel	USA	−0.50	Not applicable	Natality Detail Files, 1989 and 1992
2001	Ringel and Evans	USA	−0.70	Not applicable	Natality Detail Files, 1989 and 1995

 World Health Organization

worldwide epidemic of tobacco use among women and girls, including in countries like China, where sex differences in prevalence and health impact are high.[1,55–57]

> ***In the United States, men were found to be very responsive to changes in cigarette prices, with a long-run price elasticity of demand estimated to be –0.60. Women, however, were often found to be less responsive to cigarette price changes, a finding consistent with those of Lewit and Coate.***

Recently published studies that estimated the price elasticity of demand by gender are summarized in Table 11.1. Most of the evidence of a differential price response by gender comes from the United States, the United Kingdom, and Canada. The results from these studies are mixed. A preponderance of those conducted in North American countries concluded that women's cigarette consumption is less responsive to changes in cigarette prices than is men's. In contrast, studies in the United Kingdom have generally found women's consumption of cigarettes to be more responsive than men's to price changes.

Studies of Prevalence and Cigarette Consumption by Smokers in the United States

One of the first US studies to examine gender-specific differences in the effects of cigarette prices on consumption was conducted by Lewit and Coate in 1982.[58] Using a split-sample methodology and data from the 1976 Health Interview Survey, Lewit and Coate found cigarette demand by females to be generally not sensitive to price. In contrast, with the exception of those 26 to 35 years of age, males were found to respond significantly to price. The price elasticities of demand for males aged 20 to 25 and over 35 were estimated to be –1.4 and –0.45,

respectively. The male price coefficients were significantly larger than the male and female pooled-sample results, where the male and female price coefficients were constrained to be equal.

Chaloupka also employed a split-sample methodology to examine differences in the effects of cigarette prices on consumption by gender.[59] Using data from the Second National Health and Nutrition Examination Survey and incorporating the addictive properties of cigarette smoking, including reinforcement, tolerance, and withdrawal, Chaloupka found men to be very responsive to changes in cigarette prices, with a long-run price elasticity of demand estimated to be –0.60. Women, however, were found to be unresponsive to cigarette price changes, a finding consistent with those of Lewit and Coate.[58]

Lewit et al. examined differences in the effects of cigarette prices on smoking prevalence by gender among ninth-grade students (aged 13 to 16) in 21 North American communities in 1990 and 1992.[60] Ninth-grade boys were found to be much more responsive to changes in cigarette prices than girls were. The estimated prevalence price elasticities of demand for boys and girls were –1.51 and –0.32, respectively; however, the estimated price coefficients in the girls' equations were found not to be significantly different from zero.

Chaloupka and Pacula used data on eighth-, tenth-, and twelfth-grade students from the 1992–1994 Monitoring the Future Surveys to examine the price sensitivity of cigarette demand by sex.[61] While price was found to have a negative and significant impact on smoking prevalence rates of both young men and young women, the magnitude of the price effects was very different. The prevalence price elasticity of demand for young men was nearly twice as large (in absolute value) as that for young women: –0.928 vs –0.595.

Hersch extracted data from the 1992 and 1993 waves of the Tobacco Use Supplements to the Current Population Surveys and found that higher prices reduce cigarette demand in both men and women.[62] The estimated price elasticities of demand were similar for men and women and ranged from –0.6 to –0.4. However, when Hersch restricted the sample to individuals in the workforce, she found males to be significantly more responsive to cigarette price changes than females.

In a series of papers, Farrelly et al. pooled data from National Health Interview Surveys (NHIS) between 1976 and 1993 to investigate the cigarette-price-responsiveness of individuals with different demographic characteristics. In the first paper, Farrelly and Bray controlled for many factors thought likely to affect the demand for cigarettes, including socioeconomic and demographic characteristics, as well as year and region indicators.[35] They found that males were more responsive to changes in cigarette prices than were females. A follow-up study used the same pooled NHIS data but included state fixed effects in each model instead of region fixed effects.[63] With the state-fixed-effect specification, the authors found that women were more price-responsive than men.

The inclusion of state fixed effects eliminates time-invariant unobserved state-level heterogeneity from the model. To the extent that sentiment towards smoking within states is time-invariant during the period under investigation, the inclusion of state fixed effects in the model eliminates an omitted variable bias on the price estimates. That is, sentiment towards tobacco may be driving both changes in cigarette smoking and changes in cigarette excise taxes. Thus, not controlling for anti-tobacco sentiment may result in an omitted variable bias, producing a spurious negative relationship between price and smoking and resulting in estimated price elasticities biased away from zero. The use of state fixed effects relies on within-state variation in cigarette prices over time (as opposed to interstate differences in prices) to quantify the effect of price on consumption. For the state-fixed-effects approach to be viable, however, researchers must use multiple years of state data. One year of cross-sectional data would result in perfect multicollinearity between the state-specific prices and the dichotomous state indicators. Moreover, even if multiple years of state data are employed, there must be reasonable variation in price over time within states to avoid collinearity issues with the price variable.

Stehr used data extracted from the 1985–2000 Behavioural Risk Factor Surveillance System to investigate differences in the effects of cigarette taxes on cigarette demand by sex.[64] He included gender-specific state fixed effects in his model and concluded that women are nearly twice as responsive to cigarette taxes as men are. Specifically, the total estimated price elasticities of demand for women and for men were −0.51 and −0.26, respectively. The gender-specific state fixed effects are an attempt to control for state-specific gender gaps in smoking rate that may be

correlated with cigarette taxes. If a significant correlation exists, the omission of the gender-specific state fixed effects could lead to biased price estimates.

Studies of Smoking Transitions in the United States

As noted above, many researchers examining the influence of price on smoking prevalence have assumed that the effect of price on youth is dominated by the effect on smoking initiation, while the effect on young adults and older adults is dominated by the effect on smoking cessation. Several recent studies have attempted to directly quantify the differential impact of price on smoking initiation among youths by gender and the differential impact of price on cessation among young adults. These studies have relied on longitudinal data that track individuals' smoking behaviour and other determinants over time.

Cawley, Markowitz, and Tauras investigated the determinants of youth smoking initiation, using the first four waves (1997–2000) of the National Longitudinal Survey of Youth 1997 cohort.[65] They investigated two alternative measures of smoking initiation: one that indicated a transition from non-smoker to smoking any positive quantity of cigarettes (termed "less stringent initiation"), and one (termed "more stringent initiation") that reflected the transition from non-smoker to frequent smoker, as measured by having smoked during at least 15 of the past 30 days. While controlling for smoke-free-air laws, youth-access laws, and residence in tobacco-producing states, the authors concluded that male adolescent smoking initiation was very responsive to changes in cigarette prices, with the average price elasticity of "less stringent initiation" estimated to be −0.86 and the average price elasticity of "more stringent initiation" estimated to be −1.49. Female smoking initiation was found to be not significantly related to cigarette prices but very responsive to body-weight concerns.

A follow-up paper found results very similar to those of the earlier study, despite using a longitudinal dataset that spans a longer period.[66] The authors used data from 1988 to 2000 from the Children of the National Longitudinal Survey of Youth 1979 cohort. After controlling for smoke-free-air laws and youth-access laws, they found that cigarette prices had a negative impact on smoking initiation in all models that were estimated; however, the price coefficients were significantly different from zero in only the male equations. Specifically, the price elasticity of male "less stringent initiation" was estimated to be –1.20.

Tauras and Chaloupka examined gender differences in the impact of price on young adults' decisions to quit smoking,[67] using the longitudinal component of the Monitoring the Future Surveys and a semiparametric Cox regression to assess the probability that smokers would make a transition from smoking to non-smoking. They concluded that the likelihood of making a smoking cessation attempt for both men and women increases significantly as cigarette prices rise. The estimated price elasticity of smoking cessation ranged from 0.34 to 0.71 for women and from 0.27 to 0.92 for men, implying that a 10% increase in price raises the probability of making a cessation attempt by up to 7% for females and 9% for males.

While comprehensive tobacco control programmes have been found to be effective in reducing smoking in the overall population, some evidence suggests that women benefit in particular.

Previous Studies in the United Kingdom and Canada

One of the first studies to examine gender-specific differences in the effects of cigarette prices on consumption was conducted by Atkinson and Skegg in 1973.[68] Using aggregate-level annual data on cigarette sales in the United Kingdom from 1951 to 1970 and gender-specific shares of consumption, they found clear differences in the estimated price elasticity of demand: women have a total price elasticity of demand of –0.34, and men do not significantly respond to price changes.

Townsend, Roderick, and Cooper used biennial data on smoking from the general household survey for 1972–1990 in the United Kingdom and found that women respond more to price than men do.[21] They estimated the price elasticity of demand to be –0.61 for women and –0.47 for men.

Finally, Stephens et al. used data from Canada's National Population Health Survey to examine differential response to cigarette prices by gender and found cigarette prices to be positively associated with the odds of being a non-smoker for adults of both sexes; however, males responded more to the price change than did females.[69] The price elasticity for being a smoker for men was estimated to be –0.5, and for women it was estimated to be –0.3.

Policy Implications

Smoking and Pregnancy

Given the well-documented evidence that women who smoke or who are around smokers while pregnant expose their child to increasing health risks, it is important to quantify the impact of cigarette tax and price increases on consumption among pregnant women. The evidence on the impact of higher taxes on smoking during pregnancy comes from two studies conducted in the United States. Using data from the 1989 and 1992 Natality Detail Files, Evans and Ringel found that higher cigarette taxes reduce smoking prevalence rates among maternal smokers but do not decrease average consumption among those who continue to smoke.[70] They calculated a price elasticity of smoking prevalence of –0.50, implying that a 10% increase in the price of cigarettes will reduce the prevalence of maternal smoking by 5%. Moreover, they found that the tax-induced decreases in smoking improved birth outcomes. In particular, the average birth weight rose by approximately 400 g among women who quit smoking because of higher taxes.

In a follow-up study, Ringel and Evans examined the impact of taxes on smoking among different subpopulations of maternal smokers.[71] They extracted data from the 1989 and 1995 Natality Detail Files and found that for all subpopulations except women who did not report their education, tax increases had a significant negative effect on maternal smoking rates. They calculated an overall maternal participation price elasticity of –0.7. For all subgroups except those not reporting education, the price elasticity of participation was larger (in absolute value) than the consensus general-population participation price-elasticity estimates.

The reduction in smoking rates among pregnant women in response to a tax increase not only improves birth outcomes, but also has cost implications. Lightwood, Phibbs, and Glantz estimated that smoking cessation programmes that reduce smoking rates among pregnant women before or during the first trimester of pregnancy yield significant cost savings.[14] In particular, they found that a 1% decline in smoking prevalence among pregnant women would save US$ 21 million (in 1995 dollars) in direct medical costs alone in the first year. An annual 1% decline in smoking prevalence among pregnant women would save US$ 572 million (in 1995 dollars) in direct medical costs in the first seven years.

Many studies have found that exposure of non-smoking pregnant women to SHS results in negative consequences.[13] A recent systematic review and meta-analysis concluded that SHS exposure was associated with a 33 g reduction in mean birth weight in prospective studies and a 40 g reduction in mean birth weight in retrospective studies. The review also concluded that SHS exposure increased the risk of birth weight being below 2500 g by 22%. This review has very important implications for paternal and other household smoking during pregnancy. Independent of maternal smoking, paternal and other household smoking imposes costs and negative consequences on fetal health.

Earmarked Taxes and Tobacco Control Programmes

Earmarking a portion of the revenue generated from tobacco taxes for tobacco control programmes reinforces the effect of the higher tax on consumption. Numerous studies conducted in the United States have examined the impact of comprehensive tobacco programmes on smoking and health. The Institute of Medicine reviewed these studies and concluded that multifaceted tobacco control programmes are effective in reducing tobacco use.[72] Moreover, while such programmes have been found to be effective in the overall population, some evidence suggests that women benefit in particular. A study published by the Centers for Disease Control and Prevention found that from 1988 to 1997, lung cancer rates among women in California, the state with the longest-standing

tobacco control programme in the United States, decreased by 4.8%, whereas lung cancer rates increased by 13% among women in other parts of the country.[73] In addition, a report by Abt Associates found that between 1990 and 1999 in Massachusetts, the second state in the United States to create a comprehensive tobacco control programme using earmarked tobacco taxes, smoking among pregnant women declined by more than 50%, the greatest percentage decrease in any state over that time period.[74] Indeed, the 2001 Surgeon General's report on women and smoking concluded that pregnancy-specific tobacco control programmes, some of which are funded from earmarked revenues, benefit both maternal and infant health and are cost effective.

The evidence on the impact of higher cigarette taxes on smoking during pregnancy is clear: cigarette taxes reduce smoking prevalence rates among maternal smokers, and the impact of a tax increase is significantly larger on pregnant women than on the general population.

Other countries, including Canada, Finland, Denmark, Peru, Poland, Indonesia, the Republic of Korea, Malaysia, Romania, Thailand, and Nepal, as well as some US states, have earmarked tobacco taxes for tobacco-related education, counteradvertising, health care for underinsured populations, cancer research, and other health-related activities. Moreover, tax revenues are used in several Australian states and in New Zealand to fund athletic and art events previously sponsored by the tobacco industry.[3] While many finance ministries have concerns about the use of earmarked taxes for reasons relating to loss of control, rigidities in allocating general revenues, and the domino effect of other sectors also wanting hypothecated taxes, it has been argued that earmarked tobacco taxes can help reduce the loss of producer and consumer surplus from higher taxes.

Earmarked tobacco taxes can also be used to target lower-income populations that continue to smoke, and such transfers can help to reduce inequalities in health outcomes. For example, women's groups have called for more funds to be used to integrate tobacco control into reproductive health services, such as maternal and child health and family planning. These taxes could be used to subsidize cessation programmes and nicotine replacement therapies to assist and support continuing smokers. If women do have more difficulty quitting than men do, and if women in lower socioeconomic groups continue to smoke, supporting services for them through the use of earmarked taxes could help to reduce the burden of taxation falling on them and the resultant inequalities in health.

Health Implications

There is solid evidence from countries of all income levels that increased taxation of cigarettes is highly effective in reducing consumption.[75] Moreover, there is a strong economic rationale for governments' use of taxes to reduce smoking.[76] Studies of price-responsiveness by gender have primarily been conducted in high-income countries, and a majority of studies have concluded that males are slightly more price-responsive than females. The evidence on the impact of higher cigarette taxes on smoking during pregnancy is clear: cigarette taxes reduce smoking prevalence rates among maternal smokers, and the impact of a tax increase is significantly larger on pregnant women than on the general population. Finally, earmarking a portion of the revenue generated from tobacco taxes for tobacco control programmes reinforces the effect of the tax on consumption.

Given the relationship between pricing and demand and the significant health benefits accruing from cessation, tobacco control measures and taxation in particular can potentially avert millions of premature tobacco-related deaths. World Bank estimates of the health impact of control measures on global tobacco consumption are striking.[77] Under conservative assumptions, a sustained real price increase of 10% could lead to 40 million people worldwide quitting smoking and to deterring many more from taking it up. This price increase alone would avoid 10 million premature deaths, or 3% of all tobacco-related deaths. Four million of the premature deaths avoided would be in East Asia and the Pacific region.

While the public health community continues to appeal for higher tobacco taxes on the basis of social costs, few people would deny the justification of a tax increase based on health benefits. Given the empirical and other problems of the social cost argument, research on taxation may indeed be a very valuable pursuit in helping to convince policy-makers of the irrefutable health gains that can be achieved from increasing taxes on tobacco.

Government Perspective: Revenue Generation

Tobacco tax revenue has accounted for 3% to 5% of total government revenues in most industrialized countries, although its importance has been steadily declining.[3] Nevertheless, in some middle-income countries, tobacco tax revenue constitutes an important share of total government revenue. For example, in South Africa, with an estimated long-run price elasticity of −0.68 and where taxes now account for 40% of the price of cigarettes,[78] a permanent doubling of the cigarette tax would reduce demand by more than 27% in the long run (assuming the tax is fully passed on to consumers) and would increase cigarette tax revenues by nearly 50%.[3] Tobacco taxes would then account for nearly 2% of total government revenues. However, as already noted, because the government did not allow tobacco taxes to keep pace with inflation in the 1970s and 1980s, forgone excise revenue was substantial.

Revenue-generating potential will be highest where the demand for tobacco products is more inelastic or where tax as a percentage of price is relatively low. For most countries, there is still ample room to increase taxes and raise valuable tax revenue. A 10% tax increase will, on average, lead to a 7% increase in tobacco tax revenue. Therefore, even in countries where demand has been more elastic or where taxes are already a large share of price, tax increases would still lead to increases in government revenue, at least in the short run. Given the economic models of addiction and the fact that demand will be more responsive to price in the long run, a permanent change in price will have an effect on demand that will grow over time to almost double the short-run impact.[3] In addition, given the sensitivity of consumers—particularly youth—to price, permanent real increases in tobacco taxes will lead to greater reductions in prevalence and overall consumption. Therefore, increases in tobacco taxes will lead to greater tax revenue increases in the short run than in the long run.

Concerns About Tobacco Taxation

Regressivity

Several concerns have been expressed about using cigarette taxation as a tool for health promotion. These include policy-makers' considerations about the appropriate level of taxation and issues surrounding the efficiency and equity of taxes. Cigarette taxes impose a regressive burden on people with low incomes in places where they smoke disproportionately more than those with higher incomes. Therefore, there is a dual concern about the increasing burden of smoking-related diseases on low-income groups and the implications of price increases for low income smokers.

Tobacco taxation can violate notions of both horizontal equity (where "equals", or individuals who are identical except for their smoking behaviour, should be treated equally) and vertical equity (where rich individuals should have proportionally higher taxes because of differences in income). Vertical equity implies that individuals with the greatest ability to pay should carry the highest tax burden—in other words, marginal tax rates should be higher for the rich. Tobacco taxes clearly violate this principle in countries where poorer people smoke more than wealthy people. The disparity is worsened when income falls and tobacco taxes rise as a share of income or total expenditures. Therefore, tobacco taxes are regressive when tobacco use is more prevalent among persons with lower incomes.

However, recent evidence suggests that tobacco taxes may not be as regressive as has been feared, because rich and poor consumers do not smoke and quit at the same rates following a price increase. This has recently been shown by differences in the price elasticity of demand for different socioeconomic groups, which suggest that the regressivity normally attributed to cigarette taxation is overstated. Studies have found the price elasticity of demand to be inversely related to social class, with those in the highest social classes being less price-responsive than those in the lowest social classes.[21]

Because persons with less education, lower income, and lower SES have been found to be more price-responsive than those with more education, higher income, and higher SES, increased cigarette taxes would reduce differences in smoking among socioeconomic groups. Even though cigarette taxes may fall most heavily on lower-income smokers, increases in taxes may be progressive from a public health standpoint in that larger reductions in smoking occur among that group. The health benefits from tax-induced reductions in smoking would therefore be disproportionately larger for lower-income people. Thus, analyses that have failed to take into account the inverse relationship between elasticity and income overstate the regressive effect of tobacco taxes.

Figure 11.5. Pre-Tax Price of a Pack of Cigarettes in the European Region, 2007

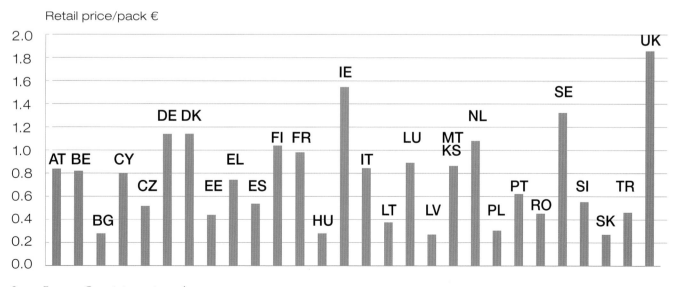

Source: European Commission, excise tax data.

However, support may be needed to reduce the regressivity of tobacco taxes for persons in lower income groups who continue to smoke and their families. In low-income families, particularly in developing countries, spending on tobacco can "crowd out" expenditures on other essential household needs, including food and education.[79] Cessation therapies and nicotine replacement products and other support services could be offered to the poor, and earmarking of tax revenues could help in subsidizing these services.

> *Manufacturers could be required to use serial numbers on each pack to facilitate tracking, while pack-marking technology could provide further information about each link in the supply chain, such as the distributor, the wholesaler, and the exporter.*

Related concerns about increased taxation include the effect it may have on cross-border shopping and smuggling and the effect it may have on the tobacco industry regarding employment and, more broadly, the macroeconomy and trade balances. These last two issues are discussed in more detail below.

The Threat of Smuggling

Differences in cigarette taxes and prices potentially lead to casual and organized smuggling and other forms of tax evasion. Worldwide, organized smuggling, which targets a significant amount of cigarettes, is the most serious illicit activity. Smugglers camouflage illicit cigarettes through trade, since the exports are free of duty from the exporting countries. Although tax differences can create a financial incentive for smugglers, this incentive already exists in the absence of taxes, because of the significant differences in pre-tax prices of cigarettes (see Figure 11.5).

The tobacco industry argues that cigarette tax increases can erode valuable tax revenues, which would be lost because of smuggling, while not reducing consumption. Sweden decreased cigarette taxes by 17% in 1998 because of a perception that smuggling led to lost cigarette tax revenues, and it saw its tax revenues fall as a result. Other countries also have chosen not to increase tobacco taxes partly out of fear of the development of a black market, given differences in tax rates across neighbouring countries.[77]

The number of studies trying to quantify the global illicit trade and examine the relationship between tobacco taxes and illicit trade is increasing. Earlier studies estimated that about 30% of internationally exported cigarettes are lost to smuggling,[3] and although the problem is acute, it has often been overstated.[80] Yurekli and Sayginsoy estimated that in 1999, 3.4% of global cigarette consumption was of illegal cigarettes,[54] whereas a study by Joossens et al. found that 11.6% of the global cigarette market is illicit.[81] Large tobacco tax increases—and significant price increases initiated by the tobacco industry—have occurred in several countries without causing dramatic increases in smuggling. Other factors, such as lack of enforcement and a general culture of corruption, may be more important contributors to the likelihood of smuggling. Many countries with high prices, including France, Norway, the United Kingdom, and Sweden, show very little evidence of smuggling, while several countries with low prices, such as Spain and Italy, have evidence of extensive smuggling.

The complicity of the tobacco industry in smuggling should also be recognized when considering the credibility of its call for reducing taxes to prevent smuggling. The tobacco industry is a clear beneficiary of smuggling, in that when smuggled cigarettes account for a high proportion of the total sold, the average price of all cigarettes, taxed and untaxed, falls, increasing sales of cigarettes overall. The tobacco industry has argued that a significant proportion of smuggled cigarettes are counterfeit cigarettes and that these counterfeit cigarettes reduce their sales.

The smuggling problem is exacerbated by the ease with which tobacco products can be transported, the huge potential profits, the informal distribution networks in many countries, the availability of tax-free and duty-free cigarettes, and the lack of enforcement in many countries.[80] Most smuggled cigarettes are well-known international brands smuggled somewhere in transit between the country of origin and the country of destination, reappearing in the country of origin at cut-rate prices, untaxed.

Any of several easy-to-implement policies, including stronger enforcement, use of tax stamps, and greater penalties for smugglers, could significantly reduce the problem.[82] Tax stamps—which must be difficult to forge—on duty-paid packs could help enforcers ensure the legality of packs. Special packaging for duty-free packs would also help.

In addition, all parties in the supply chain could be licensed, as they are in France and Singapore, for example. Manufacturers could be required to use serial numbers on each pack to facilitate tracking, while pack-marking technology could provide further information about each link in the supply chain, such as the distributor, the wholesaler, and the exporter. Manufacturers could be required to keep better records regarding the final destination of their products. Computerized control systems would enable the tracking of individual consignments and their progress at any point in time; such a system is currently in place in Hong Kong SAR. Finally, exporters could be required to label packs with the country of final destination and a health warning in the language of that country.[77]

The threat of smuggling could lead to regional coordination, enabling successful application of tobacco tax policies across countries. Multilateral agreements that take relative tax structures into account could be valuable in applying consistent tobacco control policies across regions. For example, the WHO Framework Convention on Tobacco Control (WHO FCTC), a multilateral treaty addressing global tobacco control with more than 170 Parties, includes provisions with specific obligations regarding taxation, pricing, and controlling smuggling. Specifically, Article 6 of the WHO FCTC, *Price and tax measures to reduce the demand for tobacco,* encourages Parties to adopt price and tax measures aimed at reducing tobacco consumption and to prohibit or restrict sales and importations of duty-free tobacco products. Article 15, *Illicit trade in tobacco products,* provides binding guidance on controlling illicit trade; to augment this, the Parties to the WHO FCTC are negotiating a protocol, or additional treaty, on the elimination of illicit trade in tobacco products. The presence of these issues in the WHO FCTC, a legally binding instrument, and the commitment demonstrated by undertaking a new

negotiation process for the protocol reflect the importance of coordinated action, since strong national measures taken in a single country can be undone if transnational dimensions such as smuggling are not addressed.

Impact on Employment

Although the focus of tobacco control programmes is largely on demand reduction, it is important to acknowledge that the cultivation of tobacco is important to many countries' economies. Policies regarding the supply side of tobacco production, processing, and manufacture affect millions of women workers. Much more research is needed on the economics of how gender norms and roles affect women and men differently in tobacco growing, production, and marketing. In general, rural women are the backbone of small tobacco-producing farms, performing the most labour-intensive jobs, including weeding, leaf selection, and gathering of fuel for curing. They are also the majority of bidi workers in India and, in some countries, the majority in tobacco-product manufacture.

In addition to health consequences they share with men, women face additional medical costs linked to tobacco use due to increased complications during pregnancy and low-birth-weight babies.

Tobacco is grown in more than 125 countries, and the global value of crop production is approximately US$ 25 billion. This is less than 1% of the value of agricultural production globally,[77] but in some countries the relative value is considerably higher. The Chinese government, which controls tobacco production through a state-controlled monopoly, receives about 240 billion yuan (US$ 30 billion) annually from combined profits and taxes related to production. China is the world's leading cigarette producer, manufacturing one third of the world's cigarettes. An estimated two thirds of the workers employed worldwide in

World Health Organization

cigarette production work in just three countries—China, India, and Indonesia. Tobacco leaf exports constitute an especially large part of the economy in Zimbabwe and Malawi. In Thailand, revenue from taxation of tobacco products accounts for more than 5% of total government revenue. Economic and political concerns about threats to the industry can play a major role in the debate over tobacco control policies in these countries.

One of the main concerns raised by the tobacco industry and the general public is that tobacco control policies may increase unemployment and may negatively impact the economy. Several studies have been commissioned by the tobacco industry to produce estimates of their contribution to employment, incomes, and tax revenue in order to convince legislators that tobacco control policies will harm the broader economy and cause widespread job loss.[83–85] These studies have been criticized because they calculate the gross contribution of tobacco to employment, tax revenue, and the economy. They do not take into account the fact that if people stop spending money on tobacco, they usually will spend it on other things, thus generating alternative jobs.

Several independent studies on the overall net effect of tobacco control policies on various economies indicate a very minimal but usually positive effect in the long run.[86–89] These studies take into account the compensating effect of alternative jobs that would be generated by money not spent on tobacco.[90] Independent studies also show that in most countries and over the medium and long run, even very stringent tobacco control policies will have minimal negative impact on long-run economic growth, employment, tax revenue, and foreign trade balances as expenditure switches and reallocations in the economy take place. A country's reliance on tobacco exports and its stage of development influence its view of and openness to tobacco control measures, as, in general, a few large tobacco-producing and exporting countries stand to lose more than the majority of countries that are net importers and consumers of tobacco.[91]

The impact of a fall in consumption will vary, depending on the type of economy in the country where it occurs. The small handful of net exporting economies that are heavily dependent on tobacco for foreign-exchange earnings could experience net national job losses. However, even those agrarian economies that are dependent on tobacco production and exports will have a large enough market

to ensure jobs for many years to come, despite gradually declining demand.

The overwhelming evidence suggests that the best approach is to emphasize measures that reduce demand, leaving supply to adjust to evolving changes in demand. As long as demand grows, buy-outs, price supports, subsidies, and alternative crop programmes will have minimal effect, since they will merely produce opportunities and profits for future producers of tobacco.[16] At the same time, the WHO FCTC (Articles 17 and 18) commits Party governments to supporting crop diversification, economically viable alternative activities, and sustainable livelihoods to address concerns about the effects of tobacco control on tobacco production and the environment, especially in poor developing countries.

Conclusions

This chapter provides a broad review of the economic literature on the costs of smoking and the effects of taxation, highlighting findings pertaining to women. The evidence presented on the health and economic consequences of tobacco use constitutes a robust justification for governments' use of tobacco taxes as a way to protect women's health.

Estimates of the treatment costs and productivity losses associated with diseases caused by smoking provide potentially powerful evidence for implementing tobacco control. Significant costs are also associated with SHS exposure, and the majority of victims of SHS are women and children, particularly in developing countries. Because the majority of the smokers are males, women are particularly at risk of SHS exposure at home from their partners. Moreover, since the majority of the people who work outside the home are male, women are likely to be exposed to SHS in the workplace as well. In addition to health consequences they share with men, women face additional medical costs linked to tobacco use, such as increased complications during pregnancy and low-birth-weight babies. Moreover, women face significant tobacco-related personal and economic costs, particularly in low-income countries, where they tend to have fewer resources than men.

The evidence that taxation of cigarettes is highly effective in reducing consumption is supported by more than

100 studies that examined the impact of cigarette prices on the demand for cigarettes in high-income countries. The consensus estimate from these studies is that the overall price elasticity of demand ranges from –0.25 to –0.50, implying that a 10% increase in the price of cigarettes will decrease overall cigarette consumption by between 2.5% and 5.0%. A smaller, but growing, number of studies have examined the effects of price changes in low- and middle-income countries. Recent evidence suggests that the price-elasticty estimates for these countries are approximately double those for high-income countries. That is, demand is generally found to be more elastic in low- and middle-income countries, and the average price elasticity is estimated to be about –0.8.

Economic theory predicts an inverse relationship between age and the response to changes in the price of tobacco products. A majority of the research from high-income countries confirms this prediction, finding that youth and young adults are more responsive to tobacco price changes than adults are. Some recent studies suggest that adolescents may be as much as three times as responsive to price changes as adults.

The number of studies of price-responsiveness by gender is growing. Most of these studies have been conducted in high-income, industrialized countries, and the results are mixed with respect to the influence of price. The evidence from North America generally leads to the conclusion that men's cigarette consumption is more responsive than women's to changes in price. However, recent results from the United States indicate that the magnitude of the price response by gender is sensitive to the inclusion of state fixed effects, which are designed to hold constant time-invariant state-level heterogeneity, such as smoking sentiment. Studies conducted in the United Kingdom have generally found women's consumption of cigarettes to be more responsive to price changes than men's consumption. Finally, studies from the United States have concluded that cigarette tax increases lead to significant decreases in maternal smoking rates. The price elasticity of smoking participation among pregnant women was estimated to be much larger (in absolute value) than that among the consensus general population.

Earmarking a portion of the revenue generated from tobacco taxes for tobacco control programmes reinforces the effect of the tax on consumption. Numerous studies conducted in the United States have examined the impact of comprehensive tobacco programmes on smoking

and health. These studies generally conclude that comprehensive tobacco control programmes, independent of price changes, are effective in reducing tobacco use. Comprehensive tobacco control programmes have been found to be effective in reducing smoking in the overall population, and some evidence suggests that women benefit in particular, with substantial declines in lung cancer rates and in smoking among pregnant women.

Most of the objections to increased taxes and other tobacco control policies on the supply side are based on misinformation and should not be used as arguments to dissuade governments from raising taxes. These include threats of smuggling, the idea that tobacco taxes place a disproportionate burden on the poor, the fear that higher taxes will lead to reductions in revenue, and the possibility that tax increases will lead to decreased employment and macroeconomic vitality. There is little evidence to support these claims, and the threat of not doing anything to prevent the tobacco epidemic from spreading to women and children is far greater than these concerns.

While much has been learned from previous research in industrialized countries, more research is warranted. In particular, more research is required in high-income countries to disentangle the mixed results on the effects of price on smoking prevalence and average consumption by gender. Studies should focus on the impact of unobserved heterogeneity, including sentiment towards tobacco, which may be driving some of the mixed results in research to date. Moreover, additional studies are needed from high-income countries on the gender-specific impact of cigarette prices on smoking initiation and cessation and other transitions in the smoking uptake and cessation continuums. More research is warranted on the impact of comprehensive programmes, independent of cigarette prices, on female tobacco use.

The past few decades have seen a growing recognition of the effects of smoking on women in low- and middle-income countries. Much more research must be conducted on the impact of cigarette prices on demand for cigarettes by gender in these countries. Studies that examine gender differences in the impact of price on smoking prevalence, average consumption, smoking initiation, smoking cessation, and other transitions are desperately needed. Furthermore, the differential response to price by sex should be examined for other tobacco products commonly consumed by women in some countries, e.g. chewing tobacco, hookas, bidis, and kreteks. For many of these countries, surveys will need to be conducted to collect information on tobacco consumption, SES, and demographic factors. This may not be feasible for countries with limited resources, but in countries where national health surveys are being planned, there is an opportunity for researchers to help design the surveys and collect the data needed for such analyses. Greater attention must be paid to economic research on gender with a focus on women in all their diversity, by age, ethnicity, region, occupation, and political and social status.

References

1. *WHO report on the global tobacco epidemic, 2009: implementing smoke-free environments.* Geneva, World Health Organization, 2009.

2. Rani M et al. Tobacco use in India: prevalence and predictors of smoking and chewing in a national cross-sectional household survey. *Tobacco Control*, 2003, 12:e4.

3. Chaloupka FJ et al. The taxation of tobacco products. In: Jha P, Chaloupka FJ, eds. *Tobacco control in developing countries.* Oxford, Oxford University Press, 2000, 237–272.

4. Lokshin M, Beegle K. *Forgone earnings from smoking: evidence for a developing country.* Washington, DC, The World Bank Development Research Group, 2006.

5. Sung HY et al. Economic burden of smoking in China, 2000. *Tobacco Control*, 2006, 15 (Suppl. 1):i5–i11.

6. Adams EK et al. Neonatal health care costs related to smoking during pregnancy. *Health Economics*, 2002, 11:193–206.

7. Struttman TW, Reed DK. Injuries to tobacco farmers in Kentucky. *Southern Medical Journal*, 2002, 95:850–856.

8. *The health consequences of involuntary exposure to tobacco smoke: a report of the Surgeon General.* Rockville, MD, US Department of Health and Human Services, Centers for Disease Control and Prevention, 2006.

9. Waters H et al. The economic impact of exposure to secondhand smoke in Minnesota. *American Journal of Public Health*, forthcoming.

10. Zollinger TW et al. *The economic impact of secondhand smoke on the health of residents and employee smoking on business costs in Marion County, Indiana for 2000.* Report for the Marion County Health Department, 2002.

11. Behan DF, Eriksen MP, Lin Y. *Economic effects of environmental tobacco smoke.* Schaumburg, IL, Society of Actuaries, 2005 (http://www.soa.org/ccm/content/areas-of-practice/life-insurance/research/economic-effects-of-environmentaltobacco-smoke-SOA).

12. US Census Bureau. *Current Population Survey (CPS) table creator.* Calculations using the Current Population Survey (CPS) for 2004 (http://www.census.gov/hhes/www/cpstc/cps_table_creator.html).

13. Leonardi-Bee J et al. Environmental tobacco smoke and fetal health: systematic review and meta-analysis. *Archives of Disease in Childhood—Fetal Neonatal Edition*, 2008, 93:F351–F361.

14. Lightwood JM, Phibbs CS, Glantz SA. Short-term health and economic benefits of smoking cessation: low birth weight. *Pediatrics*, 1999, 104:1312–1320.

15. Miller T et al. The economic impact of early life environmental tobacco smoke exposure: early intervention for developmental delay. *Environmental Health Perspectives*, 2006, 114:1585–1588.

16. Jacobs R et al. The supply-side-effects of tobacco control policies. In: Jha P, Chaloupka FJ, eds. *Tobacco control policies in developing countries.* New York, NY, Oxford University Press, 2000.

17. Chaloupka FJ et al. Tax, price and cigarette smoking: evidence from the tobacco documents and implications for tobacco company marketing strategies. *Tobacco Control*, 2002, 11 (Suppl. 1):i62–i72.

18. Barzel Y. An alternative approach to the analysis of taxation. *Journal of Political Economics*, 1976, 84:1177–1197.

19. Chaloupka FJ. Rational addictive behavior and cigarette smoking. *Journal of Political Economics*, 1991, 99:722–742.

20. Wasserman J et al. The effects of excise taxes and regulations on cigarette smoking. *Journal of Health Economics*, 1991, 10:43–64.

21. Townsend JL, Roderick P, Cooper J. Cigarette smoking by socioeconomic group, sex, and age: effects of price, income, and health publicity. *British Medical Journal*, 1994, 309:923–926.

22. Ross H, Chaloupka FJ. The effect of cigarette prices on youth smoking. *Health Economics*, 2003, 12:217–230.

23. DeCicca P, Kenkel D, Mathios A. *Putting out the fires: will higher cigarette taxes reduce youth smoking?* Paper presented at the Annual Meeting of the American Economic Association, Chicago, IL, 4–7 November 1998.

24. Douglas S, Hariharan G. The hazard of starting smoking: estimates from a split population duration model. *Journal of Health Economics*, 1994, 13:213–230.

25. Douglas S. The duration of the smoking habit. *Economic Inquiry*, 1998, 36:49–64.

26. Dee TS, Evans WN. *A comment on DeCicca, Kenkel, and Mathios.* Atlanta, GA, Georgia Institute of Technology (School of Economics Working Paper), 1998.

27. Chaloupka FJ, Wechsler H. Price, tobacco control policies and smoking among young adults. *Journal of Health Economics*, 1997, 16:359–373.

28. Tauras JA, Chaloupka FJ. *Price, clean indoor air laws, and cigarette smoking: evidence from longitudinal data for young adults.* Cambridge, MA, National Bureau of Economic Research, 1999 (Working Paper No. 6937).

29. Krasovsky K et al. *Economics of tobacco control in Ukraine from the public health perspective.* Kiev, Alcohol and Drug Information Center, 2002.

30. Ross H. *The Ukraine (Kiev) 1999 Global Youth Tobacco Survey: economic issues.* Washington, DC, The World Bank, 2004 (Health, Nutrition & Population Discussion Paper).

31. Karki YB, Pant KD, Pande BR. *A study on the economics of tobacco in Nepal.* Washington DC, The World Bank, 2003 (Health, Nutrition & Population Discussion Paper).

32. Kyaing NN. *Tobacco economics in Myanmar.* Washington DC, The World Bank, 2003 (Health, Nutrition & Population Discussion Paper).

33. Ross H. *Russia (Moscow) 1999 Global Youth Tobacco Survey: economic aspects.* Washington DC, The World Bank, 2004 (Health, Nutrition & Population Discussion Paper).

34. Lewit EM, Coate D, Grossman M. The effects of government regulation on teenage smoking. *Journal of Law and Economics*, 1981, 24:545–569.

35. Centers for Disease Control and Prevention. Response to increases in cigarette prices by race/ethnicity, income, and age groups: United States, 1976–1993. *Morbidity and Mortality Weekly Report*, 1998, 47:605–609.

36. *Tobacco.* Washington, DC, The World Bank (http://www.worldbank.org/tobacco/).

37. Onder Z, Yurekli A. *Cigarette taxation in Turkey: a welfare analysis.* Bilkent University, Ankara, 2009 (Working Paper).

38. Adioetomo, SM, Djutaharta T, Hendratno. *Cigarette consumption, taxation, and household income: Indonesia case-study.* Washington, DC, The World Bank, 2005 (Health, Nutrition & Population Discussion Paper—Economics of Tobacco Control Paper No. 26; http://www.worldbank.org/tobacco/discussionpapers).

39. Djutahara T et al. *Aggregate analysis of the impact of cigarette tax rate increases on tobacco consumption and government revenues: the case of Indonesia.* Washington, DC, The World Bank, 2005 (Health, Nutrition & Population Discussion Paper—Economics of Tobacco Control Paper No. 26; http://www.worldbank.org/tobacco/discussionpapers).

40. Chapman S, Richardson J. Tobacco excise and declining consumption: the case of Papua New Guinea. *American Journal of Public Health*, 1990, 80:537–540.

41. Mao ZZ, Xiang JL. Demand for cigarettes and factors affecting the demand: a cross-sectional survey. *Chinese Healthcare Industry Management*, 1997, 5, 227–229 (in Chinese).

42. Hu TW, Mao Z. Effects of cigarette tax on cigarette consumption and the Chinese economy. *Tobacco Control*, 2002, 11:105–108.

43. Hsieh CR, Hu TW, Lin CF. The demand for cigarettes in Taiwan: domestic versus imported cigarettes. *Contemporary Economic Policy*, 1999, 17:223–234.

44. Hoang VK et al. The effect of imposing a higher, uniform tobacco tax in Vietnam. *Health Research Policy and Systems*, 2006, 4:6.

45. Van der Merwe R. The economics of tobacco control in South Africa. In: Abedian I et al., eds. *The economics of tobacco control: towards an optimal policy mix*. Cape Town, South Africa, Applied Fiscal Research Centre, University of Cape Town, 1998:251–271.

46. Van Walbeek CP. The distributional impact of changes in tobacco prices. *The South African Journal of Economics*, 2002, 70:258–267.

47. Maranvanyika E. The search for an optimal tobacco control policy in Zimbabwe. In: Abedian I et al., eds. *The economics of tobacco control: towards an optimal policy mix*, Cape Town, South Africa, Applied Fiscal Research Centre, University of Cape Town, 1998:272–281.

48. Aloui O. *Analysis of the economics of tobacco in Morocco*. Washington, DC, The World Bank, 2003 (Health, Nutrition & Population Discussion Paper).

49. Sayginsoy O, Yurekli A, de Beyer J. *Cigarette demand, taxation, and the poor: a case-study of Bulgaria*. Washington, DC, 2002 (The World Bank, Health, Nutrition & Population Discussion Paper).

50. Hu TW et al. Smoking, standard of living, and poverty in China. *Tobacco Control*, 2005, 14:247–250.

51. Liu YL et al. Cigarette smoking and poverty in China. *Social Science & Medicine*, 2006, 63:2784–2790.

52. Hu T et al. Tobacco taxation and its potential impact in China. Paper prepared as part of the Bloomberg Initiative to Reduce Tobacco Use, 2009 (http://www.worldlungfoundation.org/publications.php).

53. Van Walbeek C. *Tobacco excise taxation in South Africa: tools for advancing tobacco control in the XXIst century: success stories and lessons learned*. Geneva, World Health Organization, 2003.

54. *Tax burden on tobacco*. Washington, DC, The Campaign for Tobacco-Free Kids, 2007.

55. Hesketh T et al. Smoking, cessation and expenditure in low income Chinese: cross sectional survey. *BMC Public Health*, 2007, 7:29.

56. Economic concerns hamper tobacco control in China. *The Lancet*, 2007, 370:729–730.

57. Wen WQ et al. Environmental tobacco smoke and mortality in Chinese women who have never smoked: prospective cohort study. *British Medical Journal*, 2006, 333–376.

58. Lewit EM, Coate D. The potential for using excise taxes to reduce smoking. *Journal of Health Economics*, 1982, 1:121–145.

59. Chaloupka FJ. *Men, women, and addiction: the case of cigarette smoking*. Cambridge, MA, National Bureau of Economic Research, 1990 (Working Paper No. 3267).

60. Lewit E et al. Price, public policy, and smoking in young people. *Tobacco Control*, 1997, 6 (Suppl. 2):S17–S24.

61. Chaloupka FJ, Pacula R. Sex and race differences in young people's responsiveness to price and tobacco control policies. *Tobacco Control*, 1999, 8:373–377.

62. Hersch J. Gender, income levels, and the demand for cigarettes. *Journal of Risk and Uncertainty*, 2000, 21:263–282.

63. Farrelly MC et al. Response by adults to increases in cigarette prices by sociodemographic characteristics. *Southern Economic Journal*, 2001, 68:156–165.

64. Stehr M. The effect of cigarette taxes on smoking among men and women. *Health Economics*, 2007, 16:1333–1343.

65. Cawley J, Markowitz S, Tauras JA. Lighting up and slimming down: the effects of body weight and cigarette prices on adolescent smoking initiation. *Journal of Health Economics*, 2004, 23:293–311.

66. Cawley J, Markowitz S, Tauras JA. Body weight, cigarette prices, youth access laws and adolescent smoking initiation. *Eastern Economic Journal*, 2006, 32:149–170.

67. Tauras JA, Chaloupka FJ. Determinants of smoking cessation: an analysis of young adult men and women. In: Grossman M, Hsieh C, eds. *Economics of substance abuse*. Cheltenham, Edward Elgar Publishing Ltd., 2001.

68. Atkinson AB, Skegg JL. Anti-smoking publicity and the demand for tobacco in the UK. *The Manchester School of Economic and Social Studies*, 1973, 41:265–282.

69. Stephens T et al. Comprehensive tobacco control policies and the smoking behaviour of Canadian adults. *Tobacco Control*, 2001, 10:317–322.

70. Evans WN, Ringel JS. Can cigarette taxes improve birth outcomes? *Journal of Public Economics*, 1999, 72:135–154.

71. Ringel JS, Evans WN. Cigarette taxes and smoking during pregnancy. *American Journal of Public Health*, 2001, 91:1851–1856.

72. Institute of Medicine. *State programs can reduce tobacco use*. Washington, DC, National Academy of Sciences Press, 2000.

73. Centers for Disease Control and Prevention. Declines in lung cancer rates – California, 1988–1997. *Morbidity and Mortality Weekly Report*, 2000, 49:1066.

74. Abt Associates, Inc. *Independent evaluation of the Massachusetts Tobacco Control Program. Fifth annual report: summary*. Cambridge, MA, Abt Associates, Inc., 1999.

75. Jha P, Chaloupka FJ. *Curbing the epidemic: governments and the economics of tobacco control*. Washington, DC, The World Bank, 1999.

76. Abedian I et al., eds. *The economics of tobacco control: towards an optimal policy mix*. Cape Town , South Africa, Applied Fiscal Research Centre, University of Cape Town, 1998.

77. *Curbing the epidemic: governments and the economics of tobacco control*. Washington, DC, The World Bank, 1999.

78. van der Merwe R. *Taxation of the South African tobacco industry: with special reference to its employment effects*. Cape Town, South Africa: University of Cape Town, 1997 (Dissertation).

79. John RM. Crowding out effect of tobacco expenditure and its implications on household resource allocation in India. *Social Science & Medicine*, 2008, 66:1356–1367.

80. Joossens L et al. *Cigarette trade and smuggling: project update no. 7—the Economics of Tobacco Control Project*. Cape Town, University of Cape Town, 1997.

81. Joossens L, Merriman D, Ross H, Raw M. *How eliminating the global illicit cigarette trade would increase tax revenues and save lives*. Paris, International Union Against Tuberculosis and Lung Disease, 2009.

82. Joossens L et al. Issues in tobacco smuggling. In: Jha P, Chaloupka FJ, eds. *Tobacco control policies in developing countries*. New York, Oxford University Press, 2000.

83. Deloitte & Touche Inc. *Economic contributions of the tobacco industry in the tobacco growing region of Ontario*. Guelph, Ontario, Resource Assessment and Planning Committee, 1995.

84. *The economic impact of the tobacco industry on the United States economy*. Arlington, VA, Price Waterhouse, 1992.

85. *Tobacco's contribution to the national economy*. Princeton, NJ, Tobacco Merchants Association, 1995.

86. Warner KE, Fulton GA. The economic implications of tobacco product sales in a non-tobacco state. *Journal of the American Medical Association*, 1994, 271:771–776.

87. Warner KE et al. Employment implications of declining tobacco product sales for the regional economies of the United States. *Journal of the American Medical Association*, 1996, 275:1241–1246.

88. van der Merwe R. *Employment and output effects for Bangladesh following a decline in tobacco consumption*. Washington, DC, The World Bank, 1998 (Population, Health, and Nutrition Department).

89. Collins D, Lapsley H. *The economic impact of tobacco smoking in Pacific Islands: Pacific Tobacco and Health Project*. Wahroonga, Australia, Adventist Development and Relief Agency, Australian International Development Assistance Bureau, 1997.

90. Arthur Andersen Economic Consulting. *Tobacco industry employment: a review of the Price Waterhouse economic impact report and Tobacco Institute estimates of economic losses from increasing the federal excise tax*. Los Angeles, CA, Arthur Andersen Economic Consulting, 1993.

91. Van der Merwe R. Employment issues in tobacco control. In: Abedian I et al., eds. *The economics of tobacco control: towards an optimal policy mix*. Cape Town, South Africa, Applied Fiscal Research Centre, University of Cape Town, 1998.

World Health Organization

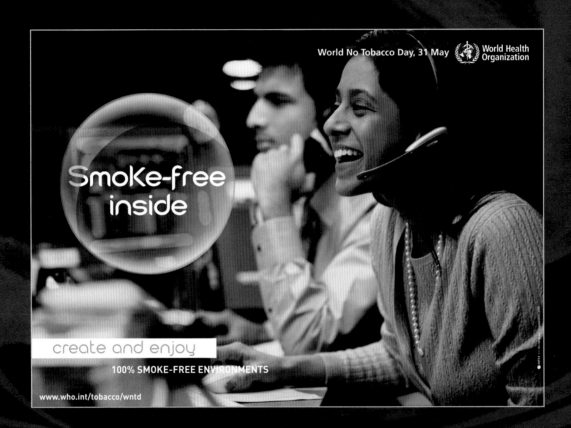

12. Women's Rights and International Agreements

Introduction

Women's right to health is a human right that has been guaranteed through international agreements.[1] It includes the right to protection against second-hand smoke in the work environment and in the home; equal access to health services, including quitting and counselling programmes; protection against misleading health messages such as "light" and "mild"; and the right to full participation in political, economic, social, and cultural decision-making.

The international community can build on existing policy documents, legislative instruments, and international initiatives to develop a gender-sensitive strategy for implementation of the WHO Framework Convention on Tobacco Control (WHO FCTC).[2] The Preamble and Guiding Principles of the WHO FCTC make reference to the Convention on the Elimination of All Forms of Discrimination against Women (CEDAW), the Convention on the Rights of the Child, and the International Covenant on Economic, Social and Cultural Rights. The provisions of the WHO FCTC, which address issues such as restrictions on advertising and promotion, warning labels, research, protection of minors, health information and education, smuggling, and liability and compensation, are comprehensive. Applied broadly to the general population, these measures may, of course, benefit women. However, the WHO FCTC also recognizes the importance of a gendered approach to the interpretation and implementation of policies, programmes, and research. The Preamble states that [The Parties to the Convention are]... alarmed by the increase in smoking and other forms of tobacco consumption by women and young girls worldwide and [are] keeping in mind the need for full participation of women at all levels of policy-making and implementation and the need for gender-specific tobacco control strategies.

The Guiding principles note that *strong political commitment is necessary to develop and support, at the national, regional and international levels, comprehensive multisectoral measures and coordinated responses, taking into considera-* *tion... the need to take measures to address gender-specific risks when developing tobacco control strategies* (Article 4, WHO FCTC).

The WHO FCTC also recognizes the importance of women's leadership, calling for emphasis on *the special contribution of nongovernmental organizations and other members of civil society not affiliated with the tobacco industry, including health professional bodies, women's, youth, environmental and consumer groups, and academic and health care institutions, to tobacco control efforts nationally and internationally and the vital importance of their participation in national and international tobacco control efforts* (Preamble, WHO FCTC).

This chapter examines how the WHO FCTC relates to other important international agreements concerning women's human rights. In particular, the issues of women, tobacco, and the WHO FCTC are analysed in the context of CEDAW.[3] In its Preamble, the WHO FCTC recalls that *the Convention on the Elimination of All Forms of Discrimination against Women, adopted by the United Nations General Assembly on 18 December 1979, provides that States Parties to that Convention shall take appropriate measures to eliminate discrimination against women in the field of health care* (Preamble, WHO FCTC).

Evolution of United Nations Agreements on Human Rights and the Convention on the Elimination of All Forms of Discrimination against Women

CEDAW is the most important legally binding international document concerning the human rights of women. It has been ratified by more than 185 countries. The importance of CEDAW and its relation to the WHO FCTC can be best understood by examining the context of its evolution. The majority of human rights agreements result from negotiations under the auspices of the United Nations. They are usually initiated in response to global concern about specific issues or tragedies such as the Second World War. In 1948, the United Nations proclaimed a Universal Declaration of Human Rights that clearly describes the "inalienable and inviolable rights of all members of the human family".[4]

 World Health Organization

This declaration marked a moral milestone in the history of the community of nations, but it lacked the force of law. Therefore, its principles have been codified in treaties, covenants, and conventions to make them legally binding on the countries and entities that became Party to them.

> *CEDAW is unique among existing human rights instruments because it is concerned exclusively with promoting and protecting women's human rights and because it operates from the premise that patriarchy is a global reality.*

Two crucial legal instruments followed the Universal Declaration of Human Rights: the International Covenant on Civil and Political Rights and the International Covenant on Economic, Social and Cultural Rights. Together, these three documents constitute what is known as the International Bill of Human Rights. Subsequent conventions have elaborated on this bill by focusing in greater detail on specific areas.

The 1960s saw an emergence in many parts of the world of a new awareness of the patterns of discrimination against women and an increase in the number of organizations committed to combating the effects of such discrimination. Although the human rights treaties had established a comprehensive set of rights to which all persons are entitled, over the years they proved insufficient to guarantee women the enjoyment of those rights. Therefore, in 1963, the United Nations General Assembly adopted a resolution requesting that the Commission on the Status of Women prepare a draft declaration combining in a single instrument international standards that articulated the equal rights of men and women. Four years later, the Declaration on Elimination of Discrimination was adopted by the General Assembly.

In 1972, five years after the adoption of the declaration, the Commission on the Status of Women considered preparing a binding instrument that would give normative force to its provisions. Finally, in 1979, CEDAW[3] was adopted, and on 3 September 1981, just 30 days after the twentieth Party had ratified it, CEDAW entered into force. Often described as an international bill of rights for women, CEDAW was the first international document to embody the concept that rights are basic values shared by every human being, regardless of sex, race, religion, culture, or age.

CEDAW is unique among existing human rights instruments because it is concerned exclusively with promoting and protecting women's human rights and because it operates from the premise that patriarchy is a global reality. It addresses the reality of deep-rooted and multifaceted gender inequality throughout the world. It also emphasizes both public- and private-sphere relations and rights and specifically underlines the almost universal difference between de jure and de facto equality of women in the world. CEDAW focuses on elements of the social traditions, customs, and cultural practices that "legitimately" violate women's rights in many societies, identifying them as elements that help perpetuate de facto inequality. CEDAW is also clear about States Parties' use of economic conditions and factors such as structural adjustment policies and programmes, slow economic growth rates, recessionary pressures, and privatization to justify discriminatory practices against women. It operates with the understanding that the States Parties' failure to remove obstacles to women's enjoyment of all their rights is discriminatory, expanding the concept of rights by holding States Parties accountable for failure to act and for abuse of power by private parties.

The idea of introducing a complaints procedure for CEDAW came about in the early 1990s with the emergence of the international women's rights movement, which called for the strengthening of the existing United Nations human rights machinery for the advancement of women. The adoption of an optional protocol to the Convention to provide a right to petition was one of the commitments made by Member States of the United Nations at the 1993 Conference on Human Rights, in Vienna, and the 1995 Fourth World Conference on Women, in Beijing. In 1995, at its fifteenth session, the CEDAW Committee adopted a suggestion (number 7) that proposed elements for a petition and an investigation procedure for complaints. Then, at the forty-third session of the Commission on the Status of Women, delegates adopted an optional protocol to CEDAW, which entered into force in 2000.

The optional protocol introduces two procedures: a communications procedure whereby individuals or groups of individuals may submit claims of violations of rights to the committee, and an inquiry procedure whereby the committee may initiate inquiries into situations of grave or systematic violations of rights. The optional protocol, ratified by 88 Parties (as of March 2008), encourages states to implement CEDAW to avoid having complaints made against them. It provides an incentive for states to provide more-effective local remedies and to eliminate discriminatory laws and practices. Moreover, it is a major tool for women, as communications concerning violations of "any of the rights set forth in the Convention" may be submitted on behalf of an individual or group of individuals. This is critical given the obstacles many women face, such as low levels of literacy, legal illiteracy, and fear of reprisals. However, although CEDAW is widely ratified, it also has the highest number of reservations of any convention. Removal of these reservations is a major goal for both nongovernmental organizations (NGOs) and governments in the coming years.

CEDAW and Women's Health

One of the rights guaranteed under CEDAW is the right to equality in the full enjoyment of health. Article 12 requires States Parties to eliminate discrimination in all aspects of women's health care, including drug addiction and related problems. According to Article 12, "States Parties shall take all appropriate measures to eliminate discrimination against women in the field of health care in order to ensure, on a basis of equality of men and women, access to health care services".

Although tobacco is not specifically mentioned in CEDAW, it is covered by Article 12 and has been interpreted by the CEDAW Committee as an issue on which governments can be held accountable. Since 1995, the CEDAW Committee has increased its efforts to hold governments accountable for accurate reporting on women and tobacco and compliance with this provision. Governments are requested to provide data on women and tobacco, along with data on drugs and alcohol. In recent years, numerous States Parties to CEDAW have improved their reporting. For example, at the forty-fourth session of the CEDAW Committee, Denmark reported a rise in lung cancer among Danish women resulting from years of tobacco use, with nearly 23% of women and 24.5%

of men smoking daily. Spain also expressed concern that young women were increasingly using tobacco.

A main assumption of CEDAW is that the maintenance of health affects the very existence of human beings and is a fundamental human need. WHO studies indicate that more than 20 million lives could be saved by the provision of necessary medicines, pharmaceuticals, and health-care education and facilitation of improved lifestyles.[1] These can all be considered included under Article 12 as part of women's right to health.

The CEDAW Committee also notes that women's health should have a high priority because women are the providers of health care to their families, and their role in health care, including childbirth and child rearing, is of great significance to national social and economic development. The Committee has worked within a framework in which health care is directly concerned with issues such as population growth, development, and the environment. If malnutrition and poverty are to be overcome, the promotion of health and education and the advancement of women's status must be considered as cardinal elements. In viewing women's enjoyment of health as an intrinsic human right, States Parties are therefore obliged to address the conditions that lead to poor health, as well as women's health status.

A human rights approach to women's health is not limited to Article 12 of CEDAW.[3] Article 7 gives women the right to participate in public life and political decision-making. The effective implementation of this right involves including women in designing and implementing national health policies and programmes. Article 2 notes that states must propose a policy to guarantee women the exercise and enjoyment of human rights and fundamental freedoms, in both the private sector and the public sector. This means that women must be fully informed about their rights, a provision that can be applied to tobacco control legislation. Article 11 refers to women's right to the protection of health and safety in working conditions, a provision that is directly relevant to passive-smoke hazards. Another example is the application of the right to life. Maternal health must be protected by implementation of special proactive measures. Further, under Article 14, States Parties are obliged to take into account the specific problems faced by rural women and, in particular, to ensure that they "have access to adequate health care facilities, including information and counselling". Article

14 also guarantees rural women the right to social services and security—a right that is increasingly relevant to rural workers in the informal sector.

According to General Recommendation 24, governments have a duty to report to CEDAW on health legislation plans, cost-effective preventive measures, and policies and to provide reliable data disaggregated by sex.

Globalization has created more jobs and new employment opportunities for women, but it has also created new forms of informal and insecure employment. Citing Article 1, the Committee has often addressed the indirect discrimination faced by women in the informal sector, regularly expressing its concern about their precarious condition and demanding statistical data from States Parties. Although the data are somewhat unreliable, there is consensus that the informal sector is steadily growing in almost all developing countries.

For example, making tobacco products is one of the major informal sector activities in Malawi and Ghana. Women tobacco workers, such as those making bidis, generally have low and unstable earnings and high risks of exposure to health hazards. It is common for women who make tobacco products at home to have no access to employment benefits or social security entitlements. They often face exploitation, and because they are isolated from each other, they are less able to join in collective bargaining.

For many poor women, street vending of tobacco products—where working conditions again are precarious—is the only occupational option. Street vendors lack legal status, and they experience harassment and evictions from their selling place by local authorities or competing shopkeepers. Reports indicate that their goods are often confiscated, and arrests are common.

In addition to creating articles, the CEDAW Committee has the power to make general recommendations that interpret and update the articles. According to General Recommendation 24, governments have a duty to report to CEDAW on health legislation plans, cost-effective preventive measures, and policies and to provide reliable data disaggregated by sex on the incidence of conditions hazardous to women's health. All data must be based on ethical and scientific research. For example, collection of data on the prevalence of tobacco use by male smokers only would constitute gender discrimination, as women's health problems would remain invisible to policy-makers. As CEDAW states:

> *States parties are in the best position to report on the most critical health issues affecting women in that country. Therefore, in order to enable the Committee to evaluate whether measures to eliminate discrimination against women in the field of health care are appropriate, States parties must report on their health legislation, plans and policies for women with reliable data disaggregated by sex on the incidence and severity of diseases and conditions hazardous to women's health and nutrition and on the availability and cost-effectiveness of preventive and curative measures. Reports to the Committee must demonstrate that health legislation, plans and policies are based on scientific and ethical research and assessment of the health status and needs of women in that country and take into account any ethnic, regional or community variations or practices based on religion, tradition or culture (General Recommendation 24, Paragraph 1, CEDAW).*

Under CEDAW, States Parties must also make appropriate budgetary provisions to ensure that women realize their rights to health care. Governments that do not provide these rights in relation to women and tobacco fail to fulfil their obligations under the Convention. General Recommendation 24 specifically notes:

> *The duty to fulfill rights places an obligation on States parties to take appropriate legislative, judicial, administrative, budgetary, economic and other measures to the maximum extent of their available resources to ensure that women realize their rights to health care (General Recommendation 24, Paragraph 17, CEDAW).*

General Recommendation 24 also outlines the need for states to promote women's health throughout the life-course:[3]

> *States parties should implement a comprehensive national strategy to promote women's health throughout their lifespan. This will include interventions aimed at both the prevention and treatment of diseases and conditions affecting women* (General Recommendation 24, Paragraph 29, CEDAW).

Under the optional protocol to CEDAW, alleged violations may be linked to state action or inaction or to the conduct of state officials in their public functions. Potential claims could include the absence of health warnings on tobacco products or the lack of information concerning the health hazards of tobacco use by pregnant women.

In addition to CEDAW, the following international agreements are also explicit on the issue of women's health:

- The International Covenant on Economic, Social and Cultural Rights (Article 12: 2a)[5]

- The Convention on the Rights of the Child (Article 24: 1d, 1f)[6]

- The Beijing Platform for Action (Articles 89 and 106)[1]

- The United Nations Declaration on Violence Against Women (Article 3f).[7]

When a Party ratifies or accedes to CEDAW and also adopts a policy document, the combination can be mutually reinforcing. The Beijing Platform for Action specifically identified tobacco as a women's health issue and called upon governments to take action. It states:

> *[Governments should] create awareness among women, health professionals, policy makers and the general public about the serious but preventable health hazards stemming from tobacco consumption and the need for regulatory and education measures to reduce smoking as important health promotion and disease prevention activities* (Paragraph 107o, Beijing Platform for Action).

> *[Governments should] increase financial and other support from all sources for preventive, appropriate*

biomedical, behavioural, epidemiological and health service research on women's health issues and for research on the social, economic and political causes of women's health problems, and their consequences, including the impact of gender and age inequalities, especially with respect to chronic and non-communicable diseases, particularly cardiovascular diseases and conditions [and] cancers (Paragraph 109d, Beijing Platform for Action).

Most of the issues in the Twelve Critical Areas of Concern in the Beijing Platform for Action[1] are also included in CEDAW. For example, paragraph 323232 entrusts the CEDAW Committee with the responsibility of monitoring the implementation of the Platform. A government or Party that has ratified CEDAW without reservation and has also signed onto the Beijing Platform for Action is doubly committed, first at the policy level, and second, according to international law. When CEDAW was drafted, the issue of women and tobacco was not widely recognized as a women's rights issue. Today, such policy and treaty agreements can strengthen the WHO FCTC with regard to emerging health issues.

Furthermore, the concept of women's health as a human right has been promoted by United Nations World Conferences, including the Conference on Human Rights, in Vienna (1993); the International Conference on Population and Development, in Cairo (1994); and the Fourth World Women's Conference, in Beijing (1995). The four United Nations World Women's Conferences and follow-up meetings, such as Beijing Plus Ten in 2005, have also produced excellent policy documents. Policy documents, however, are not legally binding, and institutional or individual discretion may determine their implementation.

Monitoring Implementation and International Mobilization

Monitoring implementation through States Parties' reports is an important tool of CEDAW. Reporting enables a comprehensive review of national legislation, administrative rules, policies, and practices, and it ensures that States Parties regularly monitor the situation with respect to each provision of the Convention. The CEDAW Committee has expressed concerns about the increase in tobacco use by women, the lack of gender-specific information and statistics (Uzbekistan, Kazakhstan, and the Netherlands in 2001), tobacco addiction (Ukraine in 2002), and women's occupational health, particularly in the tobacco-growing industry (the Republic of Moldova in 2006). A common recommendation is the provision of information and statistics on tobacco use by women (Suriname in 2002, Chile in 1999). At its twenty-first session, the Committee recommended that Spain undertake awareness-raising campaigns concerning the preventable health hazards of tobacco consumption and also that it assess the need for additional regulations and educational measures to prevent or reduce smoking by women. At its twenty-ninth session, it requested that France provide information on smoking as well as sex- and age-disaggregated data.

It is crucial to recognize the strategic importance of NGOs with regard to mobilizing international political will.

Article 18 of CEDAW obliges States Parties to submit reports on implementation of the Convention within one year of ratification and every four years thereafter. In these reports, states must indicate the legislative, judicial, administrative, or other measures they have adopted to implement the provisions of the Convention. Article 17 establishes the Committee on the Elimination of Discrimination against Women, an expert body with 23 members responsible for monitoring the progress made by states in implementing CEDAW. Since the adoption of the optional protocol, the Committee can also receive and consider complaints by individuals or groups of individuals from states that are Parties to the protocol.

The CEDAW Committee has adopted reporting guidelines to assist States Parties in the preparation of periodic reports. The Committee also considers the reports in public meetings in the presence of Party representatives, using a constructive dialogue that provides a non-judgemental approach aimed at assisting the States Parties. Following consideration of the reports, the Committee formulates and adopts concluding comments in a closed

session. The comments outline factors and difficulties affecting the implementation of the Convention for the reporting States Parties, as well as positive aspects, principal subjects of concern, and suggestions and recommendations for enhancing implementation.

Specialized United Nations agencies and other international and national organizations make important contributions to monitoring. Article 22 specifically provides for interaction between the CEDAW Committee and specialized agencies. The Committee and the pre-session working groups invite specialized agencies and other United Nations entities to provide country-specific information on States Parties whose reports are being considered. The Committee also encourages the United Nations country teams to undertake follow-up activities to support States Parties in their implementation of the Committee's concluding comments.

It is noteworthy that at its thirty-third session, in July 2005, the CEDAW Committee provided for the first time an opportunity for a national human rights institution—the Irish Human Rights Commission—to make an oral presentation. At its thirty-fourth session, in January 2006, the Committee further discussed its interaction with such institutions and confirmed its commitment to develop modalities for improved interaction.

It is crucial to recognize the strategic importance of NGOs with regard to mobilizing international political will. Although NGOs do not have formal standing under the reporting procedure, the Committee welcomes information from them, and since its early sessions, it has invited them to follow its work and provide country-specific information on States Parties. National and international NGOs are also invited to provide the pre-session working groups with country-specific information on those States Parties whose reports are being considered. Such information may be submitted in writing prior to or at the relevant session. In addition, the Committee sets aside time at each session, usually at the start, for representatives of NGOs to speak and provide information. The pre-session working groups also provide an opportunity for NGOs to give statements, usually on the first day of a working group. The Committee further recommends that States Parties involve national NGOs in the preparation of their reports and that reports contain information on NGOs and women's associations and their participation in the implementation of CEDAW and the preparation of reports.

World Health Organization

Conclusions

CEDAW is a dynamic document that is flexible enough to adapt to changing international circumstances and attitudes, while preserving its spirit and integrity. The CEDAW Committee endeavours to ensure that women benefit from globalization and that their increased participation in the labour market has an empowering effect on them. Likewise, the WHO FCTC can take up the challenge of improving the lives of women in the informal working sector by making them no longer invisible, unacknowledged, and excluded from protection and benefits.

CEDAW and the WHO FCTC share the common goal of ensuring women's rights to health as a human right. Together, these treaties can be used to commit governments to more gender-sensitive policies and legislation. Both hold governments accountable for commitments made in ratifying or acceding to them, provide a legal basis for interpretation of existing national laws or for amendments to them, and assist in the enactment of new legislation regarding women's health and tobacco. CEDAW can create an expanded human rights framework for women that is acceptable within their own cultures or under their own legal systems. This includes women's right to a safe and smoke-free environment, both in public places and in the home.

For a convention to be effective at both national and international levels, women need to be better informed about their rights under international agreements. CEDAW and the WHO FCTC can be widely disseminated to mobilize support among women's grass-roots organizations. It is also necessary to promote the active support and participation of other institutional actors, including legislative bodies, human rights lawyers, academic and research institutions, local community groups, NGOs, the media, and youth organizations. Other potential partners include national machineries for gender equality and the advancement of women and NGOs engaged in women's empowerment. Women have the right to life and therefore the right to be fully informed about Parties' obligations to protect their health.

References

1. *Platform for action,* The United Nations Fourth World Conference on Women, 1995. New York, NY, United Nations (http://www.un.org/womenwatch/daw/beijing/platform/poverty.htm, accessed 1 December 2009).
2. *WHO Framework Convention on Tobacco Control.* Geneva, World Health Organization, 2003.
3. *United Nations Convention on the Elimination of All Forms of Discrimination against Women.* New York, NY, United Nations, 1979.
4. *Universal Declaration of Human Rights.* New York, NY, United Nations, 1948.
5. *International Covenant on Economic, Social and Cultural Rights.* New York, NY, United Nations, 1966.
6. *United Nations Convention on the Rights of the Child.* New York, NY, United Nations, 1995.
7. *United Nations Declaration on the Elimination of Violence Against Women.* New York, NY, United Nations, 1993.

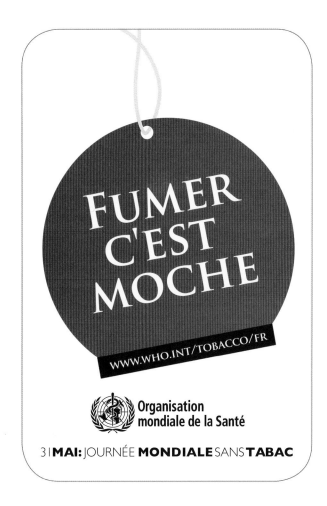

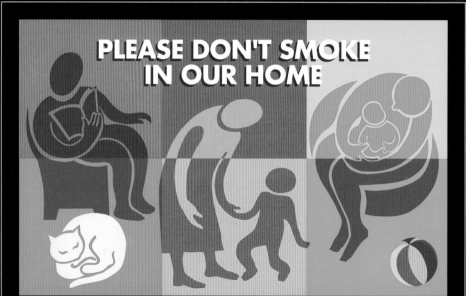

13. The International Women's Movement and Anti-Tobacco Campaigns

Introduction

For decades, the international women's movement has been mobilizing at the grass-roots level and affecting the international political agenda. Among the issues it has successfully brought to the world's attention are violence against women, consumer and environmental justice, reproductive health and sexual rights, and human rights. In recent years, the international women's movement has begun to join forces with the tobacco control movement.

The following is an historic account of women's activism in two regions where women's leadership has made a significant contribution to women's health and development. Although it deals with global trends, only two case-study regions are presented here: Asia and the Pacific, and Latin America and the Caribbean. Through an historical analysis and overview of the current situation, this chapter outlines the potential for future tobacco control actions, as well as existing social resources that promise to help prevent the rising epidemic of tobacco use among women.

A Brief History of the International Women's Movement

Women have taken strong leadership roles at the national and international levels of the women's movement throughout the world. The United Nations World Women's Conferences, which have provided opportunities to build solidarity, share visions, and articulate regional concerns, have been an important influence on the international women's movement.[1] The First United Nations World Conference on Women was held in Mexico City in 1975, the year that was designated as the International Women's Year. The Women's Tribune, consisting of about 2000 women from nongovernmental organizations (NGOs) of various countries, was held simultaneously with the United Nations Conference. The majority of the participants came from the United States and Latin America; Asian, African, and grass-roots women's groups were underrepresented. Asian women watched the heated confrontation between feminists from the industrialized northern hemisphere and the developing countries of the southern hemisphere. Issues such as women's reproductive rights were featured in debates on women and health, but otherwise, health was low on the list of priorities. In 1980, the Second United Nations World Conference on Women was held in Copenhagen, Denmark. African women were more visible at this conference, because of geographical and historical ties between Europe and Africa. The confrontation between industrialized-country and developing-country feminists was less apparent, but other political issues related to the Cold War dominated the agenda. Considered the most controversial of the global women's conferences, this one nevertheless succeeded in introducing the important Convention on the Elimination of All Forms of Discrimination against Women (CEDAW), known as the women's bill of rights. A detailed discussion of CEDAW is found in the chapter on women's rights and international agreements.

The new strength of regional women's networks was reflected at the Third United Nations World Conference on Women, held in Nairobi, Kenya, in 1985. Women's health and the environment were not major issues at that event, but women's reproductive health was an increasingly important human rights issue, and issues of poverty and education were highlighted. In the aftermath of other United Nations conferences, including one on environment and development, the Vienna Human Rights Conference, and the International Conference on Population and Development, women's NGOs concerned with health and the environment developed stronger lobbying strategies and political agendas. This momentum culminated with the Fourth United Nations World Conference on Women, held in Beijing, China, in 1995, when representatives from the industrialized and developing countries achieved an important consensus on both environmental and women's health issues.

The Platform for Action—the blueprint for women's equality in the 21st century—was adopted by the Conference in Beijing. It included 12 critical areas of concern: poverty, education, health, violence against women, armed conflicts, economy, decision-making, mechanisms for the advancement of women, women's human rights, media, environment, and the girl-child. The Platform also contained hundreds of recommendations and strategies for each area. For the first time at a United Nations Women's Conference, tobacco was recognized as a women's health issue in the general discussions and recommendations.

Founded in 1990, INWAT is a global network of more than 1700 tobacco control and women's health specialists in about 80 countries that addresses the social, cultural, health, and economic issues of tobacco as they affect women and girls.

At the parallel NGO Forum, hundreds of workshops were held on a large variety of issues, including violence against women, reproductive rights, trafficking in women, armed conflicts, feminization of poverty, and political participation. Participants at the grass-roots level shared their experiences in organizing to fight against development projects that perpetuated gender discrimination. There was also an important transformation of women's self-image, from women as victims to women as leaders and visionaries. For example, at a workshop on Asian Women's Alternatives in Action, participants from various Asian countries reported innovative and dynamic strategies and practices and showed their determination to work towards a world based on gender justice through women's empowerment. The theme of the NGO Forum, Look at the World Through Women's Eyes, reflected this newfound confidence and assertiveness.

Since that time, women's awareness of and support for tobacco control has grown. A major turning point was the gathering of nearly 500 women from 50 countries in Kobe, Japan, in November 1999, at the World Health Organization (WHO) International Conference on Tobacco and Health, Making a Difference to Tobacco and Health: Avoiding the Tobacco Epidemic in Women and Youth. Upon returning to their countries after the Conference, many women leaders carried out national campaigns and media events and joined forces with

tobacco control programmes. Anti-tobacco activities led by women's groups have grown in many countries, including Malaysia, Thailand, Bangladesh, Japan, the Lao People's Democratic Republic, Turkey, Cuba, and Brazil. At the WHO public hearings held in Geneva in 2000, women leaders from the Federation of Cuban Women, REDEH/ CEMINA (Brazil), the Centre for Human Environment in Ethiopia, the international Women's Environment & Development Organization (WEDO), and the Zuna Women's Operation Green (Zimbabwe) testified against the tobacco industry and showed their support for the WHO Framework Convention on Tobacco Control (WHO FCTC).[2,3]

A key resource and bridge between tobacco control and the women's health movement is the International Network of Women Against Tobacco (INWAT). Founded in 1990, INWAT is a global network of more than 1700 tobacco control and women's health specialists in about 80 countries that addresses the social, cultural, health, and economic issues of tobacco as they affect women and girls. INWAT also aims to promote women's leadership in tobacco control. Its publication *Turning a New Leaf: Women, Tobacco, and the Future* highlighted this theme, as well as the linkages between tobacco production and consumption and the status of women.

The InterAmerican Heart Foundation (IAHF) and INWAT organized a forum with a focus on women and tobacco during the First SRNT [Society for Research on Nicotine and Tobacco] Latin America & Second Iberoamerican Conference on Tobacco Control, held in Rio de Janeiro, Brazil, in 2007. The purpose of the forum was to provide a platform for debate and to share experiences and lessons learned about women and tobacco in the fields of advocacy, research, and policy.

The WHO FCTC negotiations provided an important opportunity for groups such as INWAT and the women's movement to work together to influence the final version of the treaty. During the negotiations in Geneva in October 2000, a women's caucus was begun as a subgroup of the Framework Convention Alliance (FCA). By 2008, FCA membership included almost 300 health, environmental, consumer, and human rights organizations from more than 100 countries. FCA plays a critical role in the treaty process, working collaboratively with governments, providing educational material and tobacco control expertise, monitoring the treaty implementation process, and helping to shape the public climate that has provided momentum for international regulation of the tobacco industry. Its board has been exemplary in its gender and regional balance.

At the founding of FCA in 1999, the women's caucus acted as a coalition of NGOs to ensure effective implementation of the WHO FCTC and provided an open forum for dialogue between NGOs, government delegates, and United Nations agencies. Its specific goal was to promote networking among leaders (both women and men) concerned with gender issues and to provide technical support to government delegations.

Throughout the WHO FCTC process, the women's caucus had daily programmes that included briefings by eminent leaders such as Judith Mackay, former chairperson of the WHO Policy and Strategy Advisory Committee; Margaretha Haglund, former president of the International Network of Women Against Tobacco; and Phetsile Dlamini, Minister for Health and Social Welfare in Swaziland. The caucus organized briefings for delegates, highlighting issues such as the exploitation of feminine imagery by multinational corporations to market tobacco to women and girls. Together with the International Alliance of Women and the Campaign for Tobacco-Free Kids, the women's caucus made numerous statements during the negotiations concerning the importance of a gender perspective on political and economic policies.

Most important, the caucus was instrumental in ensuring that the WHO FCTC made reference to treaties that would strengthen a gender perspective in its interpretation. The group prepared an NGO briefing paper that evolved into the first draft of the WHO FCTC Preamble, which eventually contained key provisions on gender and human rights. Among the priorities of the caucus were women's rights as human rights issues, as encapsulated in CEDAW, the Convention on the Rights of the Child, and the Covenant on Economic, Social and Cultural Rights.

Signs of growing awareness and activity related to the WHO FCTC beyond the arena of negotiations have been evident at other international events. It is noteworthy that in 1999 and 2000, the Commission on the Status of Women, which oversees the implementation of the Platform for Action, included the topic of women and tobacco in its working documents. Similarly, at its session

in 2000, the expert committee that oversees CEDAW requested that governments report on tobacco use under Article 12. During the Beijing Plus Five meeting in 2005, members of the CEDAW Committee spoke at a panel on the linkages between gender, women, and tobacco and CEDAW provisions. Also, at the United Nations Children's Summit, the World Association of Girl Guides and Girl Scouts, along with the Campaign for Tobacco-Free Kids, held events pointing out new and innovative ways for girls to become leaders in the anti-tobacco movement.

Ayako Kuno, one of the eight founding members of the Women's Group, wrote in the magazine Women's Revolt, *"I realized recently that most feminists smoke".*

Asian Women's Anti-Tobacco Organizations

This section describes Asian anti-tobacco organizations that, although small in membership, laid the groundwork for a stronger movement today. As taboos against women smoking in public subsided in many traditional Asian societies, well-educated, emancipated women increasingly used tobacco. Nevertheless, some health-conscious groups are prevailing in their struggle to control the tobacco epidemic among women.

The Japanese Non-Smokers' Rights Group

In 1977, around the time the Japanese Non-Smokers' Rights Group was formed, feminists in Nagoya founded the Women's Group to Eliminate Harm of Tobacco. The women's liberation movement in the early 1970s claimed the equal right to smoke, and many young feminists had started to use tobacco. However, those feminists who objected to smoking challenged this idea and insisted that both men and women should stop smoking.

Ayako Kuno, one of the eight founding members of the Women's Group, wrote in the magazine *Women's*

Revolt, "I realized recently that most feminists smoke. I felt sick of the polluted air. I myself used to look positively at women smoking because it seemed they challenged the traditional social norm based on Confucian patriarchal ideology that smoking is not women's behaviour. However, I began to question if smoking means women's liberation, because tobacco is poison and harmful to health and the environment".

The issue reappeared in 1987, when Women's Action on Smoking was formed in Tokyo by female doctors, teachers, writers, and working women who were concerned about how a male-dominated culture perpetuates women's suffering from second-hand smoke (SHS) at home and in the workplace. This group also focused its attention on rising rates of tobacco use among young women. According to Nobuko Nakano, one of the founders, the main objectives of the group were non-smokers' rights and the prevention of smoking among youth, especially girls.[4] Its members were engaged in activities to promote smoke-free education in schools, appealing to non-smokers' rights through the media and lobbying. They also established a hotline for non-smokers to address the issue of SHS in the workplace and initiated a campaign to remove tobacco vending machines. Recently, women have become more outspoken about protecting themselves and their children from SHS as a right.

In the past decade, several medical professionals in the group independently started training programmes for cessation. These programmes, carried out by women doctors, have attracted many women smokers. Also inspired by the Kobe Conference in 1999, the Japanese Nursing Association (JNA)—Japan's largest women's professional organization, with 600 000 members—campaigned to stop smoking by nurses and to make hospitals smoke-free. The rate of smoking among nurses (25.7%) was twice that of all Japanese women in 2001. JNA published booklets on quitting smoking and organized many seminars to train leaders for cessation programmes. Some progress was noteworthy: in 2006, the nurses' smoking rate dropped by 6%, although it was still high (19%). JNA is continuing its efforts to highlight nurses' important role in helping patients quit smoking and combating SHS. It is noteworthy that in other countries, such as Thailand and Brazil, nurses associations are becoming increasingly active in tobacco control and efforts to make hospitals smoke-free.

The Consumers Association of Penang

The Consumers Association of Penang (CAP), in Malaysia, an internationally recognized consumer advocacy group, started an anti-smoking campaign in 1973. Since then, it has organized numerous seminars, forums, and exhibitions and has published and distributed booklets, educational kits, posters, and stickers to inform people of the negative effects of tobacco on health, the environment, and the economy.

CAP urges women to play active roles in smoking prevention and cessation and provides concrete suggestions, including the following:

- Women health professionals can actively promote a tobacco-free lifestyle; women doctors and nurses can serve as educators and disseminators of information.

- Women in the media can reverse the social acceptability of smoking; they can promote non-smoking as an attractive and healthy lifestyle and can undo the damage done by others in the media.

- Women in politics and government can be instrumental in passing anti-smoking legislation and regulations and should advocate stricter laws.

- Women in sports should boycott sports activities sponsored by the tobacco industry, as participation in such activities implies an endorsement of smoking.

The Action on Smoking and Health Foundation of Thailand

The first project in Thailand dealing exclusively with tobacco control was the Women and Smoking Project, an NGO formed by 12 health organizations in 1986. In 1997, the Project became the Action on Smoking and Health Foundation of Thailand (ASH Thailand). Its activities include programmes designed for youth, including Smoke-Free Schools 2000. ASH Thailand cooperates closely with the National Council of Thai Women, an umbrella group that has taken strong actions against tobacco in recent years. Thai nurses have also established a national organization that works cooperatively with physicians to establish smoke-free hospitals and provide patient counselling.

A special project called "Thai Women Don't Smoke" was set up in 1995 to counter the tobacco companies' efforts to encourage women to start smoking. The project focuses on the effects of smoking on appearance and on children's health and promotes the view that smart women do not smoke. The mass media have been actively involved in the project, and ASH Thailand has worked closely with three national beauty contests: Miss Teen Thailand, Miss Thailand, and Miss Thailand World.

The Consumers Union of Korea

The Consumers Union of Korea, established in 1970, started a no-smoking campaign in 1984 to stop the spread of tobacco use among young people. The Union has 25 000 members (most of them women) and 121 member firms. Its activities and goals include:

- Demonstrations and press releases
- Street rallies on World No Tobacco Day
- Protests of tobacco-sponsored events, e.g. Marlboro concerts
- Advocating stronger warning labels
- Advocating a ban on tobacco vending machines
- The Asian Women's Health Movement.

The Asian Women's Health Movement

It is noteworthy that in the Asian region, tobacco control programmes have often worked outside the mainstream of women and health activities. This historic schism should be analysed in depth through sociological research so as to uncover more effective ways to bridge the gap in the future. Although some organizations such as the International Network of Women Against Tobacco have worked with national counterparts in the Asia region, much more work needs to be done to enlist the help of grass-roots as well as national organizations that have worked in women's reproductive health, family planning, and other public health issues—most of which currently are not advocates for tobacco control.

It is vitally important to mobilize women at the local level to participate in anti-smoking campaigns. In a number of countries, including India, Bangladesh,

Nepal, the Philippines, and Malaysia, many women's organizations are committed to the advancement of women's health and are working on important health issues.[5] The groups described in this section have not focused on issues of women and tobacco to date, but it is important to encourage their participation and involvement. Most of the organizations in the Asian women's health movement are current or potential allies for tobacco control.

> *In a number of countries, such as India, Bangladesh, Nepal, the Philippines, and Malaysia, many women's organizations are committed to the advancement of women's health and are working on important health issues.*

The Centre for Health Education, Training and Nutrition Awareness

The Centre for Health Education, Training and Nutrition Awareness (CHETNA) is an NGO based in Gujarat, India. Established in 1980 with the mission of contributing to the empowerment of disadvantaged women through health education, CHETNA (which means "awareness" in several Indian languages) has a Women and Health Programme that aims to enable women and communities to initiate, manage, and sustain comprehensive, gender-sensitive primary health care for all. Its main activity is training employees of NGOs and government in gender and health, reproductive health, emotional and mental health, ageing, and traditional health and healing practices. CHETNA uses a participatory approach, and its communications strength is its adaptation to the local social, cultural, and economic conditions of its constituents.

Buddha Bahnipati Family Welfare Project

The Buddha Bahnipati Family Welfare Project (BBP) of the Family Planning Association in Nepal formed

World Health Organization

its first women's group in 1990. Members of BBP take a comprehensive approach to improving the overall livelihood of women. They conduct informal classes on literacy, savings and credit, animal raising, and fodder production, and they operate health camps where women can learn about gynaecology, vasectomy, and dental, eye, and general-health check-ups. The purpose of the group is to help women gain confidence, security, and dignity, as well as to improve their standards of living.

Bangladesh Women's Health Coalition

The activities of the Bangladesh Women's Health Coalition (BWHC) are based on three principles: (1) each woman should be treated with respect; (2) each woman's particular needs should be carefully discussed with her by health-care professionals; and (3) each woman should be provided with sufficient information and counselling to make her own choices about her reproductive health.

BWHC operates seven clinics that offer a choice of family-planning methods. The clinics are staffed by women paramedics recruited from the community. Doctors, nurses, and attendants also provide counselling, as BWHC considers counselling crucial to overcoming class barriers between the health professionals and their clients. BWHC also organizes training programmes for government paramedics.

Gabriela

Gabriela is a national coalition of women's organizations in various sectors of the Philippines. Its Commission on Women's Health and Reproductive Rights provides community-based health services for women, men, and children. The Commission operates a women's clinic in Metro Manila and two pilot communities; in one year, it provided approximately 1500 consultations, 1100 of which were to women. The Commission's objectives are to develop women's health initiatives and to integrate these into the overall developmental efforts of the communities. Two pilot communities have already developed their own management plans. The outstanding characteristic of Gabriela's "health service to sisters in need" is that it lets women in communities organize themselves and manage by themselves.

Asian-Pacific Resource & Research Centre for Women

The Asian-Pacific Resource & Research Centre for Women (ARROW), based in Malaysia, advocates women-centred and gender-sensitive policies and programmes for women's health based on—and evolved from—comprehensive public health care. This NGO provides practical information, resources, and research findings. Its information kit, "Towards Women-Centred Reproductive Health", is an action-oriented introduction to women-centred reproductive health and is most useful for women's health projects and movements at the grass-roots level. It can also be used to advocate for government public health policy. ARROW uses a life-course approach, covering the prenatal period, girlhood, adolescence, menopause, and old age. It also addresses critical areas of women's health that have been given little attention in Malaysia, including occupational health, emotional and mental health, and violence against women.

These networks and alliances have the potential to become essential links in the worldwide movement to control tobacco and advance women's health, but stronger connections must be made between them and the tobacco control movements. It is crucial to disseminate information on the hazards of tobacco use among women to these NGOs and to foster strong leadership skills.

The Latin American and Caribbean Women's Health Movement

As in the case of the Asian women and health movement, the feminist health movement in the Latin American and Caribbean countries was initially antagonistic to tobacco control policies, because they were viewed as attempting to obstruct women's newly found "liberties". Indeed, many women considered it their "right" to smoke in public, particularly as it had been a social taboo in the past. Similar trends can be seen in North America.

It is noteworthy that the feminist movement in Latin American and Caribbean countries began simultaneously with the growth of the movement in North America and Europe. In the late 19th and early 20th centuries, important feminist leaders in Latin American countries provided leadership and stimulated activism to improve women's status and access to education, including university education. Women's rights to health and

World Health Organization

economic and political participation were the main areas of concern for the early activists.

Feminism in the Latin American and Caribbean region promoted women's autonomy and liberation. At the same time, the inclusion of women in traditional male activities changed women's lifestyles to include smoking. Feminist arguments used to improve women's status were adopted by tobacco companies, and the ideology of the movement was manipulated by tobacco advertising. Initially, advertisements associated tobacco with sophisticated and glamorous women. Images of women who succeeded in men's activities, such as Amelia Earhart, were also used. In the past decade, messages targeting women linked tobacco with liberty and pleasure.

Although the tobacco industry succeeded in courting many emancipated women, the beginnings of an opposition were forming. In 1984, representatives from 60 women's health groups who attended the First Regional Women and Health meeting in Colombia created the Latin American and Caribbean Women's Health Network (LACWHN). LACWHN is made up of approximately 2000 member groups; 80% of the members come from Latin America and the Caribbean, and the rest come from North America, Europe, Africa, Asia, and the Pacific. Its board of directors is composed of nine health activists from different countries in Latin America and the Caribbean, and its headquarters is in Santiago, Chile. One of its main activities is the publication of a quarterly journal, *Women's Health Journal*, and a special annual document, *Women's Health Collection*. For its first 10 years, LACWHN was coordinated by Isis International, a regional feminist NGO based in Santiago. In 1995, by agreement of its board of directors, LACWHN became an autonomous institution and currently functions as a foundation.

LACWHN disseminates and promotes research and studies on women's health issues and mobilizes groups and activists to advocate for and defend women's rights regarding these issues. Its activities are organized as campaigns around specific days designated to draw attention to particular health issues. The network also promotes activities by its members and disseminates health information to interested parties, such as women's groups, academic institutions, governmental health and social authorities, health and associated professionals, the private sector, journalists, and policy-makers.

A review of women's health campaigns promoted by LACWHN provides some perspective on women's health activities and their possible applications to tobacco control. The first LACWHN campaign focused on maternal mortality, and 28 May 1987 was declared the first Women's Health Day, a day set aside to emphasize that issue. National maternal mortality rates in the region and the difficulties of reducing them were the motivating factors for developing a campaign to influence political will and increase social support.

Since 1988, Women's Health Day has been adopted internationally and celebrated worldwide by women's health groups and other interested parties. Campaigns have been established on specific days to promote awareness of the issues of abortion (28 September), violence against women and girls (25 November), human rights (10 December), and HIV/AIDS (1 December).

LACWHN has organized regional training and the development of educational programmes for participants in women's health issues.

The campaign was initially a protest. Later, it began to incorporate proposals for change. Its visibility and impact grew, and the number of participating groups increased. In 1987, 100 groups from 45 countries participated, and today, more than 1500 groups participate in approximately 80 countries. Health workers have joined with women's health activist groups to diversify and expand participation.

Women's health groups have produced and published background papers providing data, analyses, and perspectives. Interactions between academic groups, as well as between health professionals and grass-roots women's organizations, have expanded conceptual boundaries, providing credibility and strengthening women's lobbying efforts. Interactions with United Nations agencies, international and national research/funding organizations, and governments have increased the impact of local and national actions. The media have been involved from the beginning, and recently, media attention has increased and heightened the campaign's visibility.[6]

 World Health Organization

The principal indicators on which to evaluate the campaign remain the numbers of participants and the alliances made, along with the programmes and actions established by health services. Small grants (from US$ 300 to US$ 1000 each) for women's groups have been distributed for local projects to improve grass-roots women's organizations.[7]

LACWHN has organized regional training and educational programmes for participants in women's health issues. These programmes were initiated in universities and academic units by LACWHN members associated with national women's health NGOs to disseminate scientific information on women's health from a gender perspective. In addition, scholarships for short training programmes at women's health NGOs have been provided to share successful women's health programmes and services, particularly programmes addressing sexual and reproductive health and violence against women.

> *One of the most important roles of global networks is lobbying and advocacy of the United Nations and other relevant international agencies.*

In 1992, LACWHN organized and promoted a regional preparatory process for the International Conference on Population and Development (ICPD), held in Cairo, Egypt, in 1994, through member meetings. The role of women's health activists and LAWCHN in the ICPD was crucial in the adoption of the ICPD Plan of Action by consensus.

In 1995, LACWHN developed a project to monitor implementation of the ICPD Plan of Action in several Latin American and Caribbean countries, with the cooperation of the United Nations Population Fund (UNFPA). Between 1996 and 1999, five countries in Latin America were monitored by women's health NGOs in partnership with United Nations agencies and governments. In the 1980s, democracies were reestablished in many Latin American and Caribbean countries, but inclusion of women in the participatory process was rare. The project to encourage women's participation in development

through the monitoring of governmental implementation strengthened democratic procedures. This project enabled many women's health leaders and activists to develop and increase their negotiation and advocacy capacities and the tools to promote national, regional, and local women's health policies and programmes. Similar experiences in other countries of the region will increase and improve women's participation.

By 2001, the majority of LACWHN's members were based in Latin America and the Caribbean. The range of themes, activities, and goals of the groups is very broad. Some groups are activist-oriented, while others provide services and sponsor academic activities. Their actions have been influential at grass-roots, local, national, regional, and international levels.

In 1997–1998, the LACWHN database included 30 categories of thematic issues, each of which was subdivided for more specific classification of members' interests and activities. All the activities are related to women and tobacco control, but they do not necessarily give the issue prominence in their programmes. The potential, however, is apparent, as their concerns include human rights, family, mental health, women's identity, life-courses, communications, legislation, environment, religions, and economic issues.

In the Andean area, where community-based organizations are a long-standing tradition, many women's groups matured decades ago and were incorporated into the network for broader interaction with other groups.[8] In the southern hemisphere, where many countries were ruled by dictatorships until the 1980s, women's groups have developed only in the past decade.

Few of the registered groups currently pursue tobacco control activities. Their primary focus is on sexual and reproductive health issues, mental health, and the impact of medical-care policies on health-care reform. Nevertheless, great potential exists for integrating anti-tobacco campaigns into these activities. There is also potential for the dissemination of research and news related to tobacco and health through LACWHN's *Women's Health Journal*.

One reason for the lack of involvement of women's groups in tobacco control has been the perception that international, regional, and national networks, as well as governments and United Nations agencies, have failed to invite them to participate in tobacco control activities. The frequent and fluid relations of LACWHN with United Nations agencies have been concerned with sexual and reproductive health matters, violence against women, and women's impact on the health-care reform process.

In Latin America and the Caribbean, there is considerable potential to expand the scope of women's health-care issues and to strengthen the social base for women's leadership in tobacco control. Increased awareness and the mobilization of women's health activists in the region are basic requirements for reaching women and girls. The advantage of having groups organized and connected through LACWHN is that it enables them to coordinate and promote tobacco control activities. The wide range of women's groups affiliated with LACWHN, in cooperation with the INWAT Latin and Caribbean Network, could ensure that information on the hazards of tobacco use reaches women and girls, including grass-roots and rural women.

Reaching Out to Other Women's Networks

One of the most important roles of global networks is lobbying and advocacy of the United Nations and other relevant international agencies. In addition to the women's NGOs that are actively involved in health promotion, a number of regional and international networks concerned with sustainable development and women's rights could be mobilized to participate in tobacco control.[9] A number of women's organizations have indicated a strong interest in joining the anti-tobacco movement. The Women's Global Network for Reproductive Rights has members in more than 110 countries and is a strong potential ally. Other important groups are the International Association of University Women, the Girl Guides Association, and Soroptimist International, which has almost 100 000 members in 119 countries. It is worth noting that Soroptimist has tobacco control as one of its official priorities.

As tobacco control efforts focus more on the WHO FCTC, the importance of including women lawyers and human rights organizations in these efforts has grown. One active regional network is the Asia Pacific Forum on Women, Law and Development (APWLD). This NGO

was an outcome of the Third World Forum on Women, Law and Development held in Nairobi, Kenya, in 1985. The Asian participants formed APWLD as a regional organization committed to enabling women to use law as an instrument of social change for equality, justice, and development.

The breastfeeding campaigns against infant formula are also important potential allies, because their organizations have had considerable experience mobilizing at an international level and calling for conventions to deal with aggressive marketing and commercial interests. In Asia, the breastfeeding campaign was launched in the 1970s, when large numbers of babies in developing countries were dying after bottle-feeding. The women's boycott of Nestle, one of the world's largest producers of infant formula, was reportedly the largest boycott in the world up to that time. The International Baby Food Action Network (IBFAN) was founded by six individuals in 1979 and had grown to 140 groups by 1989.

Women leaders offer expertise on women's perspectives and experiences, particularly in networking and building alliances.

In addition to consumer organizations, a number of international reproductive, human rights, and sustainable-development networks continue to lobby on behalf of women's health. These organizations have expressed interest in tobacco control and have occasionally contributed as advocates. Strong international networks include the Women's Global Network for Reproductive Rights and WEDO, an international advocacy network whose aim is to achieve a healthy and peaceful planet, with social, political, economic, and environmental justice for all, through the empowerment of women in all their diversity and through their equal participation with men in decision-making, from grass-roots to global arenas. It was actively involved in the Rio Summit as well as the Kobe Conference on Women and Tobacco and has played an important role in convening a "linkage caucus" that helps integrate NGO views at various United Nations conferences.

World Health Organization

Discussion

The greatest challenge facing women's organizations is that of galvanizing the leadership to prevent a rising epidemic of tobacco use among women, particularly young women. Women's groups involved in tobacco control programmes have argued that to be successful, such programmes must start from girls' and women's own experiences and take into account the broader context of women's lives. This is possible when women's leadership is prominent within tobacco control. Women's organizations should be involved in tobacco control for several key reasons:

- Working with women's groups helps to reach other groups, such as husbands and partners, as well as children, to influence their behaviour and reduce exposure to environmental tobacco smoke.

- Working with women's organizations can widen the political support for tobacco control, taking it beyond the health community. This may be particularly important when support is needed to introduce specific legislative or regulatory mechanisms.

- Women leaders offer expertise on women's perspectives and experiences, particularly in networking and building alliances.

However, several barriers should be recognized:

- An emphasis on emancipation and autonomy may provoke a hostile reaction to measures perceived as restrictive of individual freedom. Aggressive misleading advertising by tobacco companies may cause smoking to still be seen as a symbol of women's emancipation or as an important coping mechanism for women under stress. Some women's organizations are critical of traditional health education approaches aimed at changing women's smoking behaviours; they see these approaches as individualistic, victim-blaming, guilt-inducing, and disempowering.

- Funding needs have prompted some women's organizations to accept money from tobacco companies. In the United States, Philip Morris spent millions of dollars on women's causes between 1990 and 1995 and supported more than 100 women's groups in 1995.

- Many women's organizations, particularly grass-roots and community-based groups, work in a collective, non-hierarchical way. These organizations may view traditional tobacco control activities as top-down and inimical to the way they work. Information flow between national and community networks, and between international and national networks, is often limited.

Armed with a tobacco treaty—the WHO FCTC—women's health activists are promoting a comprehensive approach to women's health in which they include tobacco control activities and bring to bear important human rights treaties such as CEDAW. It is vitally important that women's leadership be enlisted at all levels in the advocacy campaign for the WHO FCTC.

Recommendations

In addition to recommendations made in other chapters, it is important to re-emphasize the importance of comprehensive tobacco control strategies such as bans on advertising and promotion of smoke-free environments, including the home.

Other measures to consider include:

1. Working closely with CEDAW and the Convention on the Rights of the Child to strengthen a gender perspective in the WHO FCTC.

2. Collaborating with women leaders working on broad social and economic issues such as the environment, human rights, labour law, religious ethics, child welfare, and fair trade laws.

3. Forming a women's watch group to monitor the WHO FCTC and the marketing practices of tobacco companies.

4. Holding regional gender, women, and tobacco conferences to strengthen regional networks against tobacco use.

5. Using new information technologies and electronic media to mobilize young women and girls in anti-tobacco campaigns.

World Health Organization

References

1. *The advancement of women.* New York, NY, United Nations, 1996.
2. *Framework Convention on Tobacco Control.* Geneva, World Health Organization, 1999 (Technical Briefing Series, WHO/NCD/TFI/99).
3. *Report of the WHO International Conference on Tobacco and Health, Kobe.* Geneva, World Health Organization, 1999.
4. Nakano N. *Report from Japan.* Paper presented at an expert group meeting in preparation for the WHO International Conference on Tobacco and Health, Kobe, 1999.
5. Matsui Y. *Women's Asia.* London, Zed Books, 1989.
6. Gomez A. Evaluating the past 8 years. *Women's Health Journal*, 1996, 31–33.
7. Berer M. A good time to return to the grassroots. *Women's Health Journal*, 1996, 39–42.
8. *The Cairo consensus: women exercising citizenship through monitoring.* Santiago, Latin American and Caribbean Women's Health Network, 1999.
9. Matsui Y. *Women's vital role in the environment movement in Japan.* Paper presented at the International Environmental Education Seminar for Women. Taipei, 1993.

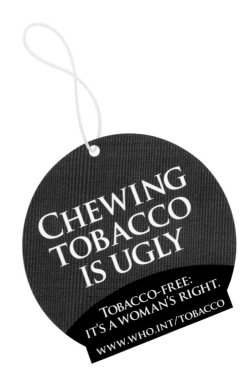